Digital Health in Focus of Predictive, Preventive and Personalised Medicine

Advances in Predictive, Preventive and Personalised Medicine

Volume 12

More information about this series at http://www.springer.com/series/10051

Lotfi Chaari
Editor

Digital Health in Focus of Predictive, Preventive and Personalised Medicine

Springer

Editor
Lotfi Chaari
IRIT-ENSEEIHT (UMR 5505)
University of Toulouse
TOULOUSE CEDEX 7, France

ISSN 2211-3495 ISSN 2211-3509 (electronic)
Advances in Predictive, Preventive and Personalised Medicine
ISBN 978-3-030-49814-6 ISBN 978-3-030-49815-3 (eBook)
https://doi.org/10.1007/978-3-030-49815-3

This Springer imprint is published by the registered company Springer Nature Switzerland AG.
The registered company address is: Gewerbestrasse 11, 6330 Cham, Switzerland

What This Book Series Is About

Current Healthcare: What Is Behind the Issue?

For many acute and chronic disorders, the current healthcare outcomes are considered as being inadequate: global figures cry for preventive measures and personalised treatments. In fact, severe chronic pathologies, such as cardiovascular disorders, diabetes and cancer, are treated after onset of the disease, frequently at near end stages. Pessimistic prognosis considers pandemic scenario for type 2 diabetes mellitus, neurodegenerative disorders and some types of cancer over the next 10–20 years followed by the economic disaster of healthcare systems in a global scale.

Advanced Healthcare Tailored to the Person: What Is Beyond the Issue?

Advanced healthcare promotes the paradigm change from delayed interventional to predictive medicine tailored to the person, from reactive to preventive medicine and from disease to wellness. The innovative Predictive, Preventive and Personalised Medicine (PPPM) is emerging as the focal point of efforts in healthcare aimed at curbing the prevalence of both communicable and non-communicable diseases, such as diabetes, cardiovascular diseases, chronic respiratory diseases, cancer and dental pathologies. The cost-effective management of diseases and the critical role of PPPM in modernisation of healthcare have been acknowledged as priorities by global and regional organisations and health-related institutions, such as the United Nations Organisation, the European Union and the National Institutes of Health.

Why Integrative Medical Approach by PPPM as the Medicine of the Future?

PPPM is the new integrative concept in healthcare sector that enables to predict individual predisposition before onset of the disease, to provide targeted preventive measures and to create personalised treatment algorithms tailored to the person. The expected outcomes are conducive to more effective population screening, prevention early in childhood, identification of persons at risk, stratification of patients for the optimal therapy planning, prediction and reduction of adverse drug-drug or drugdisease interactions relying on emerging technologies, such as pharmacogenetics, pathology-specific molecular patters, subcellular imaging, disease modelling, individual patient profiles, etc. Integrative approach by PPPM is considered as the medicine of the future. Being at the forefront of the global efforts, the European Association for Predictive, Preventive and Personalised Medicine (EPMA, http://www.epmanet.eu/) promotes the integrative concept of PPPM among healthcare stakeholders, governmental institutions, educators, funding bodies, patient organisations and public domain.

Current book series, published by Springer in collaboration with EPMA, overview multidisciplinary aspects of advanced biomedical approaches and innovative technologies. The integration of individual professional groups into the overall concept of PPPM is a particular advantage of this book series. Expert recommendations focus on the cost-effective management tailored to the person in health and disease. Innovative strategies are considered for standardisation of healthcare services. New guidelines are proposed for medical ethics, treatment of rare diseases, innovative approaches to early and predictive diagnostics, patient stratification and targeted prevention in healthy individuals, persons at risk, individual patient groups, subpopulations, institutions, healthcare economy and marketing.

About the Book Series Editor

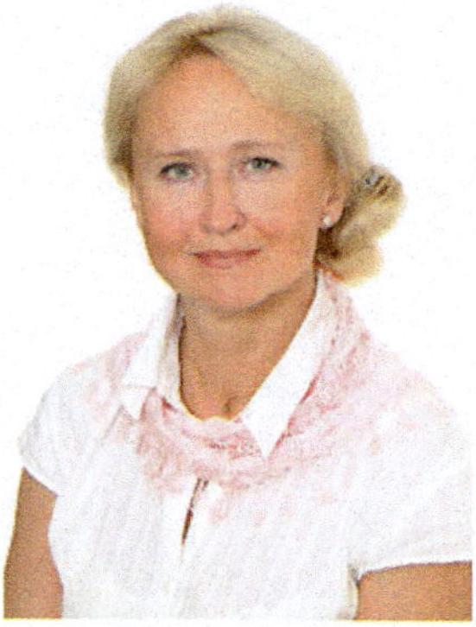

Prof. Dr. Olga Golubnitschaja

Dr. Olga Golubnitschaja Department of Radiology, Medical Faculty, Rheinische Friedrich-Wilhelms-Universität, Bonn, Germany, has studied journalism, biotechnology and medicine and has been awarded research fellowships in Austria, Russia, the UK, Germany, the Netherlands and Switzerland (early and predictive diagnostics in paediatrics, neurosciences and cancer). She is the author of more than 400 well-cited international publications (research and review articles, position papers, books and book contributions) in the innovative field of predictive, preventive and personalised medicine (PPPM) with the main research focus on pre- and perinatal diagnostics, diagnostics of cardiovascular disease and neurodegenerative pathologies, predictive diagnostics in cancer and diabetes.

She has been awarded National and International Fellowship of the Alexander von Humboldt Foundation and Highest Prize in Medicine and Eiselsberg Prize in Austria.

Since 2009, Dr. Golubnitschaja is the *Secretary General* of the European Association for Predictive, Preventive and Personalised Medicine (EPMA, Brussels) networking over 50 countries worldwide (www.epmanet.eu), *Series Editor* of *Advances in Predictive, Preventive and Personalised Medicine* (**Springer Nature**),

Editor of *Predictive Diagnostics and Personalised Treatment: Dream or Reality* (Nova Science Publishers, New York 2009) and Co-editor of *Personalisierte Medizin* (Health Academy, Dresden 2010).

She is the European Representative in the EDR Network at the National Institutes of Health, USA (http://edrn.nci.nih.gov/).

She is a regular reviewer for over 30 clinical and scientific journals and serves as a grant reviewer for national (ministries of health in several European countries) and international funding bodies.

Since 2007 until now, she has been working as the European Commission evaluation expert for FP7, Horizon 2020, IMI-1 (Innovative Medical Initiatives) and IMI-2. From 2010 to 2013, she was involved in creating the PPPM-related contents for the European Programme 'Horizon 2020'.

Currently, Dr. Golubnitschaja is Vice-Chair of the Evaluation Panel for Marie Curie Mobility Actions at the European Commission in Brussels.

Preface

Predictive, Preventive and Personalised Medicine (3PM) is a new paradigm for both bio/medical sciences and management of medical services created and promoted by the expert groups of EPMA in early twenty-first century.

On the other hand, Information Technology (IT) comprises essential tools for many aspects of societal organisation at individual and population levels, being therefore instrumental for the development and implementation of advanced 3PM concepts benefiting healthy individuals, patients, healthcare system, and the society as a whole.

Potential IT/3PM benefits could be well exemplified by the current Covid-19 Pandemic challenge, when optimal policy-making decisions could be made only by application of predictive IT algorithms for cost-effective targeted preventive measures saving lives and considering the entire spectrum of socio-economical issues related to this complex situation.

Contextually, this book addresses the IT-generated solutions for practical implementation of 3PM concepts. It presents innovative methods, algorithms and approaches which synergistically demonstrate a potential to advance 3PM concepts and implementation. A spectrum of relevant IT solutions is considered such as predictive and prognostic tools, health monitoring for targeted prevention, Internet of Things (IoT), Artificial Intelligence (AI), big data analysis and personalisation of treatment algorithms.

Toulouse, France Lotfi Chaari

Introduction

Keywords: Predictive Preventive Personalised Medicine (PPPM, 3PM); eHealth; IoT for Health; Artificial Intelligence; Big Data Analysis; Deep Learning; Health Monitoring; 3D Visualization; Covid-19 Pandemic Monitoring

Introducing Information Technology (IT) tools in today's and future medicine is being increasingly considered all over the world, especially in developed countries. Indeed, these countries are suffering the most from population aging and chronic diseases. This induces original challenges not only for healthcare but also for well-being. In this sense, Predictive, Preventive and Personalised Medicine (3PM) has been identified since more than a decade as a research avenue having huge potential for developed societies.

From Traditional to 3PM

The history of medicine[1] is rich in important events and discoveries. For centuries, medicine has regularly faced important challenges. Evolution has therefore happened relatively to historical events, but also with respect to the practice methodology. Regarding events, there is no better example than the current Coronavirus Pandemic, which is demonstrating that healthcare systems in both developed and developing countries are not adapted to such situations.

In terms of practice methodology, medicine moved from Traditional (T) practice to Complementary and Alternative Medicine (CAM) and then to Person-Centred Medicine (PCM), Individualised Medicine (IM), Stratified Medicine (SM), Personalised Medicine (PM), and more recently Predictive, Preventive and Personalised Medicine (3PM). 3PM is becoming today one of the main priorities of the European Commission (EC) to solve current health challenges [2]. Although these challenges are to a large extent due to population aging trends, chronic and severe diseases, earlier considered as being linked to the elderly, nowadays occur more and more frequently to younger generations, such as diabetes mellitus type 2, some types of aggressive cancers and 'young' stroke, among others [3,4,5,6]. Contextually, innovative population screening programmes based on advanced concepts of prediction, targeted prevention and personalisation of medical services have to be investigated.

3PM Meeting IT

Today, the paradigm of handling chronic diseases is facing a shift from reactive to Predictive, Preventive and Personalised. Recent studies clearly established this evidence in general [7] and specific chronic diseases such as heart failure [8].

This paradigm shift has been conducted by handling more patient-related data. As most of today's applications, these data may be of very large volumes. It is mostly collected from sensors either related to people's physiological state or environment.

To analyse the generated data volumes, it is not possible any more to rely on manual or operator-based tools. Hopefully, research during the last two decades in the field of IT has led to the development of many automatic and efficient tools to collect, process and analyse data. The 3PM community has therefore managed to formulate unsolved problems to be investigated using IT tools [9, 10].

IT Meeting 3PM

On the other hand, IT has completely changed our lives. Starting from homes, vehicles or even work and restaurants, we use IT tools throughout the day. On the other hand, IT today is contributing to the understanding and monitoring of the current Covid-19 Pandemic [11]. This allowed countries to adapt their prediction and prevention strategies either through non-pharmacological interventions (NPI) or personalised imagery-based testing [12]. 3PM is therefore being adopted as a paradigm to handle both the pandemic and post-pandemic phases.

In the context of healthcare, IT has a lot offer, such as patients management at hospitals, exploration tools like imagery, telemedicine, and data-driven clinical decision systems (CDS). More recently, Artificial Intelligence (AI) is being investigated deeper despite the sensitivity of the medical field [13]. Specifically, the AI community [8] has investigated solving 3PM problems. In parallel, similar contributions in the field of 3PM have been made by other scientific communities such as Internet of Things (IoT) [14].

This book addresses new contributions in the field of IT regarding 3PM. It therefore contributes to document how IT is meeting 3PM to solve current problems and give new perspectives for the future. The book's content covers tools serving personalised prediction, tools for diagnosis and prevention, monitoring, visualisation, data analytics, AI and personalized medical systems.

The reported original contributions have been presented to the second International Conference on Digital Health Technologies (ICDHT 2019). This book therefore provides one with a technical idea about future trends using IT tools for 3PM.

References

[1] Golubnitschaja, O., Baban, B., Boniolo, G., Wang, W., Bubnov, R., Kapalla, M., Krapfenbauer, K., Mozaffari, M.S., Costigliola, V: Medicine in the early twenty-first century: paradigm and anticipation - EPMA position paper 2016. EPMA J. **7**(23), (2016)

[2] Lemke, H.U., Golubnitschaja, O.: Towards personal health care with model-guided medicine: long-term PPPM-related strategies and realisation opportunities within 'Horizon 2020'. EPMA J. **5**(1), 8 (2014)

[3] Duarte, A.A., Mohsin, S., Golubnitschaja, O.: Diabetes care in figures: current pitfalls and future scenario. EPMA J. **9**(2), (2018)

[4] Kunin, A., Polivka, J. Jr., Moiseeva, N., Golubnitschaja, O.: "Dry Mouth" and "Flammer" syndromes – neglected risks in adolescents and new concepts by predictive, preventive and personalised approach. EPMA J. **9**(3), 307–317 (2018)

[5] Golubnitschaja, O., Flammer, J.: Individualised patient profile: Clinical utility of Flammer syndrome phenotype and general lessons for predictive, preventive and personalised medicine. EPMA J. **9**(1), 15–20 (2018)

[6] Polivka, J. Jr., Polivka, J., Pesta, M., Rohan, V., Celedova, L., Mahajani, S., Topolcan, O., Golubnitschaja, O.: Risks associated with the stroke predisposition at young age: facts and hypotheses in light of individualized predictive and preventive approach. EPMA J. **10**(1), 81–99 (2019)

[7] Seifirad, S., Haghpanah, V.: Inappropriate modeling of chronic and complex disorders: How to reconsider the approach in the context of predictive, preventive and personalized medicine, and translational medicine. EPMA J. **10**(3), 195–209 (2019)

[8] Barrett, M., Boyne, J., Brandts, J., Brunner-La Rocca, H.P., De Maesschalck, L., De Wit, K., Dixon, L., Eurlings, C., Fitzsimons, D., Golubnitschaja, O., Hageman, A., Heemskerk, F., Hintzen, A., Helms, T.M., Hill, L., Hoedemakers, T., Marx, N., McDonald, K., Mertens, M., Müller-Wieland, D., Palant, A., Piesk, J., Pomazanskyi, A., Ramaekers, J., Ruff, P., Schütt, K., Shekhawat, Y., Ski, C.F., Thompson, D.R., Tsirkin, A., van der Mierden, K., Watson, C., Zippel-Schultz, B.: Artificial intelligence supported patient self-care in chronic heart failure: a paradigm shift from reactive to predictive, preventive and personalised care. EPMA J. **10**(4), 445–464 (2019)

[9] Fröhlich, H., Patjoshi, S., Yeghiazaryan, K., Kehrer, C., Kuhn, W., Golubnitschaja, O.: Premenopausal breast cancer: potential clinical utility of the multi-omic based machine learning approach for patient stratification. EPMA J. **9**(2), (2018)

[10] Gerner, C., Costigliola, V., Golubnitschaja, O.: Multiomic patterns in body fluids: Technological Challenge with a Great Potential to Implement the Advanced Paradigm of 3P Medicine. Mass Spectrometry Rev. 195–209 (2019)

[11] Chaari, L., Golubnitschaja, O.: Covid-19 pandemic by the "real-time" monitoring: the Tunisian case and lessons for global epidemics in the context 3PM strategies. EPMA J. (2020) https://doi.org/10.1007/s13167-020-00207-0

[12] Xiaowei, X., Xiangao, J., Chunlian, M., Peng, D., Xukun, L., Shuangzhi, L., Liang, Y., Yanfei, C., Junwei, S., Guanjing, L., Yongtao, L., Hong, Z., Kaijin, X., Lingxiang, R., Wei, W.: Deep learning system to screen coronavirus disease 2019 pneumonia. In: arXive. 2020. https://arxiv.org/ftp/arxiv/papers/2002/2002.09334.pdf. Accessed 21 Feb 2020
[13] Davenport, T., Ravi, K.: The potential for artificial intelligence in healthcare. Future Healthcare J. **6**(2), 94–98 (2019)
[14] Schreier, G.: The internet of things for personalized health. Stud. Health Technol. Inform. **200**, 22–31 (2014)

Contents

About the Editor

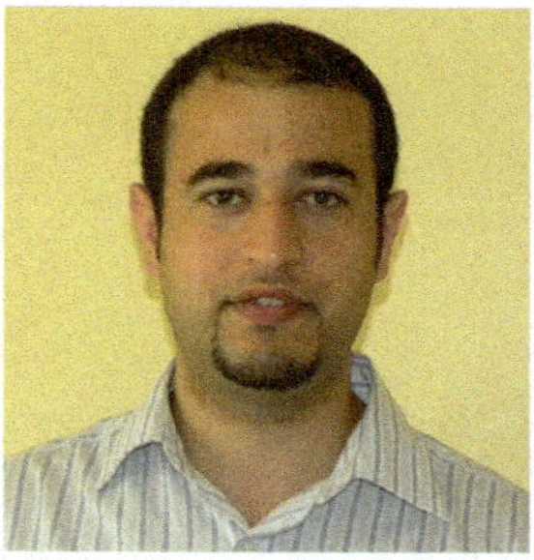

Lotfi Chaari received his PhD degree from the University of Paris-Est in France. He prepared for his PhD with the Signal and Communication Group of the Laboratoire d'Informatique Gaspard Monge (LIGM), in collaboration with NeuroSpin-CEA, the first centre in Europe dedicated to ultra-high field MRI and applications in cognitive neurosciences. He then moved to Grenoble as a Postdoctoral Fellow at INRIA with the Mistis team. In 2012, he joined the Institut National Polytechnique de Toulouse as an Associate Professor. He is also member of the IRIT laboratory. In 2017, he received the HDR dissertation from the University of Toulouse. Lotfi Chaari's research is focused on medical signal and image processing with various applications and imaging modalities. He is an expert for a number of journals of the signal and image processing as well as the medical imaging communities. He also worked as an expert for institutions like the French National Research Agency and European Commission.

Prof. Lotfi Chaari has participated in the organization of several special sessions for international conferences, is a regular member of various technical programme committees, and was the Co-founder and General Chair of the two first editions of the International Conference on Digital Health Technologies.

A New Scalable and Comprehensive Real-Time Evaluation System of Dependence

Marie-Claude Mendo, Julien Mistrzak, Vincent Peirolo, and Laurent Billonnet

1 Context

According to the latest projections of the French population, in 2050, one in three inhabitants should be more than 60 years old in France. Every country in Europe is concerned with 2.3 million of dependent elderly. In 2016, 7500 nursing homes hosted about 600,000 seniors. Other seniors have chosen or not to stay at home [1].

The French caregiver Association counts 8.3 million caregivers. To improve the daily life and the accompaniment of people in loss of autonomy, the French government has developed several plans (old age, Alzheimer's) and laws, the most recent of which is the law ASV (adaptation of society to ageing). This includes the physical environment (habitat), the social environment (family caregivers) and the traditional AGGIR grid (gerontological autonomy iso-resource groups) [2].

The AGGIR grid evaluates the level of dependence of people over 60. The GIR index found is used to adapt the Personalized Autonomy Allowance. This index goes from 1 to 6 and one is the highest level of dependence. GIR 1–4 indices allow to benefit for an assistance plan funded by the county council, including human, financial, technical (home automation for example) for the seniors and their families.

However, this tool do not take into account several parameters; such as caregivers (while they are essential for efficient home support and to maintain social link), neurodegenerative diseases (such as Parkinson and Alzheimer) or emotions and affects of the people with loss of autonomy [3].

There is also a problem of temporality between evaluations. In the current model, the AGGIR grid is evaluated only once every 2 years. The medical status and the

M.-C. Mendo · J. Mistrzak · V. Peirolo · L. Billonnet (✉)
University of Limoges, Limoges, France
e-mail: laurent.billonnet@unilim.fr

L. Chaari (ed.), *Digital Health in Focus of Predictive, Preventive and Personalised Medicine*, Advances in Predictive, Preventive and Personalised Medicine 12,
https://doi.org/10.1007/978-3-030-49815-3_1

dependence level of the user can decline in a few days, which should rationally require a new immediate evaluation.

2 How to Overcome All of These Shortcomings?

To solve all these weaknesses, we propose a global scalable system for evaluation of the people with loss of autonomy without age restriction. Based upon activity monitoring, the goal is to set up an intelligent system with sensors that can detect in real-time changes that occur after the initial evaluation using standard grids [4]. Parameters referred by the process are: transfers, movement inside and outside the house, urinary and faecal elimination, feeding, tracking and orientation in living space and time, communication, dressing and undressing. It is also possible to rate the evolution of pathologies, emotions of the user and the people around him (family, caregivers), falls and global physical activity.

According to the literature, there are different means of fall detection and activity monitoring for the elderly. One concerns "direct detection" [5] solutions, which detect a sudden change in the position of the body (drop) thanks to the accelerometers or equivalent sensors. The second refers to environmental sensors to monitor and analyse the activities (or absence of activity also called "peripheral sensing") of the person [6].

The RE-AGGIR (react) system aims to integrate the AGGIR grid and its multi-dimensional assessment into the habitat [7]:

- Feeding is one of the primary needs of life. Appetite reduction is one of the main factors in the loss of autonomy. Therefore, monitoring the diet on a daily basis can detect when the persons are no longer able to feed themselves.
- Approximately 78% of incidents and accidents usually occur overnight in seniors. So monitoring night activities must be part of our system.
- Falls are among the causes of hospitalization and mortality in the elderly. The post-fall syndrome leads to a reduction in the activities of the elder and the latter will adopt other postures to avoid falling again.
- Monitoring the grasping abilities enables to monitor the dressing and the onset of neurodegenerative diseases.
- Monitoring the outward comings and goings will allow us to know if the persons in loss of autonomy continue to have relations and/or activities outside their home thus maintaining a reasonable level of social link.
- Monitoring the attendance of the bathroom and the toilets allows having information on the hygiene of the elderly person (it is also one of the items of the AGGIR grid). Natural elimination is one of the items evaluated by the Aggir grid.

In terms of ethics and privacy respect, the system has to be practically invisible to the inhabitants since the success of our system is based first on its acceptance by the users. The data collected by the sensors will be analysed and processed intelligently by a central system. This will be connected to a monitoring interface that can issue alerts autonomously in case of emergency. The system will stay connected to the AGGIR grid's algorithm so that the GIR index can be automatically refreshed in real-time and transmitted to care services, prescribers and caregivers.

3 A Real-Time Evaluation System

3.1 Expected Benefits

Our goal is to consider the actual AGGIR grid, adding social and family environment parameters.

The re-AGGIR system has several advantages such as the daily monitoring of the evolution of pathologies in real time. It helps to reduce the delays in the intervention of professionals and prevent the loss of autonomy. It complements the remote assistance services and operates in autonomy without interaction.

RÉ-AGGIR makes it possible to re-adapt services and home support according to needs while monitoring the parameters that are part of the primary needs of the people.

Our proposal therefore consists of a panel of four types of sensors. We describe the role and implementation strategy of the different sensor types (see Fig. 1) further.

3.2 Central Unit

Pure and discrete, the design of this central unit (see Fig. 2) allows it to be placed anywhere in the house without being imposing or too intrusive. This unit collects the data of all sensors and processes it to send alerts to caregivers and professionals.

3.3 Presence Sensors

In general, a motion detector is a sensor placed at a strategic location to detect intrusions into a house. On the one hand, we use its ability to detect a presence, help daily lighting of the lamps in case of motion detection. This is essential for night walking. On the other hand, it allows monitoring the frequency of these movements.

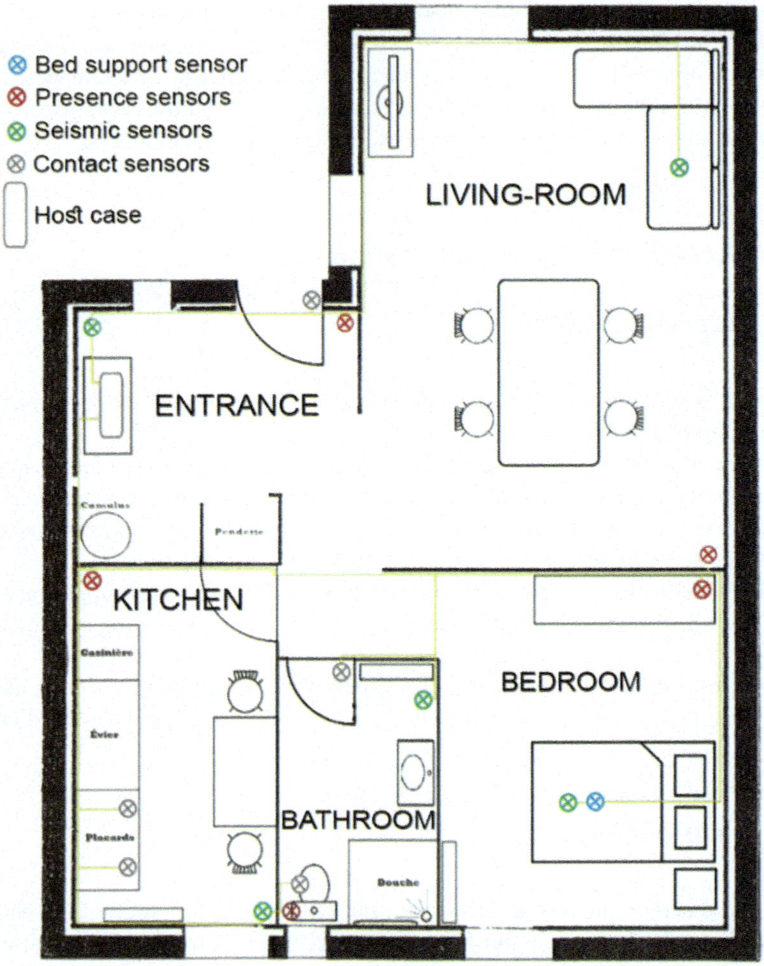

Fig. 1 Example of sensors implantation into a house

3.4 Contact Sensors

A contact sensor is a simple and effective solution for detecting for example opening of household appliances or doors/windows. In our system, it will be used to monitor three parameters: eating habits, natural elimination and hygiene, outside activities.

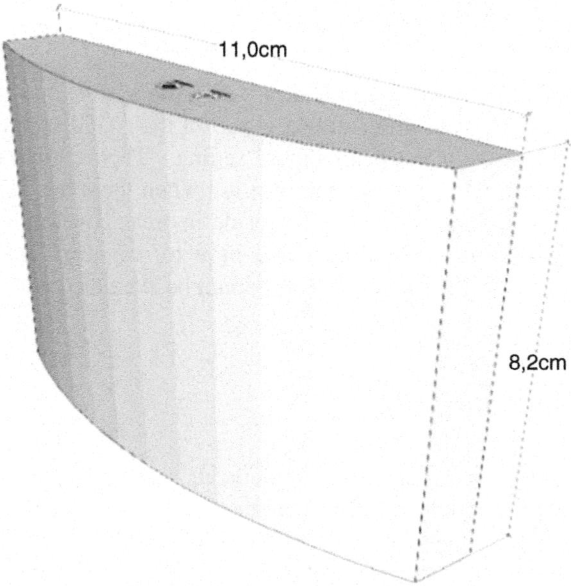

Fig. 2 Design of the central unit

3.5 *Bed Support Sensor*

Sleep cycle changes during normal aging of people. However, for the elderly, the night is the time when the risk is important. As nocturnal ambulation is a precursor to Alzheimer's disease and needs to be monitored. In this case, the contact sensors placed in the kitchen, coupled with the bed sensor, will detect and signal the action. The contact sensor will also be installed in the toilet.

The support sensor is a plate with sensors that slides under the mattress. It can detect a presence by contact with the person. Equipped with an intelligent system, He is able to differentiate the sitting position from the lying position. What makes the sleep measurement readings of the person more reliable.

3.6 *Seismic Sensor*

This sensor is the size of a two-euro coin and is placed directly on the floor of each room and in the centre. Thanks to its extreme thinness, it does not feel almost under foot when walking on it. This apparel records and analyses in real time the slightest vibrations that the soil propagates. Thanks to its precise parameterization, it is able to analyse the weight of an impact and thus to diagnose if the vibration is due to an object fallen to the ground or a person falling.

3.7 Limits of the System

Like any human work, the re-AGGIR system has some limitations, such as the grasping measurement that is part of the AGGIR grid. RE-AGGIR is going to need human help to monitor these settings. The system is not also able to identify the person who is the victim of a fall when there are several inhabitants in the house. Actually, only people who reside in areas covered by an internet network can use RE-AGGIR. The others will have to wait for network coverage throughout the territory. Finally, the affects cannot be evaluated without human aid.

4 Conclusion

Our system not only complements tele assistance services, but also secures the elderly, prevents loss of autonomy by monitoring daily changes in pathologies and facilitates the intervention of professionals. RE-AGGIR is a global evaluation system that combines discretion, comfort and technology. RE-AGGIR accompanies seniors as well as anyone without age distinction. However, for some parameters like affects, dressing / undressing, grasping, RE-AGGIR will need to use intrusive devices such as the cameras to work efficiently. It will also need a human interaction to estimate and accompany the seniors at best.

The system estimates the dependence in real time and makes it possible to adapt the different supports according to the evolution of the needs of the people with loss of autonomy. RE-AGGIR presents several advantages: the safety of the aidant, the prevention of the loss of autonomy, the serenity of the caregiver and the relatives. It is a comprehensive complement to the tele assistance services. With the increasing impact of IoT in several domains, possibilities of application extensions seems infinite.

References

1. Insee.fr https://www.insee.fr/fr/statistiques/1280826. Retrieved October 21 2018
2. Lalive d'Epinay, C., & Spini, D.: Années fragiles. Quebec University of Laval press edition, p. 146 (2008)
3. Quentin, B.: Gérontologie et société. Fondation nationale de gérontologie, 141, pp 171 (2012)
4. Guyonnet, S., & Raynaud-Simon, A.: Fragilité et nutrition, Repérage et maintien de l'autonomie des personnes âgées fragiles, (en ligne) Livre blanc.org décembre 2013, https://fragilite.org/livre-blanc.php ; reached on 10th of December 2018
5. Silvereco, Chute de la personne âgée : causes, conséquences et prévention (en ligne), octobre 2017, available on https://www.silvereco.fr/chute-de-la-personne-agee-causes-consequences-et-prevention/3187245, booked on 3rd of January 2019

6. Nexecur, Quelles sont les signes de la perte d'autonomie ? (En ligne), Enquête Santé handicap 2009, available on https://www.nexecur.fr/comment-detecter-perte-d-autonomie, reached on 25th of January 2019
7. Leduc Florence, Notre projet politique, (en ligne) Association française des aidants, available on sur https://www.aidants.fr/lassociation/notre-projet-politique, reached 28th of January 2019

An Ontology Based Authentication Framework for Healthcare Monitoring

Amira Henaien and Hadda BelHadj

1 Introduction

Nowadays, the widespread use of smart devices is producing a radical changes in our daily life activities. As one of the fields the most affected is healthcare attending more than 40% from the hole investments of the market of WoT [2, 4]. Several successful industrial or research works are developed with a very efficient design to track and monitor the health of a patient continuously and ubiquitously. The principle idea of WoT Healthcare Applications consists in involving a set of smart devices connected to daily life objects in the body of the patient or its environment. The main job of those devices is to collect the necessary data for an ubiquitous healthcare monitoring. And it may includes any sensing data about the user's health situation and the environment situation, the medical history of a patient, a device information and any health domain-specific data. It is very necessary and challenging to create new standardization and develop good practices to improve the usability, the maintainability, and the security of healthcare applications. As it is discussed in [3, 4], form this list, security is a priority. Any lost or fake information can leads to a dangerous situation and even to the death of human being. For a cardiology patient in a critical situation, any missing vital sign, as its heart beat, can delay an alert or completely loose it and deprive him from getting any aids. The wrong information or the missing data are not always technical bugs. It is absolutely possible that they are a willfully human being made errors spontaneously

A. Henaien (✉)
King Khalid University, Abha, Saudi Arabia
e-mail: aheniaen@kku.edu.sa

H. BelHadj
Laboratory of Technology and Smart Systems, Digital Research Center of Sfax, Sfax, Tunisia
e-mail: Hadda.lBnelhadj@esti.rnu.tn

L. Chaari (ed.), *Digital Health in Focus of Predictive, Preventive and Personalised Medicine*, Advances in Predictive, Preventive and Personalised Medicine 12,
https://doi.org/10.1007/978-3-030-49815-3_2

or deliberately. For this reasons, the system should be enhanced enough to protect its data. As the most first action that can be taken is a strong authentication system to limited the access using a powerful authentication methods.

Different authentication solutions are efficiently used and approved for information systems in general and medical systems in particular. However, new ubiquitous and continuous healthcare monitoring applications have a very particular type of users like: people with special needs, handicaps, old persons, new born babies. For this reason, common methods, viz, knowledge-based or possession-based methods are no more feasible. An old person with Alzaheimer probably is never able to remember the password. It is becoming necessary to create a standardized authentication technique supporting the variety of health situation of users and providing the highest guaranty of protection for the data. A technique taking on consideration the health and mental situation of a user should specify for each user his situations, specify the different possible means of authentication and associate a semantic interpretation to each one. Finally, this technique should be able to reason and interpret the best authentication technique for each user.

This paper presents a new ontology based authentication methodology for healthcare monitoring in a predictive, preventive and personalized medicine system. The main idea consists on allowing different and adapted methods of authentication depending in the health and mental situation of the user. The system allow for a caregiver or a doctor to define the different abilities and capabilities of a patient. Based on those information, the system is able to define the appropriate method to be used for the user to authenticate and is able to provide this method ubiquitously to be identified. This paper is organized as the following: Sect. 2 is a presentation of the background of this work. Section 3 is an overview of this framework. In Sect. 4 we present the main component of this framework, the knowledge management system. Finally, Sect. 5 is a conclusions and perspectives.

2 Related Work and Background

Context and Rules Based Authentication In a very general way, the process of the authentication is confirming that a specific attribute claimed by an entity in a system. This confirmation is in many cases an identification of an entity that claims using credentials. Usual identification methods are knowledge-based methods, i.e. a password, answer question, generated code, etc. Traditional authentication methods have been enhanced with different techniques, viz, location based authentication [1], bio-metric information based authentication [11], context-awareness based authentication [1, 5, 13, 14], shared authorization and authentication rules across network based authentication [17].

Security and Medicine Ontologies Ontologies are becoming a powerful tool in the development of interdisciplinary systems as e-healthcare systems since their are able to represent and interrelate many types of knowledge.

Based Context Modeling for Healthcare Applications During the last years, different medical ontologies have been proposed to summarize medicine terms and concepts, viz, Systematized Nomenclature of Medicine Clinical Terms (SNOMED CT) [15], International Classification of Diseases (ICD)-10 [9] and International Classification Nursing Practice ICNP [10]. The ontology ICNP is a formal structure containing terms and definitions providing a formal nursing terminology for the construction of nursing diagnoses, interventions, and results. Ontology is not only used for terminology, it is also involved in different healthcare applications, viz, [6] proposing a context-aware system for antihypertensive drug recommendations or [8] designing a diabetes diagnosis framework.

Ontology Based Security Approaches Besides to medicine ontologies, some security approaches have been proposed based on ontologies viz, [12] an ontology base authorization enabling semantically matching diverse authorization requests and semantic rule reasoning on requested access; [7] an ontology-based interoperation service translating security attributes from local security vocabularies into the attributes recognized by the central vocabulary. Souad et al. in [16] propose a classification into eight families of existing security ontologies for the different requirements definition.

3 Overview of the Proposed Ontology Based Authentication Framework

The proposed framework is designed to allow different types of identification. It express the abilities of a patient with a formal specification. For each user, the system determinate a personalized method of authentication. The data is collected from different devices like: body sensors worn by the user, ambient sensors surrounding the user or smart devices, as phone, tablet, etc. Body sensors are used to capture the health profile of the patient, viz, vital signs, motion, location, etc. Ambient sensor reflect an image of the patient's environment, viz, ambient temperature, lightness, existence of a caregiver, etc. Smart devices are basically used to allow the communication between the user and the system and between users, viz sending an alert to user about a patient's situation, monitoring a patient, etc. We suppose that a caregiver or doctor is authorized to enter the mental situation the abilities of the patient and edit it in case of any changes. Thus, the basis of the designed system is to provide the appropriate identification method for each user deduced from its role (Patient, Doctor, Caregiver, FamilyCaregiver, etc), the collected data of its current situation, the already described data of its mental situation and abilities and security-related knowledge. As described by Fig. 1, the general architecture of this framework is containing:

Sensing Component: a set of sensors and smart devices related directly to the user. Their role is to collect all the context data: health data, ambient data, location,

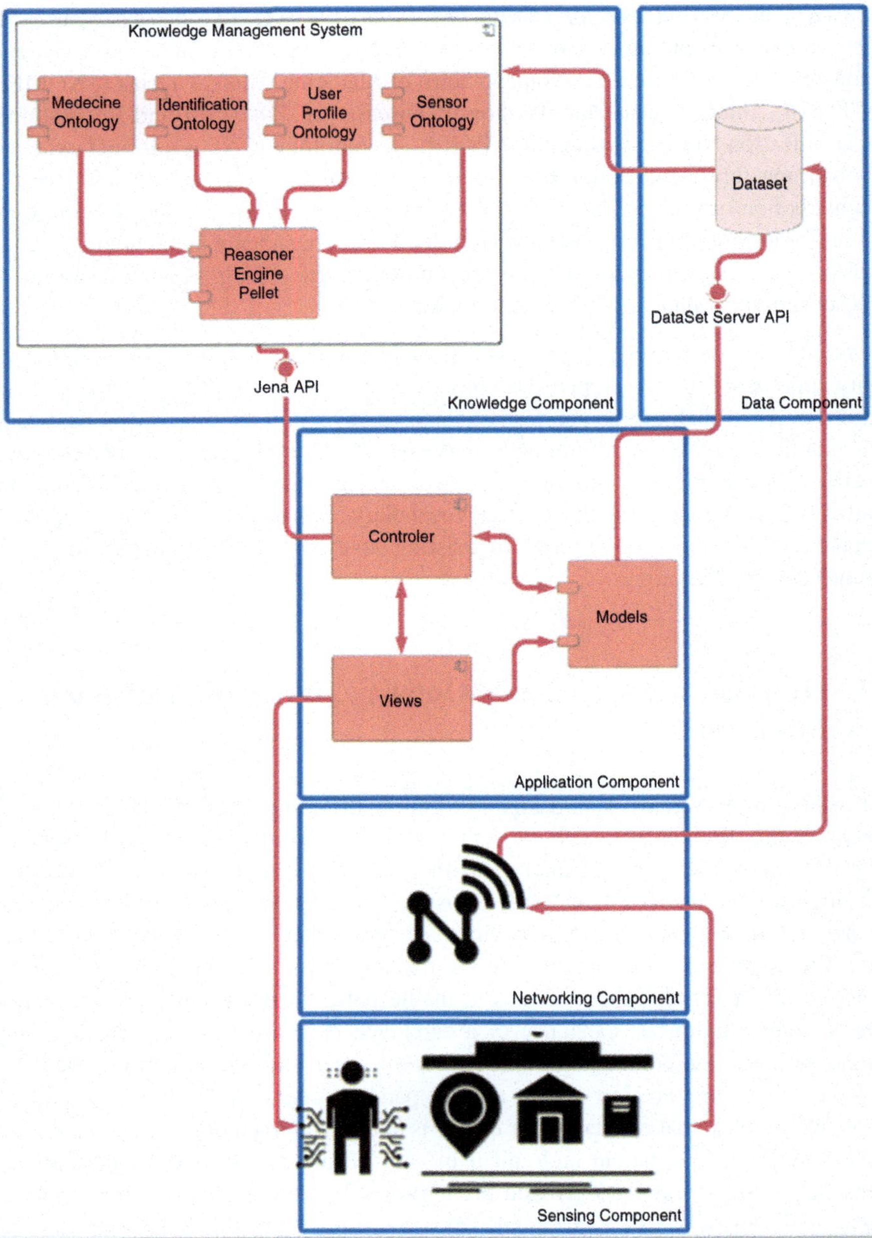

Fig. 1 General architecture of ontology based authentication framework

motion, personal information, etc. This set of sensors are related to one user and they are composing a smart platform.

Networking Component: a set of networking device allowing the communication between the different physical elements and the connection of those elements to the internet. Networking elements also allow the data exchange between the sensing layer and the knowledge component.

Data set Component: is a server hosting all the data: current data collected in real time and saved information about the user. It is providing instances enriching the ontologies from the knowledge component.

Application Component: is the implementation of all the features of the healthcare application providing all the services for ubiquitous and continuous medical monitoring. It is a MVC[1] application.

Knowledge Component: is playing a fundamental role in this architecture because it is the responsible for the knowledge base and the reasoning. It is composed of four ontologies and a reasoner engine (Pellet). This component is the responsible to provide the appropriate authentication method. The Fig. 2 explains the general process of authentication.

4 Ontology Based Knowledge Management System

The main part in the general architecture of the proposed framework, presented in Sect. 3, is the knowledge Management System. It decides the identification method associated to each user. It is composed basically from a set of ontologies: personal profile ontology, sensor ontology, medicine ontology, security ontology and a reasoner. Our ontologies are the extension of standard ontologies such as FOAF for personal profile, SSN and SOSA for sensors ontology and ICNP for medicine ontology. Those standard ontologies are merged with the security ontology containing basically a set of SWRL rules corresponding to the security rules. In the following, we present the different ontologies and the links between their entities.

Personal and health profile: we are using FOAF to present the personal profile of users. FOAF:person is representing all information related to the user, viz, account details, name, familyName, age, gender, etc. In the same time the ontology ICNP is providing an entity Individual presenting the health profile of a user as height, weight. We have specified FOAF:person equivalent to ICNP:Individual. ICNP is also describing an entity Role precising if the individual is Patient, Doctor, Caregiver, Nurse, etc. The property named hasLocation from ICNP associates a location to each patient.

Sensor ontology: The ontology SSN is providing an entity named Platform. It is a concept used to gather different entities as sensors, actuators, other platforms

[1]MVC: Model View Control

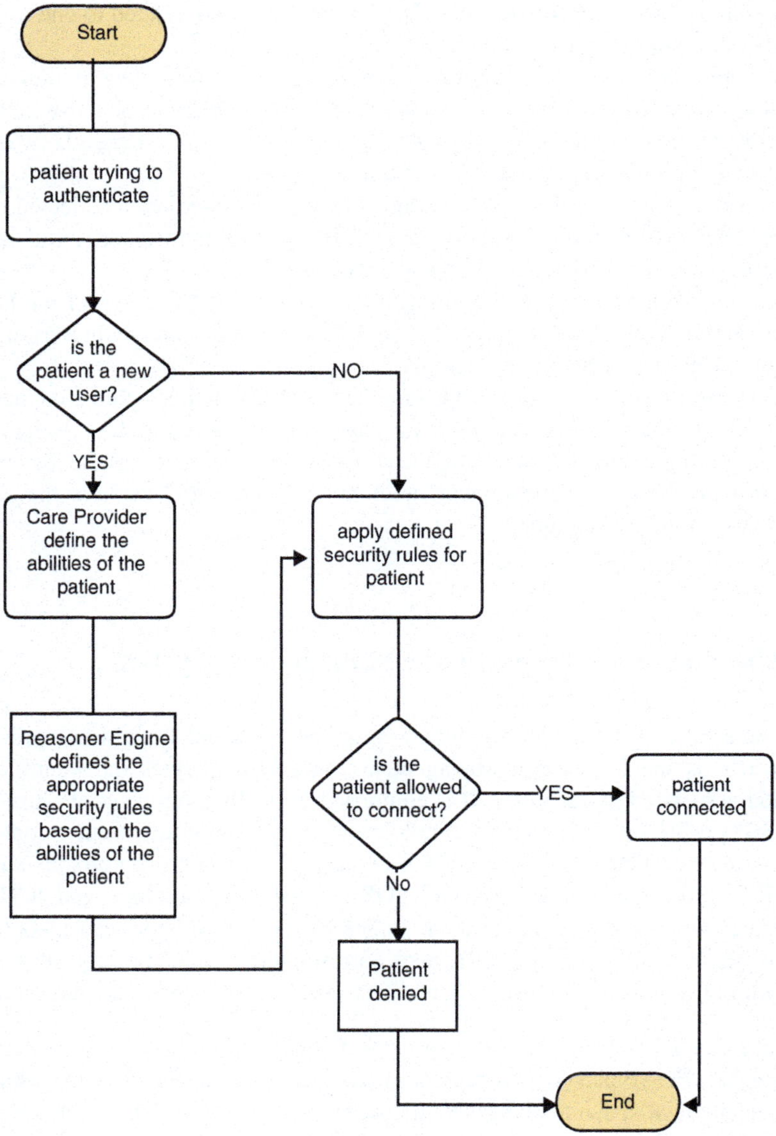

Fig. 2 Flow chart of authentication process

hosted in the same platform. SSN:Platform is associated to a user using the personalized property hasPlatform. The class SSN:Sensor is specified with two sub-classes BodySensors presenting sensors worn or attached to the body of the user and AmbientSensors presenting sensors existing in its environment. For each entity from the platform, we define its location using the same property hasLocation.

Medicine Ontology: ICNP provides an entity AbilityStatus with a set of sub-classes defining all the possible abilities of a person. Each ability contains two sub-classes an actual positive ability, in the case of safe ability, and actual negative ability, in the case of lost ability. For instance, ActualNegativeAbilityToSee is defining the disability of a patient to see. The property hasAbsoluteJudgeState is expressing the state of each ability for a user.

Security Ontology: the class IdentificationMethods contains a sub-classes for each identification methods. This list contains the different following entities: ByCareGiver, ByCornea, ByDoctor, ByEnteringPassword, ByFingerPrint, ByLocation, ByVoicePrint. The relation implementedBy related each method to its implementation. The property IdentifyBy is relating a user to his identification method.

SWRL Security Rules This ontology contains a set of SWRL rules used later by the reasoner to calculate the appropriate identification method and they are mainly authentication rules. For example, if all the abilities of a patient have ActualPositive for the hasAbsoluteJudgeState property, the authentication can be processed using classical authentication method using password, i.e. the property IdentifyBy for this patient is ByEnteringPassword. However, if a patient is blind, the property IdentifyBy for this patient is ByFingerPrint, ByCareGiver or ByDoctor.

5 Conclusions and Perspectives

This paper presents a new ontology based framework to personalize the authentication method to each user of a healthcare ubiquitous and continuous monitoring PPPM system. This new technique is very helpful for users with limited abilities or particular health situation. The identification method is defined depending on different parameters, viz, the user's personal information, his health situation, his mental situation, the possible identification methods, the available device to the user, etc. This work is based also on context and rules based authentication specified with SWRL. As a continuation of this work, we are aiming to develop the complete components constituting the system. We will also evaluate the performance of our system and compare it to other identification methods.

Acknowledgments The authors would like to express their gratitude to King Khalid University, Saudi Arabia for providing administrative and technical support.

References

1. Agadakos, I., Hallgren, P., Damopoulos, D., Sabelfeld, A., Portokalidis, G.: Location-enhanced authentication using the IoT: because you cannot be in two places at once. In: Proceedings of the 32nd Annual Conference on Computer Security Applications, pp. 251–264. ACSAC'16, ACM, New York (2016). https://doi.org/10.1145/2991079.2991090
2. Al-Fuqaha, A., Guizani, M., Mohammadi, M., Aledhari, M., Ayyash, M.: Internet of things: a survey on enabling technologies, protocols, and applications. IEEE Commun. Surv. Tutorials **17**(4), 2347–2376 (2015)
3. Alharam, A.K., El-madany, W.: Complexity of cyber security architecture for IoT healthcare industry: a comparative study. In: 2017 5th International Conference on Future Internet of Things and Cloud Workshops (FiCloudW), pp. 246–250. IEEE (2017)
4. Baker, S.B., Xiang, W., Atkinson, I.: Internet of things for smart healthcare: technologies, challenges, and opportunities. IEEE Access **5**, 26521–26544 (2017)
5. Bernal Bernabe, J., Hernandez-Ramos, J.L., Skarmeta Gomez, A.F.: Holistic privacy-preserving identity management system for the Internet of things. Mob. Inf. Syst. **2017**, 1–20 (2017)
6. Chen, D., Jin, D., Goh, T.T., Li, N., Wei, L.: Context-awareness based personalized recommendation of anti-hypertension drugs. J. Med. Syst. **40**(9), 202 (2016)
7. Ciuciu, I., Claerhout, B., Schilders, L., Meersman, R.: Ontology-based matching of security attributes for personal data access in e-health. In: OTM Confederated International Conferences on the Move to Meaningful Internet Systems, pp. 605–616. Springer (2011)
8. El-Sappagh, S., Ali, F.: Ddo: a diabetes mellitus diagnosis ontology. In: Applied Informatics, vol. 3, p. 5. SpringerOpen (2016)
9. ICD10: https://bioportal.bioontology.org/ontologies/ICD10
10. ICNP: https://bioportal.bioontology.org/ontologies/ICNP
11. Kumar, T., Braeken, A., Liyanage, M., Ylianttila, M.: Identity privacy preserving biometric based authentication scheme for naked healthcare environment. In: 2017 IEEE International Conference on Communications (ICC), pp. 1–7. IEEE (2017)
12. Poulymenopoulou, M., Malamateniou, F., Vassilacopoulos, G.: A virtual PHR authorization system. In: IEEE-EMBS International Conference on Biomedical and Health Informatics (BHI), pp. 73–76 (June 2014). https://doi.org/10.1109/BHI.2014.6864307
13. Shahzad, M., Singh, M.P.: Continuous authentication and authorization for the Internet of things. IEEE Internet Comput. **21**(2), 86–90 (2017)
14. Shone, N., Dobbins, C., Hurst, W., Shi, Q.: Digital memories based mobile user authentication for IoT. In: 2015 IEEE International Conference on Computer and Information Technology; Ubiquitous Computing and Communications; Dependable, Autonomic and Secure Computing; Pervasive Intelligence and Computing, pp. 1796–1802. IEEE (2015)
15. SNOMED CT: https://bioportal.bioontology.org/ontologies/SNOMEDCT
16. Souag, A., Salinesi, C., Comyn-Wattiau, I.: Ontologies for security requirements: a literature survey and classification. In: International Conference on Advanced Information Systems Engineering, pp. 61–69. Springer (2012)
17. Trnka, M., Cerny, T.: Authentication and authorization rules sharing for Internet of things. Softw. Netw. **2018**(1), 35–52 (2018)

DeepLCP: Towards a DeepLearning Approach to Prevent Lung Cancer

Mayssa Ben Kahla, Dalel Kanzari, and Ahmed Maalel

1 Introduction

Lung cancer is considered to be one of the leading causes of death, mainly because of the late detection of the disease's symptoms and the lack of prevention's means. According to the National Cancer Institute: lung cancer is the fourth most common cancer in France. Also, according to the International Agency for Research on Cancer: Lung cancer is the second most common cancer in Tunisia with a 14.2% incidence and 21.1% mortality. This disease has many (a) risk factors, for example personal history of disease, family history of cancer, diet, smokers, etc., and many (b) symptoms, for example chest pain, persistent cough, Spitting blood, etc. The aim of our approach is to accurately calculate the probability of having lung cancer disease based on (a) and (b) by combining two technologies; the natural language processing (NLP) [1, 2] and the convolutional neural network (CNN) [3]. This paper describes in Sect. 2 the related work in Sect. 3 our approach, named DeepLCP, and in Sect. 4 the experimental validation of DeepLCP.

M. Ben Kahla (✉)
Higher Institute of Applied Science and Technology, University of Sousse, Sousse, Tunisia

D. Kanzari · A. Maalel
Higher Institute of Applied Sciences and Technology, University of Sousse, Sousse, Tunisia

National School of Computer Sciences, RIADI Laboratory, University of Manouba, Manouba, Tunisia

L. Chaari (ed.), *Digital Health in Focus of Predictive, Preventive and Personalised Medicine*, Advances in Predictive, Preventive and Personalised Medicine 12,
https://doi.org/10.1007/978-3-030-49815-3_3

2 Related Works

Several works deal with the cancer disease using the Deeplearning [4] paradigm, we quote, for example, the work of Gruetzemacher et al. [5] which use the architecture DNN for a revolutionary image recognition method to distinguish large and small pulmonary nodules from potentially malignant lung nodules.Besides uncertainty and high cost of computation, this work achieves high false positive in the detection step. Esteva et al. [6] deal with the CNN technique to classify the skin lesion and to detect the cancer disease by giving the probability of malignancy or benignity. But, this work complains by the variance of accuracy. Park et al. [7] develops a Deep learning algorithm, called DeepNEAT-Dx, to predict the presence or absence of lung cancer in a chest X-ray. The problem of "DeepNEAT-Dx", spend 40 h to train. Also, the study by D. Yang et al. [8], presents advanced AI (artificial intelligence) technology for the early detection of lung cancer and a classification model based on the DCNN system. Bychkov et al. [9] chose to combine convolutional (CNN) and recurrent (RNN) architectures to form a deep network to predict colorectal cancer outcomes from images of tumor tissue samples. But, this work has obtained low accuracy. All these works use image as input data, furthermore, there exist other works that use text as input data, such as those of Baker et al. [10] that apply the convolutional neural network (CNN) to classify the biomedical input texts. The disadvantages of this work the Cost of calculation and complexity. Also, John et al. [11] deal with the convolutional neural network (CNN), to extract ICDO-3 topographic codes from a corpus of breast and lung cancer pathology reports. The limitation of this corpus study included pathology reports for which the truth on the ground came only from the final diagnostic section of the report We summarize the different works that deal with deep learning, associated with text or image input data, to detect the cancer disease in Table 1.

The works presented in Table 1 contain a lot of limits like precision problem, cost calculation and complexity. Moreover, we note that most of these works apply convolutional neural networks (CNN) to detect only the lung cancer. They use CNN in a delayed phase where the patient made the diagnosis by imaging. For example, [7] used CNN to detect lung cancer from CXRs images and [11] use the CNN with medical reports after diagnosis. The problem with imaging, in case of lung cancer, is that the disease can't be discover early and the remedy is hardly difficult.

3 Proposed Approach

Inspired from Zhang Y. & Wallace (2015) [12] works, our approach, aim to combine two advanced methods; the natural language processing **(NLP)** and the convolutional neuronal network **(CNN)**. As illustrated in Fig. 1, our architecture is composed of an NLP layer, CNN layers, and a disease classification output.

Table 1 Synthesis of related works

Reference	Algorithm	Architecture	Accuracy	Error rate	Input image	Input text
[5]	Maxpooling, softmax	DNN	81.08–82.10%	–	✓	
[6]	Partitioning algorithm (PA)/Inference algorithm/t-SNE (t-distributed stochastic neighbor embedding)	CNN (GoogleNet)	55.4–72.1%	–	✓	
[7]	Genetic algorithm/ DeepNEAT-Dx/ Backpropagation/SchiffMan encoding	CNN	96.00%	7.97%	✓	
[8]	–	DCNN	90–97%	10–24%	✓	
[9]	SVM/Naïve Bayes classifier/logistic regression	CNN-RNN (LSTM)	69%	–	✓	
[10]	NLP-WORD2VEC word embeddings	CNN	97.1%	2.9%		✓
[11]	Adadelta adaptive gradient descent/NLP-WORD2VEC/N-grams	CNN	71%	30%		✓

3.1 Natural Language Processing (NLP)

In the **NLP** part we use the word2vec model [13] to convert the sentences extracted from our online form to raw matrix. each sentence is a feature. The weights will choose according to the user's response and semantic transformation rules.

Semantic Transformation Rules give each information weights. All the rules defined by two doctors from hospital Farhat Hached Sousse and Hospital Taher Sfar Mahdia. We use 31 semantic rules formed by the formal Z language[14], then we implement these rules in python the construction of our raw semantic matrix. Figure 2 shows an example of these rules.

This rule means if the person answered in our online form that his gender is a man then the first column weight of VC matrix is a value of the interval [0.6..0.9]. Else if the answer is a woman then the weight of the first VC matrix column is a value

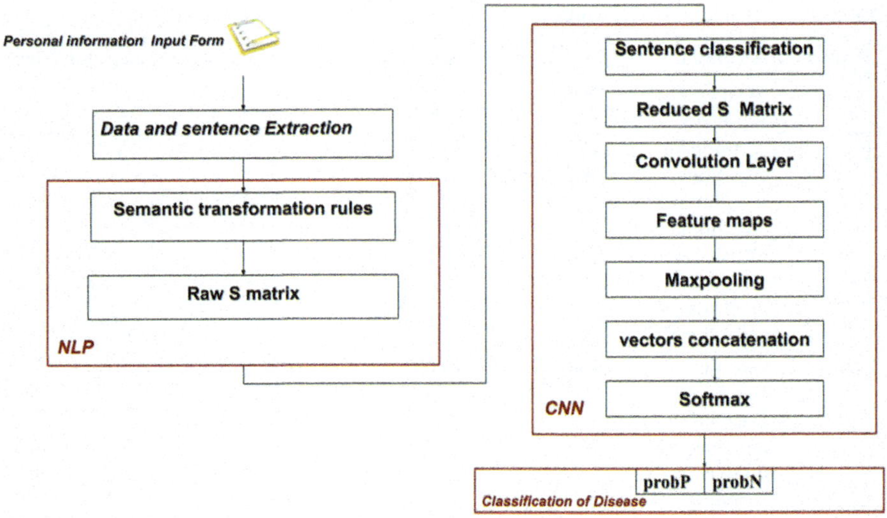

Fig. 1 DeepLCP architecture

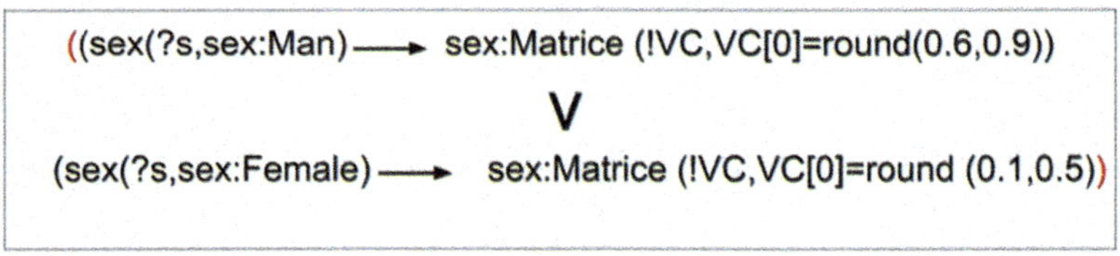

Fig. 2 Semantic transformation rules

of the interval [0.1..0.5]. These intervals are suggested by the doctor "Pr. Bouaouina Noureddine" chief radiotherapy department in the hospital Farhat hached Sousse and the doctor "Dr. Jalel Knani" Pneumologist in the Tahar Sfar Hospital because the Man have the risk of having the disease that the woman.

Raw S Matrix after the transformation we obtain the raw semantic matrix as illustrated in Fig. 3 with size [31*13].

- **31**: is the number of features.
- **13**: is the maximum number of words in the longest sentence.

3.2 Convolutional Neural Network (CNN)

In this part we apply two semantic classifications on the raw semantic matrix to obtain the reduced semantic matrix. Then we apply the CNN on this matrix to obtain the probability of detecting the disease.

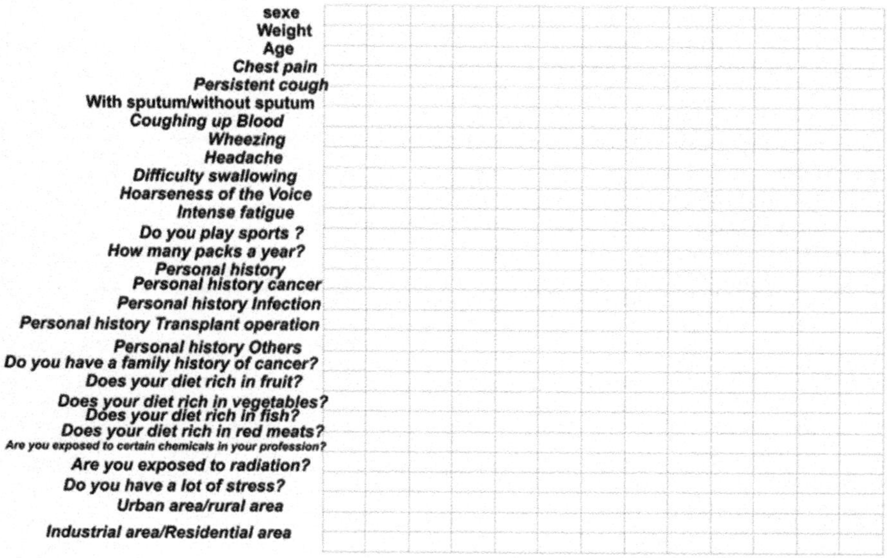

Fig. 3 Raw semantic matrix

- **Reduced S Matrix**
  To obtain the reduced semantic matrix we apply two type of classifications:
  - **Classification By Categories:** we classify data according to three categories: **Minor risk factors, Major risk factors, symptom.**
  + **Classification By Themes:** we classify data into six themes:
    * **Thoracic signs:** this matrix represents the average of the matrices "chest pain", "wheezing" and "abnormal breathlessness".
    * **Cough:** this matrix contains the average of the matrices of "persistent cough", "with/without spitting" and "spitting of blood".
    * **Feeding:** this matrix contains the average of the matrices "diet rich in fruits", "diet rich in vegetables", "food rich in fish" and "diet rich in red meat".
    * **Consumer:** this matrix contains the average of the matrices "how many packets tobacco", "passive smoking", "alcohol".
    * **Personal antecedent:** this matrix contains the average of the matrices "Cancer", "infection", "Transplant operation of an organ".
    * **Residence:** this matrix indicates either the average of the matrices "urban area" and "industrial zone", either the average of the matrices "urban area" and "residential area", either the average of the matrices "rural area" and "residential area".

After classification we obtain the reduced semantic matrix with size [18*13] as illustrated in Fig. 4.

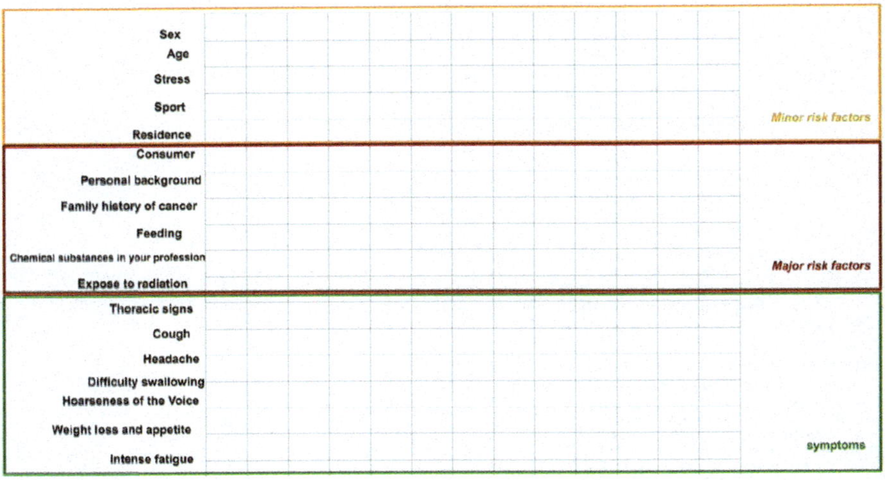

Fig. 4 Reduced matrix

We used the reduction to optimize the complexity. With the reduction will not lose any information.

- **Convolution Layer**
  In this layer we have 3 region size (5, 6, 7) and 2 filters for each region size. So, we have six filters in the total. All the filters will scan all the matrix input with stride 1 to give us one feature maps for each filter. For each feature map we will apply the maxpooling to get one value for each feature map accordingly concatenate all the maxpooling and apply the activation function "softmax".
- **Disease Classification** Our output is two probability "probP": probability of having the disease and "probN": probability of not having the disease.

4 Validation

In the validation part, we use validation set with 490 real cases divided into 315 of the patient who have the disease and 175 who haven't. Also, we use 111 real cases for test set divided into 40 patients affected by the disease and 71 who not affected. As it is shown in Figs. 5 and 6 the accuracy for our model is 94.59% with a 5.41% error rate and the test lost 15.90%.

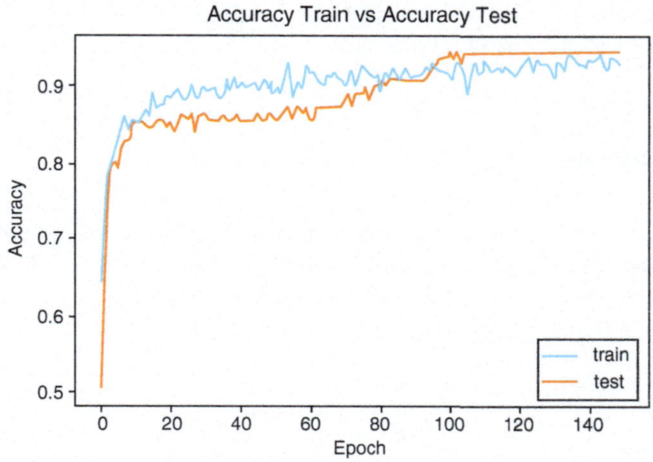

Fig. 5 Accuracy train vs accuracy test DeepLCP

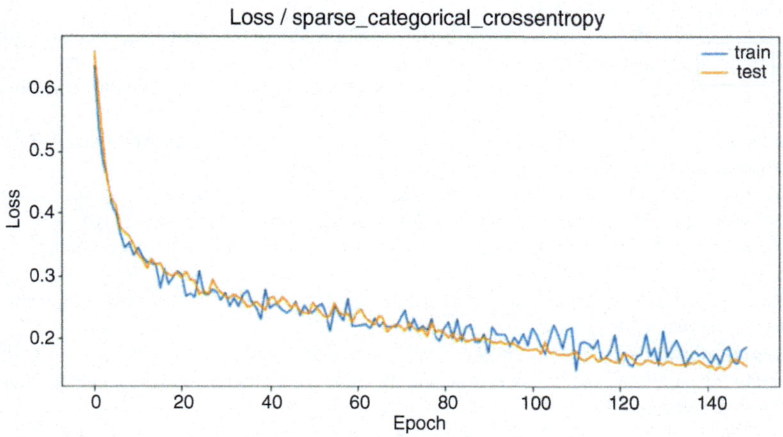

Fig. 6 Loss train vs loss test DeepLCP

5 Discussion

We tested our dataset with four machine learning algorithms:

- The **k-nearest neighbors (KNN)**: it provides a 86.48% precision rate and a 13.52% Error rate.
- The **Decision Tree algorithm**: it returns a 93.69% precision rate and a 6.31% error rate.
- The **Random Forest**: it results a 91.89% precision rate and a 8.11% error rate.
- The **Artificial Neural Network (ANN)**: it provides a 85.59% precision rate and a 14.41% error rate.

Based on these results we find that our "DeepLCP" model provides the best accuracy rate and the lowest error rate.

6 Conclusion

In this article we present a new model for the prevention of lung cancer. Our model named "DeepLCP" is a combination of NLP and CNN. In the NLP part we use semantic transformation rules. the accuracy of validation test is 94.5% which confirm that our model give an efficient result.

References

1. Otter, D.W., et al.: A survey of the usages of deep learning in natural language processing. CoRR, abs/1807.10854 (2018)
2. Towards Datascience: https://towardsdatascience.com/natural-language-processing-nlp-for-machine-learning-d44498845d5b. Last accessed 13 June 2019
3. Analytics Vidhya: https://www.analyticsvidhya.com/blog/2018/12/guide-convolutional-neural-network-cnn/. Last accessed 14 June 2019
4. Pattanayak, S.: Pro Deep Learning with TensorFlow: A Mathematical Approach to Advanced Artificial Intelligence in Python. Apress, Berkeley (2018)
5. Gruetzemacher, R., Gupta, A.: Using deep learning for pulmonary nodule detection & diagnosis. In: AMCIS, Association for Information Systems, San Diego (2016)
6. Esteva, A., et al.: Dermatologist-level classification of skin cancer with deep neural networks. Nature **542**, 115–118 (2017)
7. Michael Park, H., Monahan, C.: Genetic deep learning for lung cancer screening. Innovation Dx Inc. 23 Aug (2017)
8. Yang, D., Powell, C.A., et al.: Deep convolutional neutral networks based artificial intelligence system for pulmonary nodule detection and diagnosis in United States and Chinese dataset. In: ATS, San Diego (2018)
9. Bychkov, D., et al.: Deep learning based tissue analysis predicts outcome in colorectal cancer. In: Scientific Reports, Feb (2018)
10. Baker, S., et al.: Cancer hallmark text classification using convolutional neural networks. In: BioTxtM@COLING (2016)
11. John, X., et al.: Deep learning for automated extraction of primary sites from cancer pathology reports. IEEE J. Biomed. Health Inf. **22**, 244–251 (2018)
12. Zhang, Y., Wallace, A.: Sensitivity analysis of (and practitioners' guide to) convolutional neural networks for sentence classification. arXiv preprint arXiv:1510.03820 (2015)
13. Dataanalytics Post: https://dataanalyticspost.com/Lexique/word2vec/. Last accessed 14 June 2019
14. Bowen, J.P.: Formal Specification and Documentation Using Z: A Case Study Approach. International Thomson Publishing, London/Boston, June (2003)

A Sleep Monitoring Method with EEG Signals

Yessrine Abichou, Siwar Chaabene, and Lotfi Chaari

1 Introduction

One of the crucial issues in the development of cognitive and clinical neuroscience is undoubtedly the ability to track over time and to precisely locate human brain activity. Sleep detection is one of the most active research topics in biomedical signal processing. This involves the acquisition and recording of a set of physiological signals, followed by visual analysis to establish the diagnosis. Assessing sleep disorders is also an important step to prevent further physical and mental complications. This could be done for instance to predict and prevent sleep apnea.

Several methods for sleep exploration have been proposed during the last decades. The basic examination, called polysomnography, allows to group the recording of several variables by mentioning for example the electrical activity of the brain, the activity of the muscles of the face and the chin, sometimes muscles legs, the activity of eyeballs and also the electrical activity of the heart.

This study is mainly based on the electroencephalogram (EEG) signal which presents the result obtained by a recording of electrical signals transmitted by means of electrodes applied on the scalp. This recording is a potential difference between the electrodes excited by the neurons.

In 2009 with Li et al. [7], the EEG signals are analyzed with the Hilbert-Huang transformation, the energy frequency distribution of the EEG is used as a function

Y. Abichou · S. Chaabene
MIRACL laboratoty, University of Sfax, Sfax, Tunisia

Digital Research Centre of Sfax, Sfax, Tunisia

L. Chaari (✉)
University of Toulouse, IRIT-ENSEEIHT, Toulouse, France
e-mail: lotfi.chaari@enseeiht.fr; lotfi.chaari@toulouse-inp.fr

L. Chaari (ed.), *Digital Health in Focus of Predictive, Preventive and Personalised Medicine*, Advances in Predictive, Preventive and Personalised Medicine 12,
https://doi.org/10.1007/978-3-030-49815-3_4

parameter for each sleep stage. This method gave a classification rate of 81.7% using the k nearest neighbor method. In 2010, Tagluk et al. [9] used frequency analysis, specifically using the power spectral density. An artificial neural network technique is the used for classification. This system gave a recognition rate up to 76.8%.

In 2012, Fraiwan et al. [2] used Hilbert transformations and continuous wavelet transformations to extract the characteristics with an accuracy rate of 83%, relying on a random forest classification method.

In 2013, Lajnef et al. [6] used variance, Skewness, Kurtosis and energy permutations as features, and the SVM classification method was considered achieving an accuracy level of 92%. The performance of the method was evaluated using polysomnographic data of 15 subjects (electroencephalogram (EEG), electro oculography (EOG) and electromyogram (EMG) recordings.

In 2015 Kayikcioglu et al. [5] reached a 91% classification rate with LPC (Partial Least Squares Regression) using an auto-regressive method. The results were compared with those of other classifiers, such as k nearest neighbor (k-NN), linear discriminant (LDC) and Bayes classifiers.

More recently, Alickovic et al. [1] used the decomposition based on iterative filtering with SVM as classifier. This system achieved a classification rate of 91.1%.

In this work, a feature-based method for EEG data classification is proposed with additional features and a dimension reduction strategy.

The rest of this paper is organized as follows. Section 2 formulates the problem. The proposed method is then presented in Sect. 3, while experimental results are drawn in Sect. 4. Finally, conclusions and future work are given in Sect. 5.

2 Problem Formulation

The EEG signal is complex, its inspection gives inaccurate information; to improve its sensitivity, the plot is cut into short observation windows. Each window undergoes a mathematical analysis intended to extract quantitative parameters. In this paper,the parameters extracted from EEG signal in order to identify the recognition of the state through a study of classifications. Secondly, we go on to describe the method used in our work that specifies the performance of our research.

3 Proposed Method

The basic structure of the method proposed in this paper is given in Fig. 1. It can be seen that it has three main modules: the first is Data Preparation; the second is feature extraction; the third is dimension reduction; and finally classification. In this section, we provide detailed explanation of each module.

We performed a windowing with a frame in 2 s. Then we varied the size of the window (3 s). The best results were obtained for the size of 2 s. So we decided to

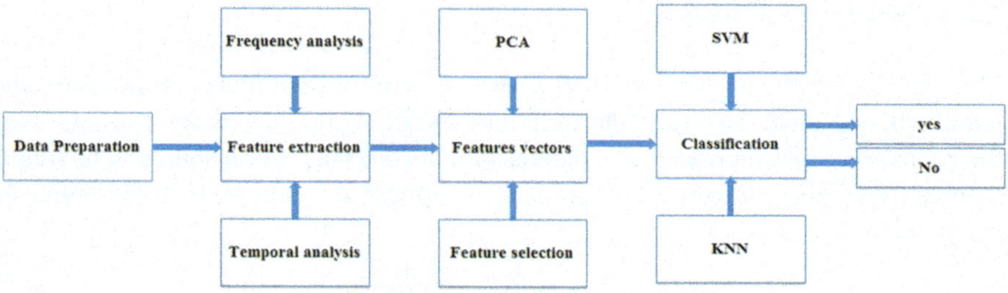

Fig. 1 Structural diagram of the proposed method for sleep monitoring

decrease the frame to have a better result we advocated to 1 and 0.5 s. Which leads to deduce that the window a second is the one that suits the most.

3.1 Feature Extraction

The main interest in signal processing is to extract as much information as possible on the temporal or frequency structure of these signals. It is therefore necessary to break down the signal on functions well localized in both time and frequency.

3.1.1 dwt

The discrete wavelet transform analysis the signal at different frequency bands with different resolutions by decomposing the signal with a rough approximation and detailed information. The basic principle of the discrete wavelet transform is to separate the signal into two components, one representing the shape of the signal, the other representing its details. The general appearance of a function is represented by its low frequencies, the details by its high frequencies.

3.1.2 Energy

The most traditional features among wavelet-based methods is the measurement of energy in each sub-band. Mathematically, it is presented as follows:

$$ED_i = \sum_{j=1}^{N} |D_{ij}|^2. \tag{1}$$

$$EA_i = \sum_{j=1}^{N} |A_{ij}|^2. \tag{2}$$

3.1.3 Shannon's Entropy

The entropy here is a reflection of the amount of information present at each sub-band, where X is a discrete scalar random variable with realizations $x_1,\ldots, x_n$ and the probability distribution $p_1,\ldots, p_n$ measure his disorder. For a source X having n symbols, a symbol i having a probability pi to appear, the entropy H of the source X is defined as:

$$H(x) = -\sum_{i=1}^{n} p_i log_2 p_i. \tag{3}$$

3.1.4 Variance

Variance is the measure of the dispersion of a set of data points around their mean value, it is defined as follows:

$$v(x) = \frac{\sum_{i=1}^{n}(x_i - \overline{x})^2}{n}. \tag{4}$$

avec $\overline{x} = \sum_{i=1}^{n} p_i x_i$ et n: total number of data points.

3.1.5 Mean

We can define the mean M of a data vector X as follows:

$$M = \frac{1}{n}\sum_{i=1}^{n} x_i. \tag{5}$$

3.1.6 Minimum

This is the minimum value of an X data vector.

3.1.7 Maximum

This is the maximum value of a data vector X.

3.1.8 Energy Ratio

Each of the brainwaves (delta, theta, alpha and beta) occupy a quantity of the energy of the EEG signal. We proceed to a quantitative study of the energetic ratios of each of the waves compared to the global energy of the signal. The energy ratio is calculated by the ratio between the wave energy (E_0) and the total energy of the signal (E_s).

$$RE = \frac{E_0}{E_s}. \quad (6)$$

3.1.9 Frequency Analysis

The frequency characteristics of a time series can be written by calculating its power spectral density (DSP).

$$DSP(v) = \lim_{N_k \to \infty} \frac{1}{2N_k+1} E(|FFT(v)|^2). \quad (7)$$

3.2 *Dimension Reduction*

3.2.1 PCA

Which consists of replacing the initial set of data with a new reduced set constructed from the initial set of characteristics.

3.2.2 Feature Selection

Which consists in selecting the most relevant characteristics from the dataset of the variables describing the phenomenon studied.

3.3 *Classification*

3.3.1 SVM

Is a binary classification method by supervised learning. This method relies on the existence of a linear classifier in an appropriate space. Since this is a two-class classification problem, this method uses a learning dataset to learn the model's parameters.

3.3.2 KNN

Is a method based on memory, which unlike other statistical methods, requires no learning. It works according to the intuitive principle that the closest objects are most likely to belong to the same category. Thus, with the k nearest neighbors method, forecasts are based on a set of prototype examples that are used to predict new data.

4 Experimental Results

4.1 Data Set

Our database is a record taken from the "Physio Bank" [3], in the form EDF "European Data Format"; EDF is a file that contains separate lines according to the samples. It can have several sampling frequencies as it can contain several signals; in our case he can present an EEG and an EOG together. This database is registered for eight Caucasian people (men and women) between the ages of 21 and 35, healthy (who do not have trouble sleeping) and without medication. The records are named sc4002e0.rec, sc4012e0.rec, sc4102e0.rec, sc4112e0.rec, st7022j0.rec, st7052j0.rec, st7121j0.rec, st7132j0.rec. These signals are recorded through the electrode FpzCz (E1), PzOz (E2) against C4-A1 and C3-A2 according to the alternative placement of the electrodes during the automatic detection of sleep. Four recordings are obtained by four volunteers during 23 h: 45 min during their normal lives, while using a modified tap tape cassette. The other four recordings lasted one night of sleep in a hospital, while using a 100 Hz sampling rate miniature telemeter with a frequency response equal to −3 dB per point, a 14-bit representation per sample, and a total noise equal to −2V p-p.

4.2 Experimental Setup

According to the exploitation of the Daubechies wavelet decomposition method (db5) we found the 5 brain waves: alpha, theta, gamma, beta, delta (please see Figs. 2 and 3).

The calculation of these parameters is done on each EEG rhythm, that is to say for each wave we will calculate the 7 features (energy, variance, maximum, minimum, average, entropy, energy ratio).

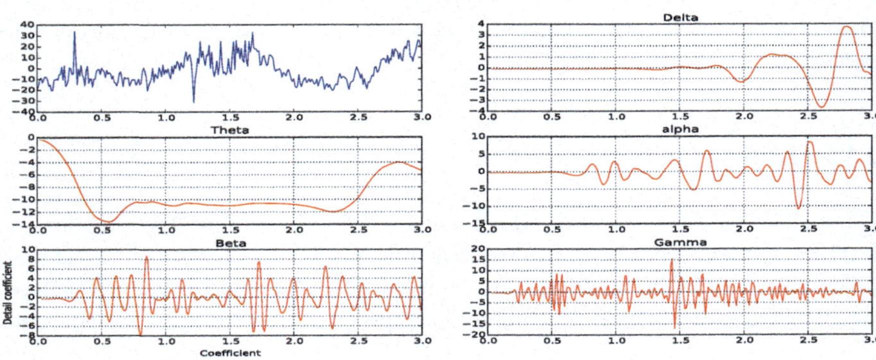

Fig. 2 Decomposition with a window of 3 s

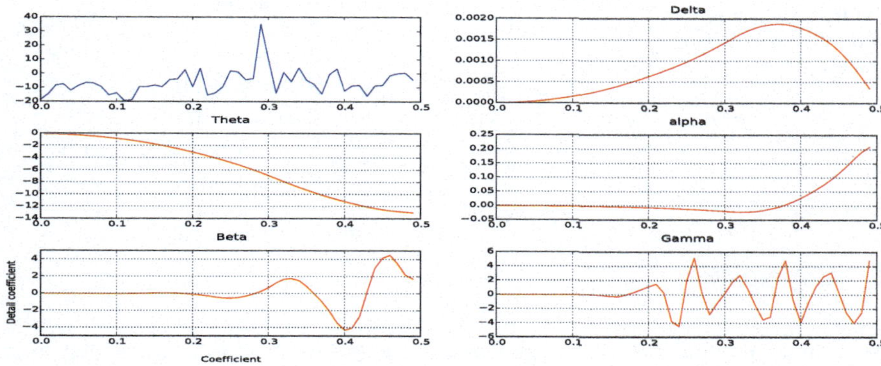

Fig. 3 Decomposition with a window of 0.5 s

Table 1 Best accuracy obtained

	OneClassSVM	KNN
Without reduction	84%	82.5%
PCA	91.5%	79.7%
SF	**93%**	88.2%

From the FFT, we calculated the DSP of our signal. We used this method to subdivide the signal into subband and we started with 2 then 3 then 4 and finally 5 bands. In order to grasp the exact choice we had to try with all the frequencies proposed in the classification.

The following table shows the results without and with reduction. This table shows that we have succeeded, on two levels of reduction, in improving the recognition rate and reducing by more the number of characteristics used. By reducing the characteristics, a small subset of examples containing only those that seem to influence the class separation capability can be selected from the training set. Our contribution comes within this framework. The proposed method makes it possible to significantly reduce the number of characteristics of the database then to make an offline learning. The results obtained show the performance of this solution using the OneClassSVM classification method with electrode 2 (Table 1).

4.3 Comparison with the Existing Methods

Our detection results are compared with those of the literature to better position our algorithm with other recent methods of sleep detection. The choice of articles to make the comparison was based on the methods used and their similarities to our algorithm (Table 2).

Table 2 Comparison of performance of previous studies

Methods	Accuracy
Li et al. [7]	81.5%
Hassan et al. [4]	87.5 %
sharma et al. [8]	90%
Kayikcioglu et al. [5]	91 %
Proposed method	93 %

5 Conclusion

This study proved that statistical features can be used with standard accuracy. This proposed methods provides convincing classification accuracy of 93% using statistical parameters of EEG signal. Future work will focus perform parallel analysis using electro oculography (EOG) and electrocardiography (ECG).

References

1. Alickovic, E., Subasi, A.: Ensemble SVM method for automatic sleep stage classification. IEEE Trans. Instrum. Meas. **67**(6), 1258–1265 (2018)
2. Fraiwan, L., Lweesy, K., Khasawneh, N., Wenz, H., Dickhaus, H.: Automated sleep stage identification system based on time–frequency analysis of a single EEG channel and random forest classifier. Comput. Methods Prog. Biomed. **108**(1), 10–19 (2012)
3. Goldberger, A.L., Amaral, L.A., Glass, L., Hausdorff, J.M., Ivanov, P.C., Mark, R.G., Mietus, J.E., Moody, G.B., Peng, C.K., Stanley, H.E.: Physiobank, physiotoolkit, and physionet: components of a new research resource for complex physiologic signals. Circulation **101**(23), e215–e220 (2000)
4. Hassan, A.R., Bashar, S.K., Bhuiyan, M.I.H.: On the classification of sleep states by means of statistical and spectral features from single channel electroencephalogram. In: 2015 International Conference on Advances in Computing, Communications and Informatics (ICACCI), pp. 2238–2243 (2015)
5. Kayikcioglu, T., Maleki, M., Eroglu, K.: Fast and accurate pls-based classification of EEG sleep using single channel data. Expert Syst. Appl. **42**(21), 7825–7830 (2015)
6. Lajnef, T., Chaibi, S., Ruby, P., Aguera, P.E., Eichenlaub, J.B., Samet, M., Kachouri, A., Jerbi, K.: Learning machines and sleeping brains: automatic sleep stage classification using decision-tree multi-class support vector machines. J. Neurosci. Methods **250**, 94–105 (2015)
7. Li, Y., Yingle, F., Gu, L., Qinye, T.: Sleep stage classification based on EEG Hilbert-Huang transform. In: 2009 4th IEEE Conference on Industrial Electronics and Applications, pp. 3676–3681 (2009)
8. Sharma, R., Pachori, R.B., Upadhyay, A.: Automatic sleep stages classification based on iterative filtering of electroencephalogram signals. Neural Comput. Appl. **28**(10), 2959–2978 (2017)
9. Tagluk, M.E., Sezgin, N., Akin, M.: Estimation of sleep stages by an artificial neural network employing EEG, EMG and EOG. J. Med. Syst. **34**(4), 717–725 (2010)

Numerical Simulation of Venous System Blood Flow for Hepatic Donor Patient and Portal Hypertension's Proposed Measurement

Safa Ben Cheikh Souguir, Raouf Fathallah, Asma Ben Abdallah, Badii Hmida, and Mohamed Hedi Bedoui

1 Introduction

Concerning hepatic blood flow, clinicians require reproducible and non-invasive methods. In clinical practice, we quote two useful non-invasive methods in hepatic flow measurement despite their known limitations such as Doppler ultrasound (US) and Phase-contrast magnetic resonance imaging (PC-MRI). However, results in the literature suggest that these methods may in some cases show diverse analysis. Furthermore, in velocity measured by US doppler, there is great errors' percentage that may reach 20% in reference to blood velocity estimation [1]. In this case, a comparative study was done in order to set the variability of parameters using these methods [2, 3].

Nowadays, Numeric simulation of blood circulation opens up predictions and perspectives for doctors in terms of performing a surgery. Virtual simulation provides useful biomechanical models for clinicians in different blood flow systems. However, like any technic or method, the virtual simulation will be used with well-defined conditions in order to be verified in terms of capability and performance.

Little work has been done to study blood flow in the portal vein. The work reported in the literature has mentioned the hemodynamic simulation of blood flow in different organs such as the cerebral arterial circle [4], the carotids [5]

S. B. C. Souguir (✉)
National Engineering School of Sousse, Sousse, Tunisia

Laboratory Technology and Medical Imaging, Monastir, Tunisia

A. B. Abdallah · M. H. Bedoui
Laboratory Technology and Medical Imaging, Monastir, Tunisia

B. Hmida
Medical Imaging Services, CHU Fattouma Bourguiba, Monastir, Tunisia

L. Chaari (ed.), *Digital Health in Focus of Predictive, Preventive and Personalised Medicine*, Advances in Predictive, Preventive and Personalised Medicine 12,
https://doi.org/10.1007/978-3-030-49815-3_5

and cardiovascular system [6] etc. The numerical simulation of venous system was rarely approached due to its complex geometry as well as its difference of elasticity with respect to the arterial system.

The purposes of this research will focus mainly on studying the normal venous blood circulation in the liver of a female donor through the determination of blood's pressure and velocity by the chosen hypothesis and condition, validating results, understanding the phenomenon of portal hypertension [7] that can be seen in several pathologies such as cirrhosis or thrombosis, as well as proposing portal pressure's measure related to a young receiver patient before and after chirurgical intervention.

2 Methods

We propose to simulate the 3D blood flow of the venous system based on 2D database. Our approach is as follows: We segmented series of anatomical images about the venous system, along with a 3D reconstruction extracting iso-surfaces. Subsequently, from the generated 3D triangular mesh, we modelled the volume of our structure by the "Reverse Engineering" method. Finally, we prepared a CFD study Fig. 1.

2.1 *Segmentation and 3D Reconstruction*

The anatomical structure was obtained from native cuts using a thoraco-abdominopelvic CT scan of liver donor patient before the chirurgical inter-

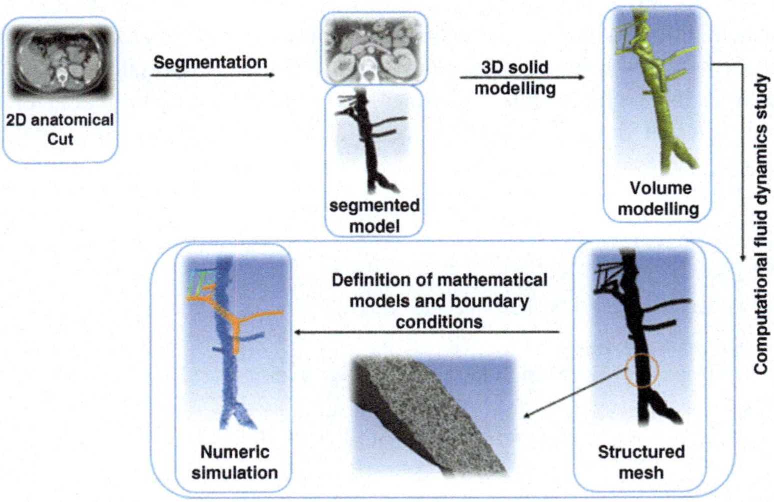

Fig. 1 Methods and approach

vention. We identified different veins and segmented the 2D anatomical cuts (0.7 × 0.7 × 1.25 mm) after injection of the contrast medium. Indeed, for each anatomical section we surround the concerned veins and control the appearance of the following line using AMIRA software. The segmentation has been validated by radiologist experts.

2.2 3D Volume Modelling

the next step is to prepare a volume model through the Reverse Engineering method which used to generate a three-dimensional digital model from 2D data [8]. This method consists of designing a series of parallel curves relating to the generated 3D triangular mesh and connecting them with surface sections in order to obtain a closed surface. It is noteworthy to mention; this surface model has been transformed into a volume model by filling the material.

2.3 CFD Study

In this section, we performed a CFD study consisting of the following steps:

2.3.1 Finite Elements Mesh

In CFD analysis, the flow domain is subdivided into smaller subdomains. For this geometry, a structured mesh has been conducted in which domain has been discretized into purely tetrahedral elements.

This figure depicts a mesh quality study about the size and number of geometric primitives which forms the tetrahedral mesh after choosing one of these five meshes composed of 2,138,653 elements from which the pressure is almost constant. This volume mesh allowed us to have a reliable result along with optimizing the calculation time Fig. 2.

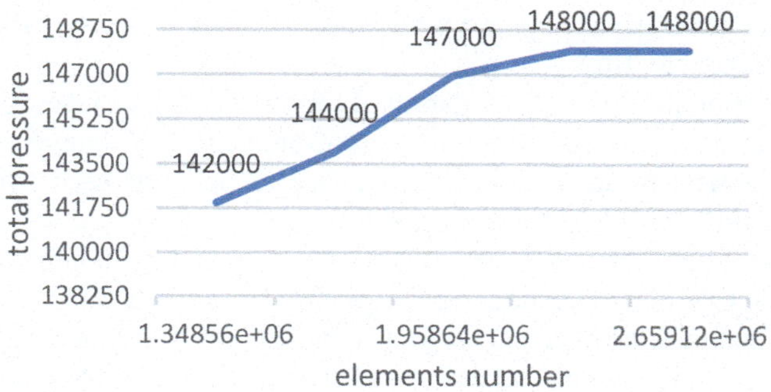

Fig. 2 Pressure variation according to the number of elements

2.3.2 Parameter Definition: Mathematical Model and Boundary Conditions

The flow is assumed to be isothermal so the energy equations have been neglected, while the Navier Stokes equations of continuity and momentum equations 1 and 2 have been solved numerically under stable conditions and for an incompressible fluid.

$$\frac{\partial \rho}{\partial t} + div \rho \vec{V} = 0 \quad (1)$$

$$\rho \frac{\partial \vec{V}}{\partial t} + \overline{\overline{grad}}\, \vec{V}.\rho \vec{V} = \rho \vec{F} - \overrightarrow{grad}\, p + \mu \left(\Delta \vec{V} + \overrightarrow{grad}\, div\, \vec{V} \right) \quad (2)$$

V: Vector fluid velocity, p: momentum, F: External forces exerted on the fluid, ρ: density of the fluid.

We use the hypothesis of a perfectly rigid wall. Blood is a non-Newtonian fluid its viscosity depends on mechanical shear stress. Several models can describe this behaviour between mechanical stress and deformation. Recently, comparative research has been conducted in order to identify the most useful model within blood circulation. Power Law model was recommended which defined by the following Eq. (3) and parameters [9].

$$\mu = \mu_0 (\dot{\gamma})^{n-1} \quad (3)$$

γ: Shear rate, n: power-law index, $\mu_0$initial Viscosity.

Blood density usually depends on the sex and age group of human beings. We took on average density equal to 1060 kg / m3. The flow is defined laminar since the Reynolds coefficient Re (4) does not exceed 1500.

$$R_e = \frac{\rho V D}{\mu} \quad (4)$$

ρ: density (kg.m-3), μ: Dynamic viscosity, V: Characteristic velocity (m / s), D: Largest vein diameter (m).

Due to the complexity and orientation of venous system's shapes, the flow must be considered as turbulent. That is why we examined both laminar and turbulent cases. Although there are numerous turbulence models, we used two turbulence models named K Epsilon and K Omega [10].

In addition, we know that the definition of boundary conditions plays an indispensable role in the numeric experience. We have affected the entry velocities of the veins that feed the liver and vena cava. In CFD study, the input velocity values are obtained from in vivo measurement and are specified in Table 1. For the output values, we used a flow ratio of 1 at the level of the right atrium.

Table 1 Boundary Conditions

Veins	Velocity	Diameter
Left iliac vein	14 (cm/s)	13 (mm)
Right iliac vein	14 (cm/s)	13 (mm)
Left renal vein	15 (cm/s)	8 (mm)
Right renal vein	15 (cm/s)	8 (mm)
Superior mesenteric vein	18 (cm/s)	11 (mm)
Splenic vein	16 (cm/s)	7 (mm)

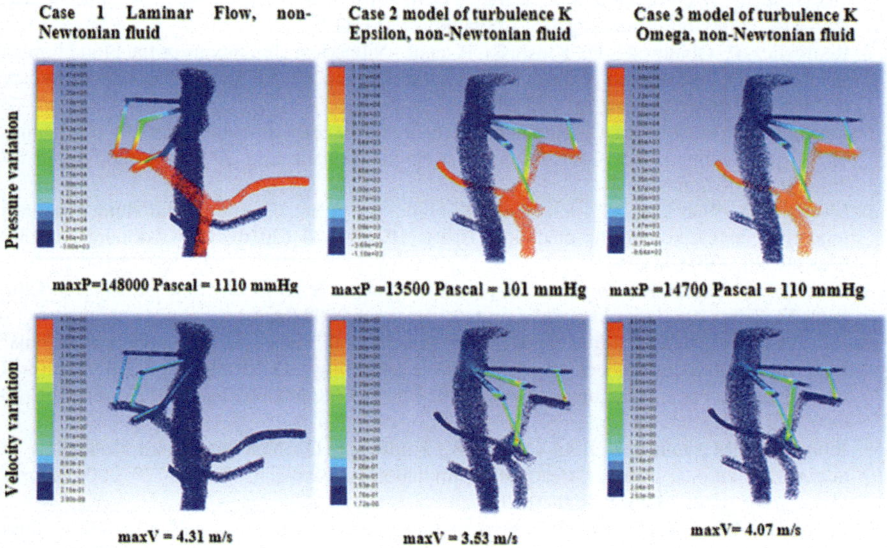

Fig. 3 Results of virtual simulation

3 Results and Conclusions

Regarding the figure below, it is concluded that the laminar model diverged from measured data. In contrast, turbulence models provide an accurate result. Indeed, virtual velocity in the portal vein is 20 cm/s, this result shows a significant correlation with the result measured by Us Doppler which is between 15 and 20 cm/s. Maximum pressure is concentrated at the liver while maximum velocity appears in capillaries situated between sus-hepatics veins and portal branches. Moreover, this research opens perspectives on studying the phenomena explaining portal hypertension through a mechanical model starting by data acquisition, segmentation, 3D reconstruction and numerical simulation. Indeed, there is a growing need for clinicians to detect portal hypertension by measuring hepatic pressure gradient using numeric simulation. Furthermore, we are going to simulate a hepatic pressure gradient for a receiver patient suffering from portal hypertension after and before chirurgical interventions, and to determinate wall shear stress in order to predict variceal bleeding risk (Fig. 3).

References

1. Carlisle, K.M., Halliwell, M., Read, A.E., Wells, P.N.: Estimation of total hepatic blood flow by duplex ultrasound. Gut. **33**, 92–97 (1992). https://doi.org/10.1136/gut.33.1.92
2. Hepatic vascular flow measurements by phase contrast MRI and doppler echography: A comparative and reproducibility study – Yzet – 2010 – J. Magnet. Reson. Imaging – Wiley Online Library. https://onlinelibrary.wiley.com/doi/full/10.1002/jmri.22079. Accessed 9 Jun 2019
3. Annet, L., Materne, R., Danse, E., et al.: Hepatic flow parameters measured with MR imaging and Doppler US: correlations with degree of cirrhosis and portal hypertension. Radiology. **229**, 409–414 (2003). https://doi.org/10.1148/radiol.2292021128
4. Reorowicz, P., Obidowski, D., Klosinski, P., et al.: Numerical simulations of the blood flow in the patient-specific arterial cerebral circle region. J. Biomech. **47**, 1642–1651 (2014). https://doi.org/10.1016/j.jbiomech.2014.02.039
5. Lancellotti, R.M., Vergara, C., Valdettaro, L., et al.: Large eddy simulations for blood dynamics in realistic stenotic carotids. Int. J. Numer. Methods Biomed. Eng. **33**, e2868 (2017). https://doi.org/10.1002/cnm.2868
6. Morris, P.D., Narracott, A., von Tengg-Kobligk, H., et al.: Computational fluid dynamics modelling in cardiovascular medicine. Heart. **102**, 18–28 (2016). https://doi.org/10.1136/heartjnl-2015-308044
7. Lebrec, D., Moreau, R.: Hypertension portale : avancées et perspectives. Gastroenterol. Clin. Biol. **33**, 799–810 (2009). https://doi.org/10.1016/j.gcb.2009.04.001
8. Yu C-C., & Cheng, H-Y.: Study of biomechanical behavior on temporomandibular joint during jaw movement using reverse engineering 3D technology (2018). https://www.ingentaconnect.com/content/asp/jbte/2018/00000008/00000012/art00012. Accessed 20 Oct 2019
9. Johnston, B.M., Johnston, P.R., Corney, S., Kilpatrick, D.: Non-Newtonian blood flow in human right coronary arteries: steady state simulations. J. Biomech. **37**, 709–720 (2004). https://doi.org/10.1016/j.jbiomech.2003.09.016
10. Zhang, J., Zhang, P., Fraser, K.H., et al.: Comparison and experimental validation of fluid dynamic numerical models for a clinical ventricular assist device. Artif. Organs. **37**, 380–389 (2013). https://doi.org/10.1111/j.1525-1594.2012.01576.x

Medical Decision-Making: Incompressible Blood Flow Simulation for the Coronary Artery and Bifurcation Stenosis with CFD Module

Houneida Sakly, Mourad Said, and Moncef Tagina

1 Background

Recently, cardiovascular disease is considered dramatically increased. The common type of death that is mainly due to heart disease or stroke, which is caused by the accumulation of plaques on the endothelial walls of the coronary arteries [1]. The coronary artery disease (CAD) induces to a reduction in the oxygen level at the myocardium and this has been related to the antecedents of cardiovascular disease such as myocardial infarction, stroke and unstable angina [2]. Despite the diversification of risk factors, in particular high cholesterol, diabetes and hypertension, being of a systemic nature, the plaques are located at specific sites of the coronary artery where an endothelial shear disorder occurs [3–5]. In recent years, the additional explanation that has been shown for plaque formation is blood pressure/shear stress [6, 7].

The appearance of atherosclerosis that is based on observation plays a role in the identification of blood behavior. According to the distribution of vascular inflammation and plaques near the lateral branches or arterial stenosis, the blood trajectory n It is not uniform and at the slightest curvature of curvatures where blood flow is relatively low [8, 9]. The inflow of blood flow on the vessel wall is caused by shear stress is reflected via the behavior of endothelial cells. The shear stress leads to shear deformation of the cells and subsequently the inflammatory component and the progression of the plaque [10].

H. Sakly (✉) · M. Tagina
COSMOS Laboratory -National Institute of Computer Sciences – Campus University of Mannouba, Mannouba, Tunisia
e-mail: houneida.sakly@esiee.fr

M. Said
Radiology and Medical Imaging Unit, International Center Carthage Medical, Monastir, Tunisia

L. Chaari (ed.), *Digital Health in Focus of Predictive, Preventive and Personalised Medicine*, Advances in Predictive, Preventive and Personalised Medicine 12,
https://doi.org/10.1007/978-3-030-49815-3_6

The main objective in our study is to analyze the impact of CFD modules on a 3D artery model for a blood flow of normal physical characteristic and detect if there are anomalies via velocity value study and pressure.

2 Related Works

The detection of coronary stenosis is crucial for decision making in coronary revascularization. With the advancement of digital fluid dynamics (CFD), flow accuracy is limited due to the adopted modeling approach. To overcome this problem, a new non-invasive method based on CFD is proposed [11]. The study in [12] focuses on examining the effects of hyperemic flow, such as velocity, shear wall in 3D coronary artery models with and without stenosis on the hydrodynamic parameters. 3D coronary artery models suffer from a > 50% shrinkage of the light surface to simulate the hyperemic flow condition. In contrast, the decrease in pressure was found downstream of the stenosis relative to the coronary artery without stenosis. The analysis provides a view of the distribution of shear stress and pressure drop across the walls to understand the effect of hyperemic flow under both conditions. The research developed in [13] shows the effectiveness of 3D modeling of the artery on the Coronary CT Angiography-derived Fractional Flow Reserve via the Machine Learning Algorithm versus Computational Fluid Dynamics technique. The severity of the stenosis is assessed relative to invasive angiography and angiographic stenosis and does not necessarily apply with hemodynamic accuracy when the fractional flow reserve is used as a reference. In this context, Machine Learning algorithms improve the performance of CTA by correctly reclassifying hemodynamically no significant stenosis and CFD-based CT [14]. The study of the correlation between left coronary bifurcation angle and coronary stenosis as assessed by coronary angiography coronary angiography (CCTA) analysis generated by digital fluid dynamics (CFD) [15]. MV *et al* [16] proposes a reconstruction of the right coronary artery from the angiogram of a patient. The flow analyzes were performed using the Digital Fluid Dynamics (CFD) method focusing on the geometry of the stenosis characterized by areas of stasis, multidirectional velocity, and high wall shear stress. A clinical review was proposed by JM *et al* [1] for the prognostic indications for quantifying the severity of coronary artery disease and invasive and non-invasive imaging technologies to quantify the anatomical parameters of coronary stenosis. The application of image-based CFD simulation techniques [17, 18] to elucidate the effects of hemodynamics in vascular physiopathology on the initialization and progression of coronary artery disease. At this stage Blood flow presents the key for localization and progression of coronary heart disease [19]. CFD simulation based on 3D luminal reconstructions is used to analyze local flow fields and flow profile due to changes in vascular geometry. It helps to identify the risk factors for the development of coronary heart disease [20].

2.1 *Methods and Materials*

A 3D model of the artery has been reconstructed with a geometry that contains 4 nodes, 6 edges, 4 faces. The Hex-dominant algorithm for only CFD module has been adopted with internal meshing mode and moderate finesses. The Blood-type fluid parameterization was set with a Newtonian model viscosity, (ν) Kinematic viscosity = 0.00004 m^2/s, (ρ) Density = 1056 kg/m^3. A second 3D for this bifurcation model is composed of two nodes, 6 edges, 6 faces, 1 volumes. The mesh was generated with Max global cells = 100,000,000, Resolve feature angle = 30, Solver iterations = 150, Relax iterations = eight. Therefore, the boundary conditions is defined as follows: Pressure inlet = 1184 (Pa), the turbulence kinetic energy = 0.00375 (m^2/s^2) and the specific dissipation rate = 3.375 (1/s) for the blood fluid.

3 CFD Studies on Coronary Artery Disease

In order to predict the flow field, particle transport and related phenomena in the region of interest, the numerical methods are used by computational fluid dynamics to solve the set of main equations (continuity and Navier-Stokes equations) for blood flow). The CFD procedure includes the pre-processing phase, which essentially contains the construction of the geometry (artery) to represent the domain of interest, discretization of the domain with meshes as well as the description of the physical model and the boundary conditions. The post-processing part is dedicated for the presentation of the results and the numerical resolution of the equations. The coronary arteries are very curved and are mobile and deformable; this is why the flow study is considered a hard task which leads to in-depth studies on CFD to analyze coronary artery disease in recent decades. To minimize the numerical diffusion and to reduce the number of elements, the generation of the coronary artery model consists of defining the fluid and structural domains that are meshed with hexahedral cells.

4 Results and Discussion

4.1 *Dedicated for Coronary Artery Analysis*

A model of coronary stenosis acquired with CT with a maximum diameter 3.27 mm, minimum diameter 1.08 mm, length 29.66 mm, and a main tortuosity 0.11 mm presented in Fig. 1a was selected. The reconstruction of the 3D model was generated in Fig. 1b.

In order to minimize the numerical diffusion and to reduce the number of elements we adopted the geometry of the artery in Fig. 2. For the generation of

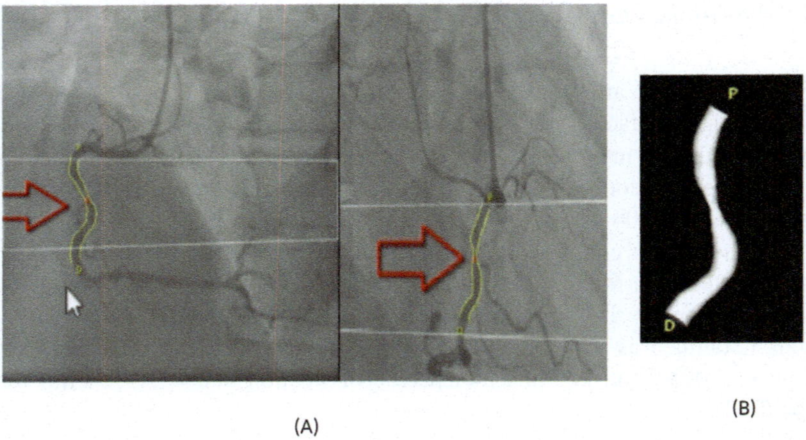

Fig. 1 Reconstruction of the 3D coronary artery model

Fig. 2 Model of the artery in 3D

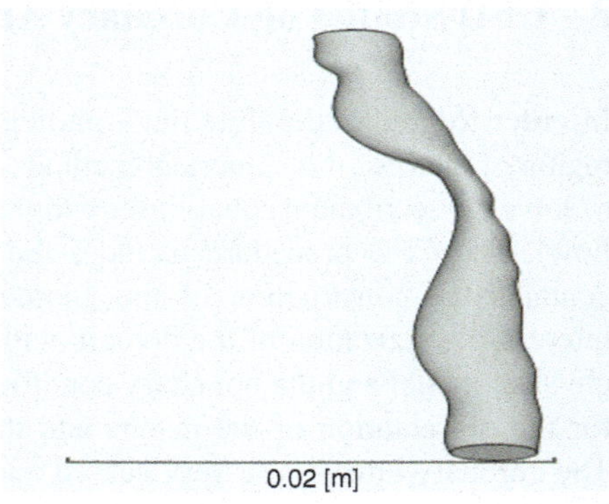

the model of coronary artery, the fluid and structural domains are in mesh with the hexahedral cells.

The next step is to define the meshing mode. We have used an internal meshing, which is typically used for pipe flow and valves. It will place the mesh inside the body and attempt to generate multiregional and will surround the materiel point and extend until the boundaries of the artery as shown in Fig. 3.

The mesh quality are depicted in Table. 1 as follows after finishing parallel processing:

Due to the variation of the blood flow with the cardiac cycle, the flow in the coronary artery is unstable. The inflow and outflow conditions allow the observation of the hemodynamic changes of the arterial system, including the coronary artery. Therefore, the boundary conditions is defined as follows: velocity inlet and outlet = 0.2 m/s and arterial pressure = 76 mmHg in the diastole phase [21]. The fluid solver completed the parallel computation for execution time = 318.52 s and ClockTime = 340 s and the residual simulation is presented as follows in Fig. 4.

Fig. 3 Mech of the artery

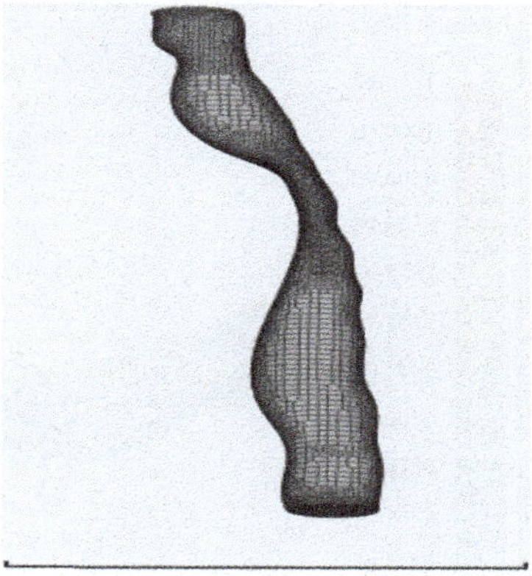

Table 1 Mesh quality metrics

Mesh quality metrics	
Median	1.043005289846296
Min	1.0000000202514494
Max	59.82625634572443
Average	2.7749034006189257
Standard deviation	3.3558916335140054

0-th percentile: 1.0000000202514494
20-th percentile: 1.006279489227181
40-th percentile: 1.0199218383015278
60-th percentile: 1.1554712432086376
80-th percentile: 6.693254767354305
100-th percentile: 59.82625634572443

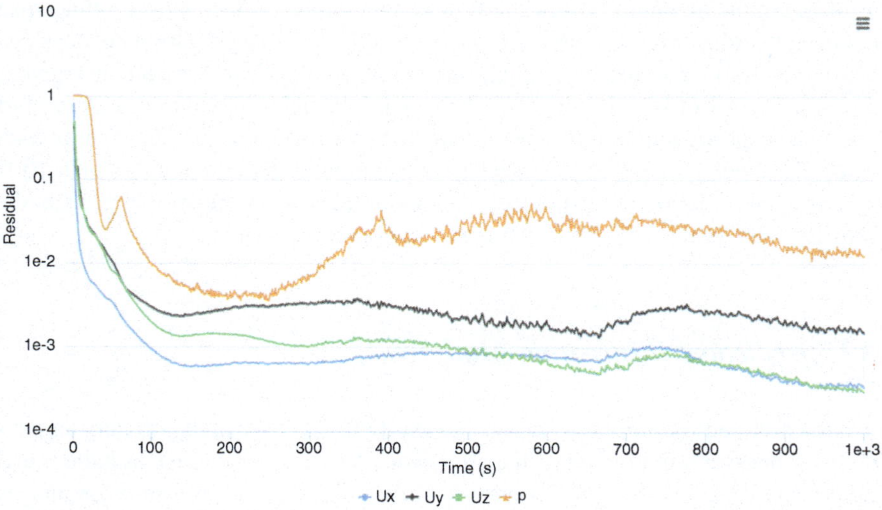

Fig. 4 The residual simulation

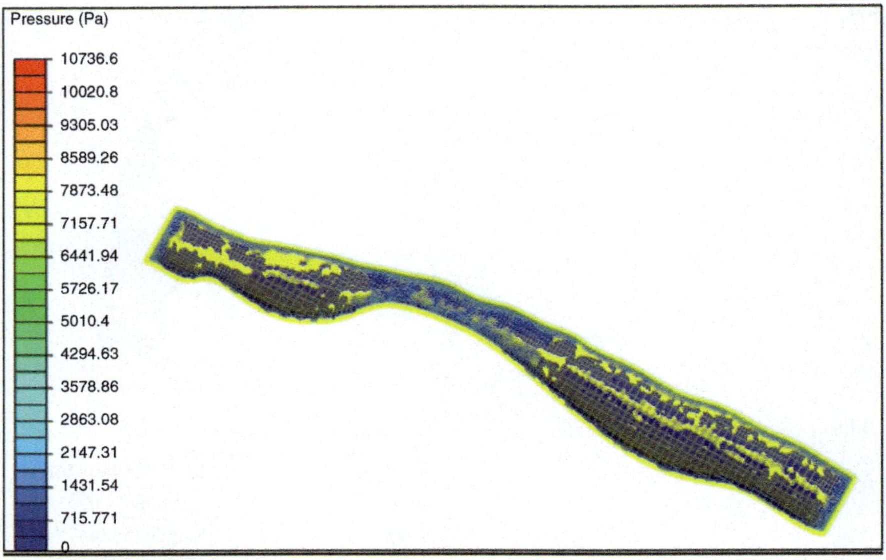

Fig. 5 Simulation of the pressure

The inlet and outlet boundary conditions are based on a physiological flow rate and pressure of the aorta. The average blood flow in the left coronary artery is estimated to be about 57 ml / min, reaching a maximum of 105 ml/min during the diastolic phase according to average human coronary blood flow data that are available in the literature [22–24]. A flow simulation is conducted over a time-span of several cardiac cycles, which are represented by time steps. The time steps can be divided into a number of coupling iterations, with each time step converged to a residual target of less than 1×10^{-4} by approximately 100 iterations. A total of 600 time steps are required to achieve satisfactory convergence for fluid simulation when all velocity component changes from iteration to iteration are less than 10^{-6} [25, 26]. The solution field simulation shows a decrease in pressure as well as the velocity value in the stenotic segment as shown in Figs. 5 and 6.

4.2 *Dedicated Bifurcation Analysis*

In a research setting, coronary arterial analysis (QCA) is used after coronary angiography or intervention to evaluate the effectiveness of treatments such as ballooning, stenting, or drug therapy. For coronary device studies, QCA is performed on images acquired before treatment, immediately after treatment and follow-up. The main dedicated laboratories usually perform the analysis for independent analysis. The most important search parameters, calculated using QCA, are: the acute luminal gain; MLD which gives insights on the acute efficacy of the device and is defined as

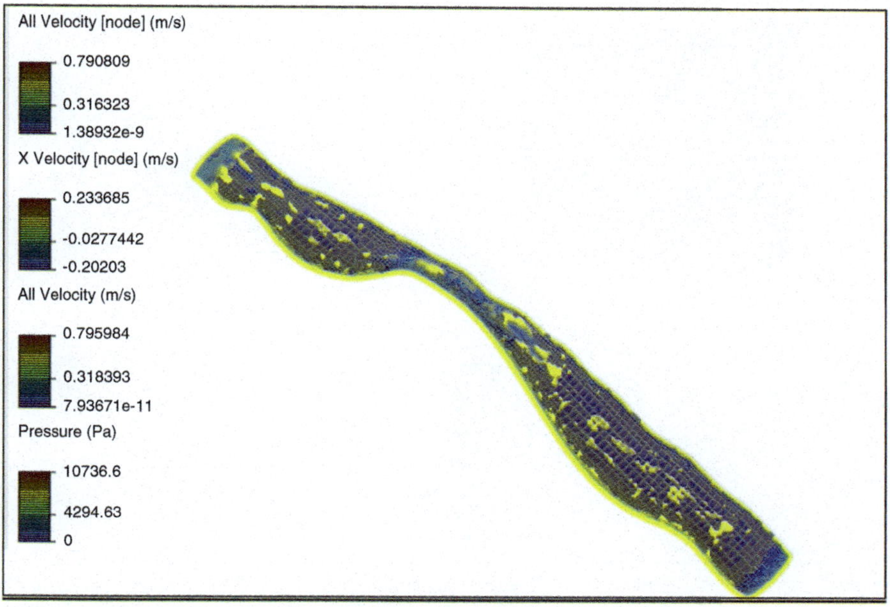

Fig. 6 Simulation of the velocity

post-procedural, the luminal loss which is the estimator for restenosis and defined as post-procedural MLD and the binary angiographic restenosis which is the incidence of percent diameter stenosis>50% [27].

By adopting the same methodology for the conception of coronary artery QCA offers a dedicated bifurcation analysis option to overcome the major challenges in quantifying bifurcation lesions as seen in Fig. 7:

The processed model is a pathological case with occlusion 60%. A second 3D for this bifurcation model is composed of two nodes, 6 edges, 6 faces, 1 volumes. The mesh was generated with Max global cells = 100,000,000, Resolve feature angle = 30, Solver iterations = 150, Relax iterations = eight. Therefore, the boundary conditions is defined as follows: Pressure inlet = 1184 (Pa), the turbulence kinetic energy = 0.00375 (m^2/s^2) and the specific dissipation rate = 3.375 (1/s) for the blood fluid. The final processing of the Solver finished with the initial residual = 8.49079723516e-07, Final Residuel = 8.49079723516e-07, average solving K: 7.12500637921e-05, Execution Time = 1923.11 s and Clock Time = 2075 s as showed in Fig. 8.

The results of analysis of the arterial bifurcation with the CFD modules represent a considerable advantage, because now, for these cases also, the previous and subsequent data can be compared and these patients can be included. Due to blood reflux in the stenotic segment, velocity as well as pressure take up significantly negative values, which may give indications for detecting the position of the stenosis as indicated in Fig. 9.

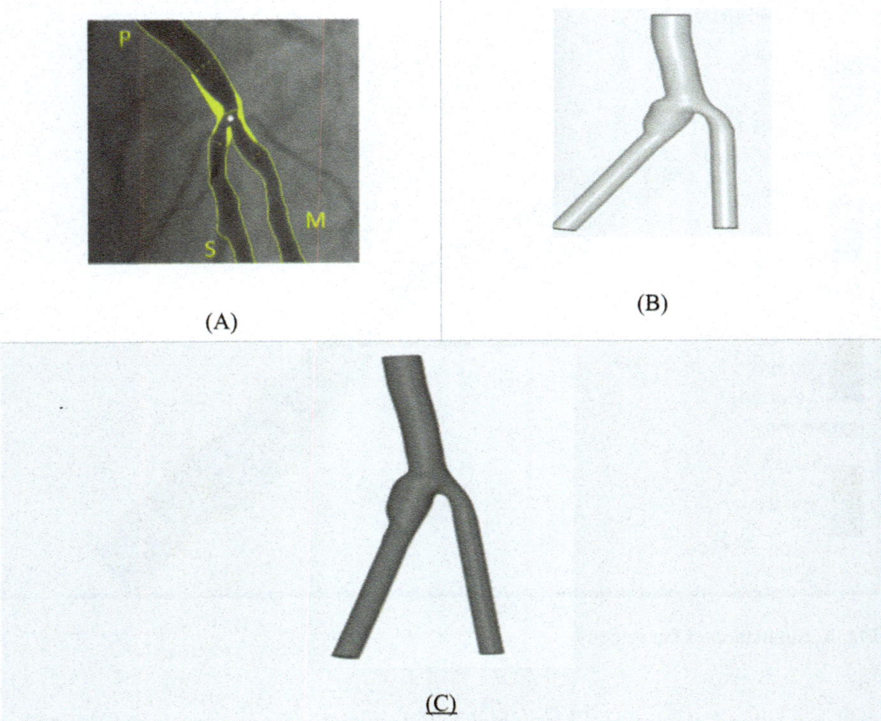

Fig. 7 (**a**) Reconstruction of the 3D bifurcation model;(**b**) Model of the bifurcation in 3D; (**c**) Mech of the bifurcation

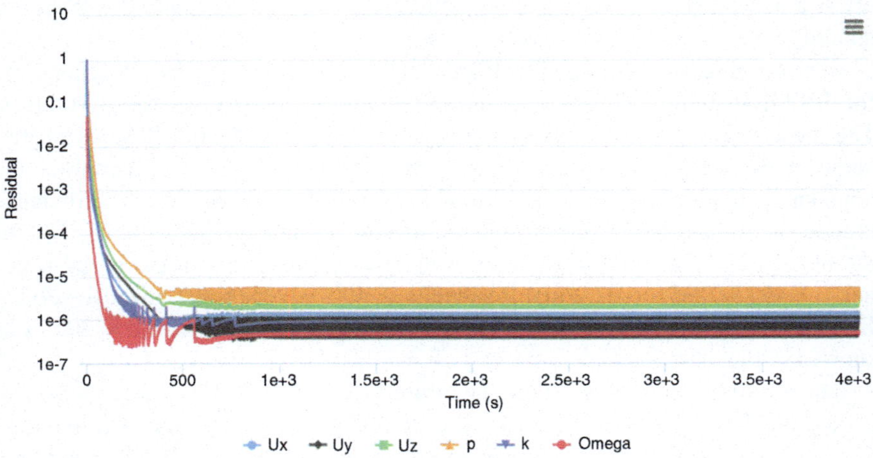

Fig. 8 Convergence plot of the solution

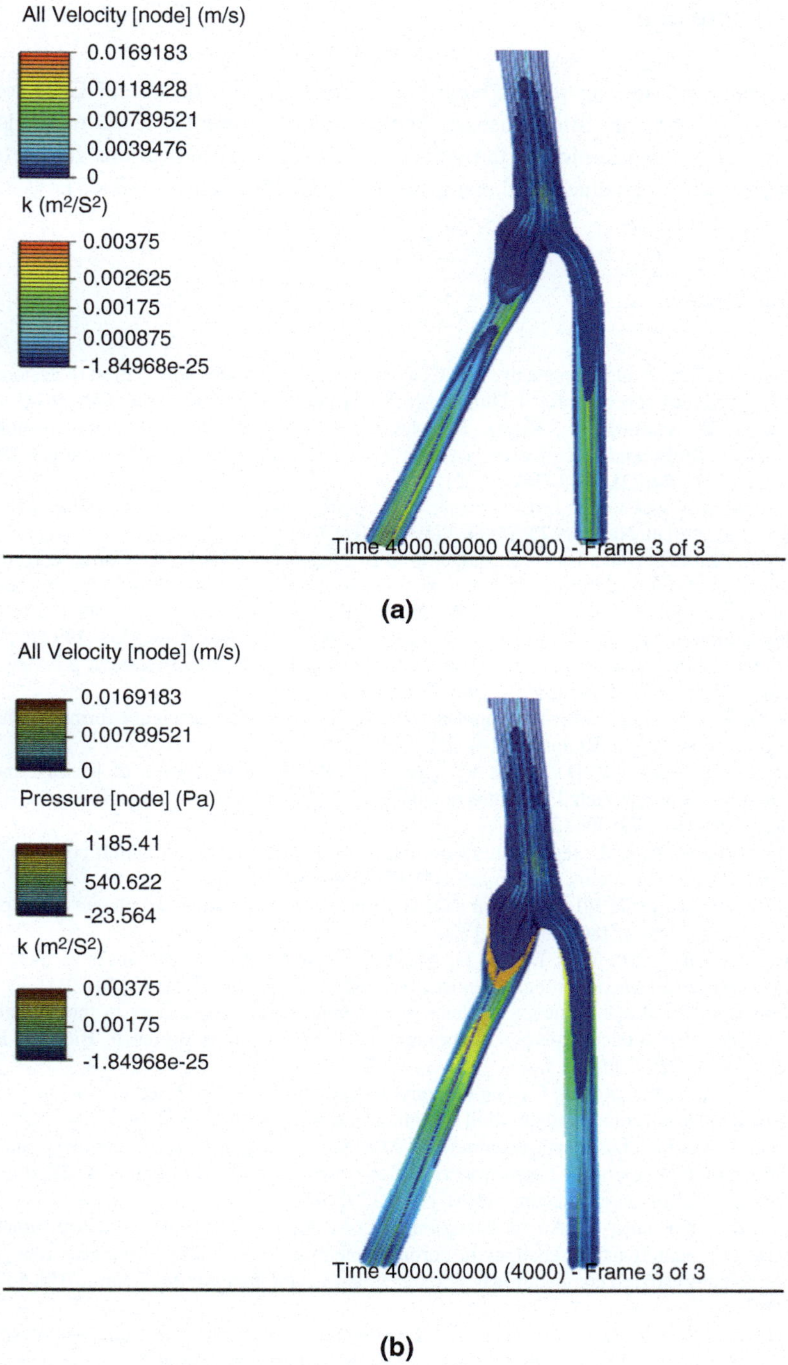

Fig. 9 (**a**) simulation of the velocity (**b**) simulation of the pressure

5 Conclusion

In summary, promising results have been depicted with the use of CFD for the diagnosis of coronary artery disease. With the advancement of CFD methods and image processing techniques, the detection of additional indications for coronary heart disease will be elucidated using specific CFD applications [28–31].

References

1. Zhang, J.-M., et al.: Perspective on CFD studies of coronary artery disease lesions and hemodynamics: a review. Int. J. Numer. Methods Biomed. Eng. **30**(6), 659–680 (2014)
2. Heitzer, T., Schlinzig, T., Krohn, K., Meinertz, T., Münzel, T.: Endothelial dysfunction, oxidative stress, and risk of cardiovascular events in patients with coronary artery disease. Circulation. **104**(22), 2673–2678 (2001)
3. Caro, C.G., Fitz-Gerald, J.M., Schroter, R.C.: Arterial wall shear and distribution of early atheroma in man. Nature. **223**(5211), 1159–1160 (1969)
4. Friedman, M.H., Hutchins, G.M., Bargeron, C.B., Deters, O.J., Mark, F.F.: Correlation between intimal thickness and fluid shear in human arteries. Atherosclerosis. **39**(3), 425–436 (1981)
5. Lutz, R.J., Cannon, J.N., Bischoff, K.B., Dedrick, R.L., Stiles, R.K., Fry, D.L.: Wall shear stress distribution in a model canine artery during steady flow. Circ. Res. **41**(3), 391–399 (1977)
6. Shaaban, A.M., Duerinckx, A.J.: Wall shear stress and early atherosclerosis: a review. AJR Am. J. Roentgenol. **174**(6), 1657–1665 (2000)
7. Wang, Y., et al.: High shear stress induces atherosclerotic vulnerable plaque formation through angiogenesis. Regen. Biomater. **3**(4), 257–267 (2016)
8. Davies, P.F., Polacek, D.C., Shi, C., Helmke, B.P.: The convergence of haemodynamics, genomics, and endothelial structure in studies of the focal origin of atherosclerosis. Biorheology. **39**(3–4), 299–306 (2002)
9. Chaichana, T., Sun, Z., Jewkes, J.: Computation of hemodynamics in the left coronary artery with variable angulations. J. Biomech. **44**(10), 1869–1878 (2011)
10. Helderman, F., et al.: Effect of shear stress on vascular inflammation and plaque development. Curr. Opin. Lipidol. **18**(5), 527–533 (2007)
11. Xie, X., Zheng, M., Wen, D., Li, Y., Xie, S.: A new CFD based non-invasive method for functional diagnosis of coronary stenosis. Biomed. Eng. Online. **17**(1), 36 (2018)
12. Kamangar, S., et al.: Influence of stenosis on hemodynamic parameters in the realistic left coronary artery under hyperemic conditions. Comput. Methods Biomech. Biomed. Engin. **20**(4), 365–372 (2017)
13. Tesche, C., et al.: Coronary CT angiography-derived fractional flow reserve: Machine learning algorithm versus computational fluid dynamics modeling. Radiology. **288**(1), 64–72 (2018)
14. Coenen, A., et al.: Diagnostic accuracy of a Machine-learning approach to coronary computed tomographic angiography-based fractional flow reserve: result from the MACHINE consortium. Circ. Cardiovasc. Imaging. **11**(6), e007217 (2018)
15. Sun, Z., Chaichana, T.: An investigation of correlation between left coronary bifurcation angle and hemodynamic changes in coronary stenosis by coronary computed tomography angiography-derived computational fluid dynamics. Quant. Imaging Med. Surg. **7**(5), 537–548 (2017)
16. Caruso, M.V., De Rosa, S., Indolfi, C., Fragomeni, G.: Computational analysis of stenosis geometry effects on right coronary hemodynamics. Conf. Proc. Annu. Int. Conf. IEEE Eng. Med. Biol. Soc. IEEE Eng. Med. Biol. Soc. Annu. Conf. **2015**, 981–984 (2015)

17. Zhang, J.-M., et al.: Numerical simulation and clinical implications of stenosis in coronary blood flow. Biomed. Res. Int. **2014**, 514729 (2014)
18. Papafaklis, M.I., et al.: Functional assessment of lesion severity without using the pressure wire: coronary imaging and blood flow simulation. Expert. Rev. Cardiovasc. Ther. **15**(11), 863–877 (2017)
19. Javadzadegan, A., Moshfegh, A., Qian, Y., Ng, M.K.C., Kritharides, L., Yong, A.S.C.: The relationship between coronary lesion characteristics and pathologic shear in human coronary arteries. Clin. Biomech. Bristol. Avon. **60**, 177–184 (2018)
20. Sun, Z.: Coronary CT angiography: beyond morphological stenosis analysis. World J. Cardiol. **5**(12), 444–452 (2013)
21. Vignaux, O.: Imagerie cardiaque: scanner et IRM, 2nd ed. Elsevier Masson (2011)
22. Vlachopoulos, C., O'Rourke, M., Nichols, W.W.: McDonald's blood flow in arteries: theoretical, experimental and clinical principles, 6th edn. CRC Press, London (2011)
23. Berne, R. M., Levy, M. N.: Cardiovascular physiology. The C.V. Mosby Company, (1967)
24. Boutsianis, E., et al.: Computational simulation of intracoronary flow based on real coronary geometry. Eur. J. Cardio-Thorac. Surg. Off. J. Eur. Assoc. Cardio-Thorac. Surg. **26**(2), 248–256 (Aug. 2004)
25. Siauw, W.L., Ng, E.Y., Mazumdar, J.: Unsteady stenosis flow prediction: a comparative study of non-Newtonian models with operator splitting scheme. Med. Eng. Phys. **22**(4), 265–277 (2000)
26. Elhadj, S., Akers, R.M., Forsten-Williams, K.: Chronic pulsatile shear stress alters insulin-like growth factor-I (IGF-I) binding protein release in vitro. Ann. Biomed. Eng. **31**(2), 163–170 (2003)
27. Ramcharitar, S., et al.: A novel dedicated quantitative coronary analysis methodology for bifurcation lesions. Euro Intervent. J. Eur. Collab. Work. Group Interv. Cardiol. Eur. Soc. Cardiol. **3**(5), 553–557 (2008)
28. Frauenfelder, T., et al.: Flow and wall shear stress in end-to-side and side-to-side anastomosis of venous coronary artery bypass grafts. Biomed. Eng. Online. **6**, 35 (2007)
29. Knight, J., et al.: Choosing the optimal wall shear parameter for the prediction of plaque location-a patient-specific computational study in human right coronary arteries. Atherosclerosis. **211**(2), 445–450 (2010)
30. Wellnhofer, E., Osman, J., Kertzscher, U., Affeld, K., Fleck, E., Goubergrits, L.: Flow simulation studies in coronary arteries–impact of side-branches. Atherosclerosis. **213**(2), 475–481 (2010)
31. Chaichana, T., Sun, Z., Jewkes, J.: Impact of plaques in the left coronary artery on wall shear stress and pressure gradient in coronary side branches. Comput. Methods Biomech. Biomed. Engin. **17**(2), 108–118 (2014)

Accurate Left Ventricular Segmentation Based on Morphological Watershed Transformation Towards 3D Visualization

Khouloud Boukhris, Ramzi Mahmoudi, Badii Hmida, and Mohamed Hédi Bedoui

1 Introduction

Cardiac magnetic resonance imaging (cMRI) represents the golden reference method for assessing the LV function and analyzing the myocardial diseases [1], using mainly short-axis cine images. With the aim of obtaining full exploitation of the information contained in these MRI images, the automated extraction and segmentation of the myocardium contours, which are often drawn manually by cardiologists, are proving to be crucial [2].In this paper, we propose to compare a set of existing methods dealing with ventricular segmentation in short axis cine MR images, in order to prove the accuracy of our proposed method. This comparison was also assessed against manual segmentations performed by cardiologist. The main issue with an accurate LV segmentation is to ensure its faithful 3-D reconstruction. This paper is organized as follows: Sect. 2 describes the previous work aiming to segment the heart cavities. Sects. 3 and 4 are dedicated to introduce then evaluate the proposed segmentation process to extract the LV myocardium. Section 5 depicts resulting 3D visualization. Finally, Sect. 6 presents the conclusion.

K. Boukhris (✉) · M. H. Bedoui
Faculty of Medicine of Monastir, Medical Imaging Technology Lab – LTIM-LR12ES06, University of Monastir, Monastir, Tunisia

R. Mahmoudi
Faculty of Medicine of Monastir, Medical Imaging Technology Lab – LTIM-LR12ES06, University of Monastir, Monastir, Tunisia

Gaspard-Monge computer-science laboratory, Paris-Est University, Mixed Unit CNRS-UMLV-ESIEE UMR8049, BP99, ESIEE Paris City Descartes, 93162 Noisy Le Grand, France

B. Hmida
Radiology Service- UR12SP40 CHU Fattouma Bourguiba, Monastir, Tunisia

L. Chaari (ed.), *Digital Health in Focus of Predictive, Preventive and Personalised Medicine*, Advances in Predictive, Preventive and Personalised Medicine 12,
https://doi.org/10.1007/978-3-030-49815-3_7

2 Review of Ventricular Segmentation Methods in cMRI

Cardiac Magnetic Resonance Imaging (cMRI) is used to help visualizing the internal structures of the human heart in order to highlight the medical management of patients. MRI cardiac planes include short axis, horizontal long axis (four-chamber view), and vertical long axis (two-chamber view) [3]. Various segmentation methods have been proposed by different researchers using generally the short-axis view [4]. These existing methods can be divided into two main categories: "segmentation based on no or weak prior" and "segmentation based on a strong prior". Approaches based on no or weak prior are very contingent upon the gray-level histograms and the thresholding techniques. These approaches include image-based methods [5–7], pixel classification and deformable models [8, 9]. However, approaches based on strong prior are characterized by the use of statistical models which are mainly divided into three categories: deformable models based segmentation with strong prior, Active shape ("ASM") [10, 11] and active appearance models ("AAM") [12] and atlas based ones [9, 13, 14].

3 Proposed Method Based on Watershed Transform

Since the early work of Serge Beucher [15], the watershed transform has been successfully applied in thousands of applications, including medical ones. Our approach is based mainly on the watershed transformation method [16] and considers prior properties. The set of prior knowledge that will allow an accurate segmentation are: topology (the left ventricular myocardium LVM is delimited by two surfaces: endocardium and epicardium), geometry (the endocardium cannot exceed the epicardium) and brightness (the endocardium is a very bright object). Our proposed method to automatically segment the LVM in 3D + t short-axes images is composed of two consecutive steps: endocardium segmentation, followed by the epicardium segmentation. Thereafter, the myocardium extraction (LVM) consists in applying the ensemblist difference between the epicardial and the endocardial civility. The segmentation of the endocardium is performed by geodesic dilations. Its recognition is ensured by extracting a connected set of pixels that belongs to the endocardium (thanks to its brightness). The delineation is then performed by dilating this marker in a mask made to be a candidate that belongs to the endocardium. The epicardium segmentation is consequent to the endocardium one preserving certain anatomical constraints. We propose to separate the myocardial cavity from the ventricular background. To achieve this goal, we propose to dilate the endocardium contour in order to obtain the first epicardial marker (EPm).To extract the EPm, the idea is to dilate the endocardium segmented cavity (ENC) as much as possible by ensuring that the resulting set is included in the real ENC, according to the prior:

$$Epicardium\_Boundary \cap Endocardium\_Boundary = \emptyset \qquad (1)$$

The next step consists of finding a marker for the left ventricular background (LVBm) that does not belong to the myocardium: composed of several tissues including the liver, the stomach, the right ventricle and the lungs. In order to extract the LV background marker (LVBm), we propose a second dilatation, based on the prior that the myocardium thickness cannot exceed a certain threshold. Then, the delineation is performed by the topological watershed transformation approach cited in [16] using the above-selected markers as inputs. The delineation is followed by a smoothing post-processing using shape filters coming from mathematical morphology. Thus, in order to obtain the final segmentation, we use the alternating sequential filter (ASF) [17] to regularize the epicardial boundary (Ep) and to restore a correct shape of the intensity information. The ASF is a sequence of intermixed morphological openings and closings by balls of an increasing size.

4 Validation of the Proposed Segmentation

In our experiment, we used 4D cine MR images of 20 patients to segment. For the evaluation, the same dataset was manually segmented by two different experts, called below Exp1 and Exp 2.

4.1 Point to Surface Measurement

Given two surfaces S and S′ represented by two polygons, the point-to-surface measurement (P2S) defined in [18] estimates the mean distance between the vertices of these surfaces (S and S′).

From our proposed segmentation, the endocardial and the epicardial surfaces (EndoS and EpiS) were used to compute the P2S in order to compare them with those obtained by other groups on their own datasets [6, 9, 11, 12, 14, 19–22]. In Table 1, different distance measures similar to P2S where used: APD (Average Perpendicular distance), Hausdroff distance and image volumes. The comparison demonstrates that the distance (P2S) evaluation results averaged favorably across our proposed method and those obtained by previous works. The P2S was computed from the segmentations resulting from our proposed method and the two experts. In order to assess the inter-observer variability, the P2S of both experts is also provided as shown in Table 2.

The obtained results are convergent (PM vs.exp. and exp. vs. exp) with a distance that does not exceed 2 mm, thus evidencing the reliability of the proposed segmentation.

Table 1 Literature values of left ventricle delineation errors

	Distance (mm)	
	EndoS	EpiS
Mitchell and al [11]	2.75	2.63
Kaus and al [19]	2.28	2.62
Lötjönen and al [14]	2.01	2.77
Van Assen and al [12].	1.97	2.23
Lorenzo-Valdes and al [9]	1.88	2.75
Jolly and al [6]	2.48	2.91
Ying-Li Lu and al [20]	2.07	1.92
Huaifei Hu and al [21]	2.3	2.2
Irshad and al [22]	2.1	3.1
Proposed method	1.52	1.75

Table 2 Results of the P2S(mm) measurements from our proposed method (PM)

		PM VS. EXP1	PM VS.EXP2	EXP1 VS.EXP2
End-diastolic time	EndoS	1.62	1.52	1.46
	EpiS	1.81	1.60	1.62
End-systolic time	EndoS	1.45	1.30	1.44
	EPIS	**1.82**	**1.42**	**1.63**

4.2 *False Negative and False Positive Volume Fraction*

These two measures are recommended by [18] to characterize the delineation accuracy. Considering Struth the set of image pixels containing 'true' delineations of the LV and Spm the segmentation to be compared to the ground truth to be evaluated, we set False Negative Ejection Fraction FNEF and False Positive Ejection Fraction FPEF:

$$FPVF\,(Spm, Struth) = \frac{|\ Spm \backslash Struth\ |}{Struth} \tag{2}$$

$$FNVF\,(Spm, Struth) = \frac{|\ Struth \backslash Spm\ |}{Struth} \tag{3}$$

Figure 1 illustrates the meaning of these measures: A false positive volume fraction (FPVF)indicates the amount of pixels falsely extracted to be considered as a fraction of the true delineation (considered as the reference segmentation) and the false negative volume fraction (FNVF) depicts the fraction of pixels that was missed. These metrics were computed for the three segmented areas: the epicardium, the endocardium and the myocardium. Table 3 depicts their mean values between the proposed method PM and the two experts at end-systolic and end-diastolic time. In order to achieve an accurate assessment, these measures were also provided between

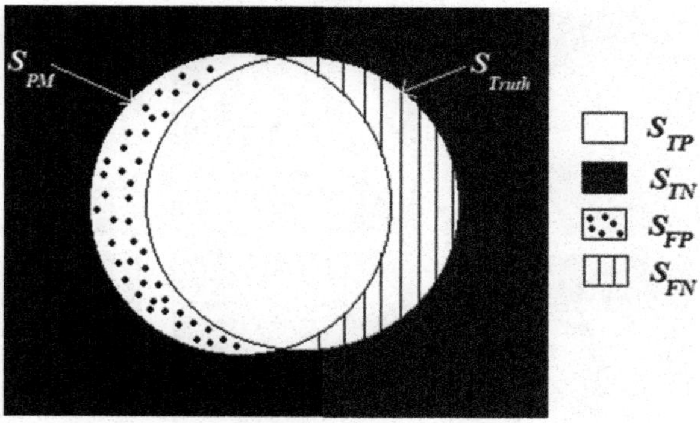

Fig. 1 Illustration of the accuracy factors from a binary case segmentation

Table 3 FPVF and FNVF values for the segmentation of the endocardium, the epicardium and the myocardium at end-systolic and end-diastolic time

		PM vs. exp1	PM vs.exp2	Exp1 vs. exp2	Exp2 vs. exp1
End-systolic-time					
Endocardium	FPVF	0.04	0.05	0.15	0.02
	FNVF	0.12	0.07	0.03	0.14
Epicardium	FPVF	0.08	0.14	0.06	0.09
	FNVF	0.21	0.06	0.10	0.12
Myocardium	FPVF	0.02	0.10	0.25	0.09
	FNVF	0.04	0.22	0.14	0.08
End-diastolic-time					
Endocardium	FPVF	0.06	0.12	0.09	0.12
	FNVF	0.12	0.23	0.21	0.10
Epicardium	FPVF	0.09	0.11	0.09	0.06
	FNVF	0.14	0.02	0.13	0.07
Myocardium	FPVF	0.04	0.08	0.18	0.21
	FNVF	0.03	0.13	0.09	0.04

the two experts. The inter-expert segmentations results (exp1 vs.exp2 and exp2 vs. exp1) compare well to those obtained between the proposed method and expert segmentations (PM vs. exp1 and PM vs. exp2). The Dice metric can be expressed in terms of true positives (TP), false positives (FP) and false negatives (FN) as:

$$Dice\,(A, B) = (2 * TP)\,/\,(2 * TP + FP + FN) \tag{4}$$

Comparing our method to both experts, the best segmentation result had a Dice Metric of 0.96 and the worst a DC of 0.73.

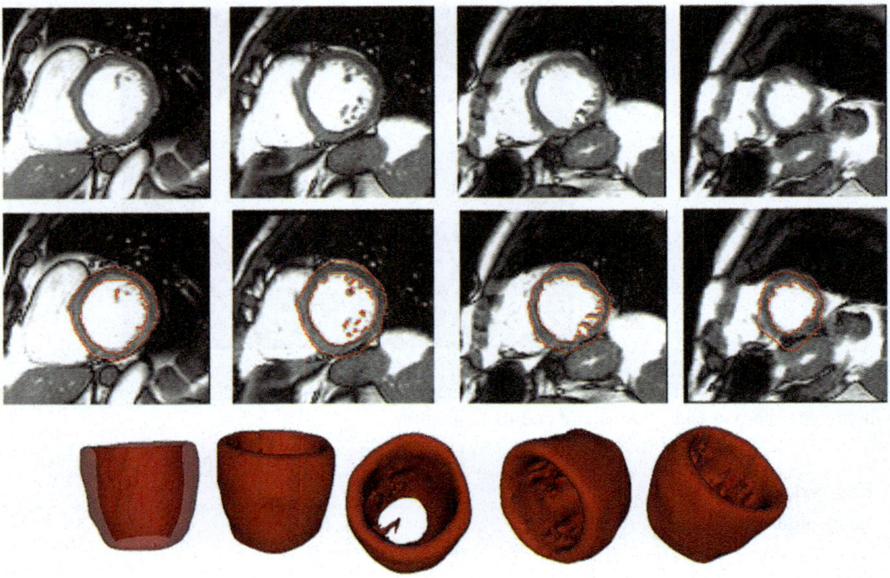

Fig. 2 Illustration of the myocardium segmentation results: The first row shows the pseudo slices from apical to basal direction without any contours. The second row depicts the extraction of myocardial contours. The third row shows the extracted mesh from different corners

5 The 3D Visualization

Searching for a means to display the segmentation results proved to be important. To achieve it, we start by generating meshes from the binary images resulting from the proposed segmentation. The ability to visualize the LV meshes would be a significant advantage. To generate these meshes we applied the method defined in [23] using the marching cube algorithm [24].The ensuing step consists on applying Laplacian smoothing steps [25] on these resulting meshes and save them in the vtk format [27]. Figure 2 depicts an example of myocardium segmentation ranging from apical to basal plane and the extracted mesh from different corners.

6 Conclusion

The purpose of this work was to provide an automatic and accurate LV myocardial segmentation method for 3D cine-MRI images. Extraction of the LV endo- and epicardium has provided accurate and consistent results. Our Proposed method has achieved a mean Dice metric of 0.87 for the endocardium and 0.82 for the epicardium. Therefore, we focused on the volumetric object reconstruction (3D visualization) by exporting the endocardial and the epicardial extracted contours as 3D surface meshes [24]. This reconstruction is ensured throughout a complete cardiac cycle (from systole to diastole) to allow dynamic visualization of the LV.

References

1. Olimulder, M.A.G.M., Van Es, J., Galjee, M.A.: The importance of cardiac MRI as a diagnostic tool in viral myocarditis-induced cardiomyopathy. Netherlands Heart J. **17**(12), 481–486 (2009)
2. Buser, P.T., et al.: Noninvasive evaluation of global left ventricular function with use of cine nuclear magnetic resonance. J. Am. Coll. Cardiol. **13**(6), 1294–1300 (1989)
3. Ginat, D.T., et al.: Cardiac imaging: Part 1, MR pulse sequences, imaging planes, and basic anatomy. Am. J. Roentgenol. **197**(4), 808–815 (2011)
4. Petitjean, C., Dacher, J.-N.: A review of segmentation methods in short axis cardiac MR images. Med. Image Anal. **15**(2), 169–184 (2011)
5. Katouzian, A., Prakash, A., Konofagou, E.: A new automated technique for left-and right-ventricular segmentation in magnetic resonance imaging. 2006 International Conference of the IEEE Engineering in Medicine and Biology Society. IEEE (2006)
6. Jolly, M.: Fully automatic left ventricle segmentation in cardiac cine MR images using registration and minimum surfaces. MIDAS J. Cardiac MR Left Ventricle Segment. Challenge. **4**, 59 (2009)
7. Lin, X., Cowan, B.R., Young, A.A.: Automated detection of left ventricle in 4D MR images: experience from a large study. In: International conference on medical image computing and computer-assisted intervention. Springer, Berlin/Heidelberg (2006)
8. Pednekar, A., et al.: Automated left ventricular segmentation in cardiac MRI. IEEE Trans. Biomed. Eng. **53**(7), 1425–1428 (2006)
9. Lorenzo-Valdés, M., et al.: Segmentation of 4D cardiac MR images using a probabilistic atlas and the EM algorithm. Med. Image Anal. **8**(3), 255–265 (2004)
10. Pennell, D.J., et al.: Clinical indications for cardiovascular magnetic resonance (CMR): consensus panel report. J. Cardiovasc. Magnet. Reson. **6**(4), 727–765 (2004)
11. Mitchell, S.C., et al.: 3-D active appearance models: segmentation of cardiac MR and ultrasound images. IEEE Trans. Med. Imaging. **21**(9), 1167–1178 (2002)
12. Van Assen, H.C., et al.: SPASM: a 3D-ASM for segmentation of sparse and arbitrarily oriented cardiac MRI data. Med. Image Anal. **10**(2), 286–303 (2006)
13. Zhuang, X., et al.: Robust registration between cardiac MRI images and atlas for segmentation propagation. Medical Imaging 2008: Image Processing. Vol. 6914. International Society for Optics and Photonics, (2008)
14. Lötjönen, J., et al.: Statistical shape model of atria, ventricles and epicardium from short-and long-axis MR images. Med. Image Anal. **8**(3), 371–386 (2004)
15. Beucher, S.: Use of watersheds in contour detection. In: Proceedings of the International Workshop on Image Processing. CCETT (1979)
16. Mahmoudi, R., Akil, M., HédiBedoui, M.: Concurrent computation of topological watershed on shared memory parallel machines. Parallel Comput. **69**, 78–97 (2017)
17. Couprie, M., Bertrand, G.: Topology preserving alternating sequential filter for smoothing two-dimensional and three-dimensional objects. J. Electr. Imaging. **13**(4), 720–731 (2004)
18. Udupa, J.K., et al.: A framework for evaluating image segmentation algorithms. Comput. Med. Imaging Graph. **30**(2), 75–87 (2006)
19. Kaus, M.R., et al.: Automated segmentation of the left ventricle in cardiac MRI. Med. Image Anal. **8**(3), 245–254 (2004)
20. Lu, Y.-L., et al.: Automatic functional analysis of left ventricle in cardiac cine MRI. Quant. Imaging Med. Surg. **3**(4), 200 (2013)

21. Hu, H., et al.: Automatic segmentation of the left ventricle in cardiac MRI using local binary fitting model and dynamic programming techniques. PLoS One. **9**(12), e114760 (2014)
22. Irshad, M., et al.: Automatic segmentation of the left ventricle in a cardiac MR short axis image using blind morphological operation. Eur. Phys. J. Plus. **133**(4), 148 (2018)
23. Lachaud, J.-O., Montanvert, A.: Deformable meshes with automated topology changes for coarse-to-fine three-dimensional surface extraction. Med. Image Anal. **3**(2), 187–207 (1999)
24. Lorensen, W.E., Cline, H. E.: Marching cubes: a high resolution 3D surface construction algorithm. ACM siggraph computer graphics, nol. 21. No. 4. ACM (1987)
25. Vollmer, Jörg, Robert Mencl, and Heinrich Mueller. "Improved laplacian smoothing of noisy surface meshes." Computer Graphics Forum. 18 3. Oxford/Boston: Blackwell Publishers Ltd, 1999
26. Wesarg, S.: AHA conform analysis of myocardial function using and extending the toolkits ITK and VTK. International Congress Series, vol. 1281. Elsevier (2005)

A Smart Search Functionality for a Memory Prosthesis: A Semantic Similarity-Based Approach

Fatma Ghorbel, Wafa Wali, Elisabeth Métais, Fayçal Hamdi, and Bilel Gargouri

1 Introduction

In the context of the VIVA[1] project (*«Vivre Paris avec Alzheimer en 2030 grace aux nouvelles technologies»*), we are proposing a memory prosthesis, called Captain Memo [1], to help Alzheimer's patients to palliate mnesic problems. Data are structured semantically using an ontology, called PersonLink[2] [2]. It is a multilingual ontology for storing, modeling and reasoning about interpersonal relationships and describing people. This prosthesis supplies a set of services. Among these services, one is devoted to "remember things about people", i.e., retrieving information about a person (e.g., preferences, gifts exchanged and shared events). However, these particular users, living in a form of uncertainty, can substitute words having the same meaning and have an increased difficulty in naming things. For instance, they may enter "the brothers having the same birthday" instead of "the twins".

[1] http://viva.cnam.fr/

[2] http://cedric.cnam.fr/isid/ontologies/files/PersonLink.html

F. Ghorbel (✉)
CEDRIC Laboratory, Conservatoire National des Arts et Métiers (CNAM), Paris, France

MIRACL Laboratory, University of Sfax, Sfax, Tunisia

W. Wali · E. Métais · F. Hamdi
CEDRIC Laboratory, Conservatoire National des Arts et Métiers (CNAM), Paris, France
e-mail: wafa.wali@fsegs.rnu.tn; wafa.wali@fsegs.rnu.tn; faycal.hamdi@cnam.fr

B. Gargouri
MIRACL Laboratory, University of Sfax, Sfax, Tunisia

L. Chaari (ed.), *Digital Health in Focus of Predictive, Preventive and Personalised Medicine*, Advances in Predictive, Preventive and Personalised Medicine 12,
https://doi.org/10.1007/978-3-030-49815-3_8

Captain Memo aims to offer a smart search functionality. It is able to deal with all kinds of input e.g., full sentence, sentence fragments or keyword, natural language text. It takes into account that the user may substitute the words/sentences that express the same meaning. To address this issue, we estimate the semantic similarity score between the user's search filed entry and the saved personal data of the user.

Several approaches for sentences similarity estimation have been proposed. However, they are applied only to the English language. Moreover, many knowledge elements, e.g., the semantic class, the thematic role and the relationship between them, are not taken into account when measuring the sentences similarity.

In this paper, we propose a multilingual semantic similarity-based approach to estimate the similarity between the user's search filed entry and the patient's saved personal data. Compared to related work, it is mainly based on semantic information notably the synonymy relationships between words and syntactico-semantic information especially semantic class and thematic role. It supported three languages: English, French and Arabic. It is mainly proposed to be integrated in Captain Memo. However, it can be used on others applications.

The remainder of the paper is structured as follows. Section 2 details some related work. The approach is presented in Sect. 3. Section 4 discusses some experimental results. Finally, in Sect. 5, we conclude and we give perspectives.

2 Related Work

Several approaches have been proposed to measure the semantic similarity between sentences. We classify them into *(i)* syntactic-based, *(ii)* semantic-based and *(iii)* hybrid approaches. An example of a syntactic-based approach is [3]. An example of a semantic-based approach is [4]. An example of a hybrid approach is [5].

However, these approaches are applied to the English language and they do not support the specific particularities of the French and Arabic languages. Moreover, they estimate the semantic similarity based only on the syntactic structure of sentence notably word order or the syntactic dependency and the synonymy relationship between terms. They do not take into consideration the semantic arguments notably the semantic class and thematic role in computing the semantic similarity.

3 Proposed Approach

The proposed approach allows estimating a semantic similarity score between the user's search input sentence (USIS) and the others saved in data tier (DTS). It supports three languages: English, French and Arabic. It includes an extension of previous strategies by taking into account the most important linguistics and the syntactico-semantics information. Compared to related work, it also takes into account the semantic arguments notably the semantic class and thematic role.

It is composed of two modules: *(i)* "Preprocessing" and *(ii)* "Similarity Score Attribution".

3.1 Preprocessing

Before estimating the similarity score between USIS and DTS, three sub-steps are proposed:

- Tokenization: USIS and DTS are decomposed into authentication tokens (words). This step filters the answers and tags the words into their part of speech and labels them accordingly. WordNet [6] handles only relationships between noun-noun and verb-verb. The other parts of speeches are not taken onto account. Therefore, to reduce the time and space complexity of the approach, we only consider nouns and verbs to calculate the similarity.
- Removal of the punctuation signs: For the two sentences, all punctuation signs are removed.
- Lemmatization: morphological variables are reduced to their base form using the Stanford Morphological analyzer [7].

3.2 Similarity Score Attribution

To estimate the similarity score between USIS and DTS, three similarity level are measured: lexical, semantic and syntactico-semantic.

The lexical similarity score (SL(USIS, DTS)) is computed using the lexical units that compose the two sentences to extract the words that are lexically the same. It is computed based on the Jaccard coefficient [8].

$$SL\,(USIS, DTS) = MC/\,(MA_{USIS} + MA_{DTS} - MC) \tag{1}$$

MC is the number of common words between USIS and DTS; MA_{USIS} is the number of words contained in USIS; and MA_{DTS} is the number of words contained in DTS.

The measurement of the semantic similarity is reinforced by means of the WordNet database in order to extract the synonyms of each sentence's words. Also, we use the NOOJ platform [9] to determine the named entities. We also use the OpenCyc ontology to extract common sense facts (for instance, twins have the same birthday).

The computing process of the semantic resemblance between USIS and DTS involves primarily the creation of a set of joint words from the two sentences $W = \{W_1 \ldots W_m\} = SW_{USIS} \cap SW_{DTS}$. For each sentence, only the words returned by the "Preprocessing" component are taken into consideration. Then, we calculate the semantic vector $V = \{V_{USIS}, V_{DTS}, W\}$. For each $W_i \in W$, if $W_i \in SW_{USIS}$,

V_{USIS} is set as one (case1). In the other case ($W_I \notin \in SW_{USIS}$), a set of semantic similarity scores between W_i and all the words contained in SW_{USIS} are estimated ($SIM(W_I,SW_J)$). The closest word to W_J in the answer is the one that has the highest semantic similarity score. T_{USIS} is set to this score. To estimate the semantic similarity scores, we rely on synonymy link of the WordNet database.

$$SIM\,(W_I, SW_J) = MC/\,(MW_I + MSW_J - MC) \tag{2}$$

where, MC is the number of common words between the two synonym sets; MW_I is the number of words contained in the W_I synonym set and MSW_J is the number of words contained in the SW_J synonym set.

On the basis of the semantic vector previously calculated, the semantic similarity score (SM(USIS, DTS),) is computed by applying the Cosine similarity.

$$SM\,(USIS, DTS) = (V_{USIS}.V_{DTS})\,/\,(||V_{USIS}||\,.\,||V_{DTS}||) \tag{3}$$

The estimation of the syntactico-semantic similarity score consists of extracting the characteristics of the semantic arguments of USIS and DTS from the VerbNet database for the French and English languages [10] and LMF Arabic dictionary for the Arabic language [11]. As a consequence, a syntactic parser is used to identify, on the one hand, the syntactic behavior of the sentences and, on the other hand, the semantic predicates from the databases which is very rich in semantic predicates. Moreover, the meanings of the lexical entry (such as the verb of the sentence) and the predicative representation that connects the syntactic behavior and the semantic predicate pre-defined in the first stage are looked up in the databases. Then, when the predicative representation is caught, the semantic arguments will be extracted. Once the pairs of semantic argument have the same thematic role and semantic class, they are considered similar. After that, the degree of the syntactico-semantic similarity between two elements of each pair of the sentence is computed based on the common semantic arguments of the elements of the pair of sentences, which are called SSM(USIS,DTS) by using the Jaccard coefficient.

$$SSM\,(USIS, DTS) = ASC/\,(\,AS_{USIS} + AS_{DTS} - ASC) \tag{4}$$

Where, ASC is the number of common semantic arguments between USIS and DTS; AS_{USIS} is the number of semantic arguments contained in USIS; and AS_{DTS} is the number of semantic arguments contained in DTS.

The similarity score between USIS and DTS (SS(USIS,DTS)) is a USIS and DTS is a weighted sum of the three mentioned scores.

$$\begin{aligned} SS\,(USIS, DTS) =& SL\,(USIS, DTS)\,.\alpha + SM\,(USIS, DTS)\,.\beta \\ &+ SSM\,(USIS, DTS)\,.\gamma \end{aligned} \tag{5}$$

We propose to use the automatic learning in order to define the appropriate coefficients α, β and γ.

4 Experimentations

A Java-based prototype is implemented based on the proposed approach.

4.1 Integration in Captain Memo

The prototype is integrated in Captain Memo. A set of similarity scores are estimated between the user's search input sentence and all saved data. To consider that the data having the higher similarity score is right, it ought to be greater than 0,9. Figure 1 shows an example of the system's response for the following user's search entry: "the brothers having the same birthday".

4.2 Evaluation

We evaluated the efficiency of the proposed approach in determining the correctness of the responses given by the user. This evaluation was done in the context of Captain Memo. A total of 20 Alzheimer's patients $\{P_1 \dots P_{20}\}$ and their associated caregivers $\{C_1 \dots C_{20}\}$ were recruited to participate in this study. All caregivers are first-degree relatives. Most Alzheimer's patients were living in a nursing home

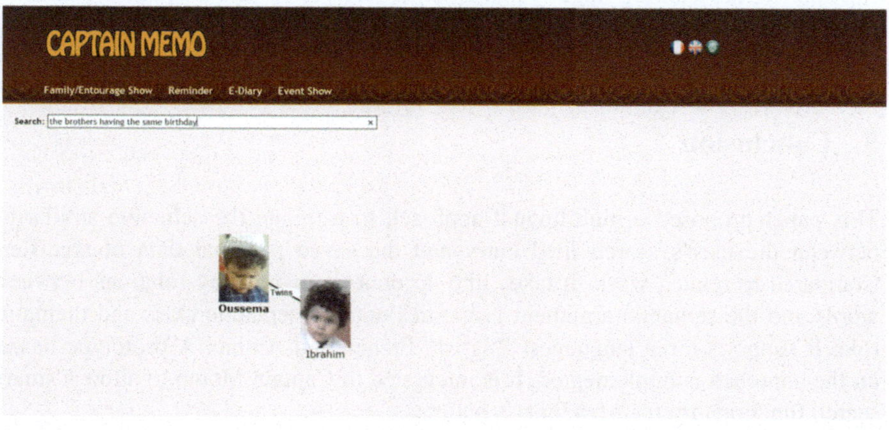

Fig. 1 An example of the system search's response

in Sfax/Tunisia. We asked each patient's legal sponsor for the consent letter. We excluded participants with overt behavioral disturbances, sever aphasia and sever auditory and/or visual loss.

The evaluation consisted of one test session for each patient. Its duration depends on the cognitive performance of the Alzheimer's patient. At mean, it was about 1 h. At the beginning of each session, we gave a brief introduction and a live demo of Captain Memo. Each patient uses the search functionality about 20 times. We classify these attempts according to the length of user's search filed entry. For each patient P_i, two scenarios had been tested:

- The first scenario, called "One or a part of sentence scenario", represents only user's search filed entries formed only by one or a part of sentence. $T_{S1/i}$ represents the total of the search's results related to the patient P_i and recorded as true responses. $GS_{S1/i}$ represents the "gold standard" responses. There are given by the caregiver C_i.
- The second scenario, called "Two or more sentences scenario", represents only user's search filed entries responses formed by two or more sentences. $T_{S2/i}$ represents the total of the search's results related to the patient P_i and recorded as true responses. $GS_{S2/i}$ given by the caregiver C_i represents the "gold standard" responses. There are given by the caregiver C_i.

For each scenario, we compare the generated response against the golden standard ones. The exact Precision measures Pi@S1 $((|T_{S1/i} \cap GS_{S1/i}| / |T_{S1/i}|))$ and Pi@S2 represent respectively, the precision values related to the first and second scenarios of the patient P_i. The results obtained are encouraging. The means of the Precision measures related to the first scenario is estimated to 82,98 and the one related to the second scenario is estimated to 74,58. We noticed that the analysis of short sentences presents the highest measures of precision. As the sentence gets longer, there will be a more complex calculation, which reduces the system's performance. We believe that these results can be improved. In fact, we think that we can improve the learning stage by adding other features besides the lexical, semantic and syntactico-semantic features.

5 Conclusion

This paper proposed a multilingual approach to estimate the semantic similarity between the user's search filed entry and the saved personal data of the user. Compared to related work, it takes into account the synonymy relations between words and the semantic argument properties notably semantic class and thematic role. It supports three languages: English, French and Arabic. A prototype based on the approach is implemented. It is integrated in Captain Memo to allow a smart search functionality for Alzheimer's patients.

We plan to extend the proposed approach to be able to deal with spelling mistakes ungrammatical text entries.

References

1. Métais, E., Ghorbel, F., Herradi, N., Hamdi, F., Lammari, N., Nakache, D., Ellouze, N., Gargouri, F., Soukane, A.: Memory prosthesis. Non-pharmacol. Therapies Dementia. **3**(2), 177–180 (2015)
2. Herradi, N., Hamdi, F., Metais, E., Ghorbel, F., Soukane, A.: PersonLink: an ontology representing family relationships for the CAPTAIN MEMO memory prosthesis. In: ER 2015 (Workshop AHA). Lect. Notes Comput. Sci. **9382**, 3–13 (2015)
3. Li, Y., Mclean, D., Bandar, Z.A., O'Shea, J.D., Crockett, K.: Sentence similarity based on semantic nets and corpus statistics. Knowl. Data Eng. IEEE Trans. **18**(8), 1138–1150 (2006)
4. Kozlowski, M.: Opi: Semeval-2014 task 3 system description. SemEval. **2014**, (2014)
5. Md Arafat Sultan, Steven Bethard, Tamara Sumner. Dls@ cu: Sentence similarity from word alignment. In Proceedings of the 8th International Workshop on Semantic Evaluation (SemEval 2014), pp. 241–246 (2014)
6. Miller, G.A.: Wordnet: a lexical database for english. Commun. ACM. **38**(11), 39–41 (1995)
7. Manning, C.D., Surdeanu, M., Bauer, J., Finkel, J., Bethard, S.J., McClosky, D.: The Stanford CoreNLP natural language processing toolkit. In: Association for Computational Linguistics (ACL) System Demonstrations. pp. 55–60 (2014),
8. Jaccard, P.: Etude comparative de la distribution orale dans une portion des Alpes et du Jura. Impr. Corbaz (1901)
9. Silberztein, M., V_aradi, T., Tadi_c, M.: Open source multi-platform NooJ for NLP. In: Proceedings of COLING 2012: Demonstration Papers. pp. 401–408. The COL-ING 2012 Organizing Committee, Mumbai, India (2012)
10. Schuler, K.K.: VerbNet: A Broad-Coverage, Comprehensive Verb Lexicon. PhD thesis, University of Pennsylvania (2006)
11. Khemakhem, A., Gargouri, B., Ben Hamadou, A., Francopoulo, G.: Iso standard modeling of a large arabic dictionary. Nat. Lang. Eng. 1–31 (2015)

An Efficient Image Retrieval Using Medical-Dependent Features

Hajer Ayadi and Mouna Torjmen-Khemamkhem

1 Introduction

Facing the explosion in the amount of medical images, the image indexing and retrieval systems have seen an evolution to provide access to biomedical literature and satisfy the user information needs. In traditional text-based image retrieval (TBIR) approaches, the image meta-data (document) is represented as a bag of words and frequencies, that are used to compute its relevance score according to a given query. While this traditional approach served as a building block to several well-known retrieval models (e.g. vector model and language model), it is no longer satisfied due to the limits dealing with noun phrases, synonyms, abbreviations and variants of terms mismatch problems. Moreover, the semantic relatedness between query terms and document terms need to be considered. To overcome these linguistic problems, several research and indexing studies known as "concept-based" have appeared [5]. The conceptualization is known as a step leading to a higher level of abstraction of text content, as well as a method to bridge the gap between surface linguistic form and meaning. However, this kind of approach is extremely time consuming, rendering it less effective. This issue was the subject of several indexing and retrieval studies such as "MDF-Feature-based" approach [1]. Recently, exploiting features within the retrieval process has received high attention in the information retrieval (IR) domain. The key benefits of using medical-dependent features(MDF) in TBIR are the following: First, they are specific for TBIR. In fact, they display the textual specificity for image retrieval as they denote a set of imaging modality (e.g. x-ray, MRI), image dimensionality (e.g. micro, macro), and so on. Second, they are specific to the medical domain as they contain a

H. Ayadi (✉) · M. Torjmen-Khemamkhem
ReDCAD Laboratory, National School of Engineering of Sfax, Sfax University, Sfax, Tunisia
e-mail: hajer.ayadi@redcad.org; mouna.torjmen@redcad.org

L. Chaari (ed.), *Digital Health in Focus of Predictive, Preventive and Personalised Medicine*, Advances in Predictive, Preventive and Personalised Medicine 12,
https://doi.org/10.1007/978-3-030-49815-3_9

set of medical terminology (e.g. Ultrasound, Dermatology). This paper investigates the performance of MDF based medical image indexing and retrieval according to both criteria: efficiency and effectiveness. Our main findings are: (1) the MDF based approach gives accuracy results comparable to those found by concept based approach, meaning that MDF based approach may be applied to any medical image collection; and (2) the MDF approach has several strengths compared to literature indexing approaches, especially as regards space-time occupancy. The remainder of this paper is organized as follows. In Sect. 2, we describe the related work. We present the MDF based image retrieval approach in Sect. 3. In Sect. 4, we set up our experimental environment. In Sect. 5, the experimental results are presented and discussed. Finally, we conclude our work briefly and discuss directions for future research in Sect. 6.

2 Related Work

In the literature, several text-based image retrieval (TBIR) approaches have been proposed. Their success highlight the area of image retrieval thanks to the relatively mature techniques of traditional information retrieval(such as query expansion, simple bag of words (BoW)). The largest number of medical retrieval systems which deal with annotated images exploits only the keywords of these images to search for relevant images in large collections. The standard approach is to represent the text as a "bag-of-words" and to associate a weight for each word using the Term Frequency-Inverse Document Frequency (TF-IDF) method [2]. Authors in [3] propose to extend the probabilistic Latent Semantic Analysis model to integrate the textual information from medical images. However, in [13] authors propose to extract textual information from patients records, such as the patient age, sex and medical history. Then, they use these textual attributes into retrieval process to search the possibly incomplete medical cases consisting of several images together with semantic information.

In many cases, the use of external resources, such as ontologies and thesaurus, significantly enhances the performance of TBIR systems. In [5], authors proposed a conceptual model to resolve the word sense ambiguity problem using the semantic relations between extracted concepts, through MetaMap[1] tool and UMLS Metathesaurus. In [7], the authors investigate the use of a query expansion strategy process using an advanced PubMed search. They conclude that the query expansion using external resources in PubMed improves the recovery efficacy. The query expansion was carried out, in [4], using the Mesh and UMLS ontologies and showed that using these ontologies improves the retrieval performance. Authors in [8], used conceptual language modeling with the additional use of the UMLS (Unified Medical Language System) metathesaurus to compute the similarity between a

[1] https://metamap.nlm.nih.gov/

given query and a document by simply computing the log-probability of the concept set of the document.

3 MDF Based Retrieval

In this section, we incorporate the MDFs into the retrieval process. First, we detail the set of MDFs; second, we present the used method to extract MDFs from documents/queries; finally, we applied the retrieval process based on MDF.

3.1 *Medical-Dependentent Features*

As our work falls into medical image retrieval field, we use MDFs [1, 15], which help in improving the retrieval performance. These features are detailed as follows:

- Radiology = {"Ultrasound Imaging", "Magnetic Resonance Imaging", "Computerized Tomography", "X-Ray", "2D Radiography", "Angiography", "PET", "Combined modalities in one image"}
- Microscopy = {"Light Microscopy", "Electron Microscopy", "Transmission Microscopy", "Fluorescence Microscopy"}
- Visible light photography = {"Dermatology", "Skin", "Endoscopy", "Other organs"}
- Printed signals and waves = {"Electroencephalography", "Electrocardiography", "Electromyography"}
- Generic Biomedical Illustrations = {"modality tables and forms", "program listing", "statistical figures", "graphs", "charts", "screen shots", "flowcharts", "system overviews", "gene sequence", "chromatography", "gel", "chemical structure", "mathematics formula", "non-clinical photos", "hand-drawn sketches"}
- Dimensionality = {"macro", "micro", "small", "gross", "combined dimensionality"}
- V-Spec = {"brown", "black", "white", "red", "gray", "yellow", "blue", "colored"}
- T-spec = {"finding","pathology", "differential diagnosis"}
- C-spec = {'Histology"}

3.2 *MDFs Extraction Procedure*

Although many approaches in the literature, such as conceptual approaches, have shown excellent retrieval results, most of them are very time and storage space consuming. In this work, we use the MDF based retrieval approach which saves both indexing time and space occupancy. Usually, the indexes encode the whole internal representation of documents. However, this work addresses an indexing approach that is restricted on the occurrence of features values in the collection. Extracting features from both documents and queries requires several different operations. First, all features, represented with terms, pass through a snowball stemmer. The resulting stems are then recorded in the stemmed feature list. Each term in the image metadata ($docID$) passes through the same stemmer and is checked against the stemmed feature list. If this list already contains the stem of interest, this term is considered an MDF/value. Then, it is recorded in the image-feature list with the same identifier ($docID$). The representation of the text "Radiographic findings of osteomyelitis" using medical-dependent-features is "{2D Radiography, finding}". After this processing, the dataset considered in the retrieval process is a set of MDFs.

3.3 Retrieval Process

In this section, we present an approach for image retrieval based on MDFs. It is presented in three steps: first, we compute the relevance score that measures the similarity between a document and a query. This is the baseline score which represents the correspondence degree between document and query based on terms; second, we measure the relevance score of query and document representations through MDFs by using the same baseline model; finally, we combine the MDF score with the baseline score to form the new retrieval score ($MDF - BM$). In particular, we propose modeling the MDF-BM score by a simple and classic linear combination (Eq. 1). Before combining the two scores, we need to normalize the initial and feature based scores as follows:

$$MDF - BM = \alpha * \frac{BMScore}{max(BMScore)} + (1 - \alpha) * \frac{MDFScore}{max(MDFScore)} \quad (1)$$

Where α is a balancing parameter [0..1], $BMScore$ represents the initial ranking score for the image, and $MDF - BM$ is the MDF score of the same image, by using the same baseline. The normalized score is obtained by dividing the relevance score for a given document d by the highest relevance score in the whole collection.

4 Experimental Setting

4.1 Datasets and Evaluation Metrics

To evaluate the MDF based image retrieval, we use two ImageCLEF collections in medical Image Task: 2009 [10] and 2010 [11] presented in Table 1. In ImageCLEFmed datasets, each image has a textual annotation that may contain a caption,

Table 1 MedicalClef dataset

	MedicalCLEF dataset	
	2009	2010
# Total queries	25	16
# Total images	74,902	77,495

a link to the HTML of the full text article [16] and also the article title [10]. In this paper, we use both image caption and article title to evaluate the retrieval models. For measuring the IR effectiveness, we used three evaluation measures that are commonly used in Medical ImageCLEF: the Mean Average Precision (MAP), the precision at the top ranking results (P@5, P@10, P@15, etc.), and the Binary Preference (Bpref).

4.2 *Review of Baseline Models*

In order to show the effectiveness of the MDF based retrieval, we conduct comparative study with different models such as classic text-based model (BM25) which is used as baseline, and concept based model. Our experiments are conducted using the classic information retrieval system Terrier (Terrier 3.5) and its implementations.

4.2.1 Text-Based Image Retrieval

As a text-based model, we use the probabilistic model BM25 [14] as shown in Eq. (2).

$$RSV(q,d) = \sum_{t \in (q \bigcap d)} \frac{t_f}{t_f + nb * k_1} * \log(\frac{N - df_t + 0.5}{df_t + 0.5}) * q_{tf} \tag{2}$$

Where q is a query, d is a document, t_f is the term frequency in the document, df_t is the document frequency of the term t, N is total number of documents in the collection, q_{tf} is frequency of term t in the query, $k_1 = 1.2$ is a defaults parameter and nb is the normalization factor which may be calculated as: $nb = (1 - b) + b * \frac{t_l}{Avgt_l}$. With t_l is the number of terms in the document, $Avgt_l$ is the average number of terms in the document and b are default parameters. Also we have compared the specific feature based image retrieval model with the Dirichlet language model "DLM" [9] and Bo1 Pseudo-relevance feedback "Bo1-prf" [6]. In order to build a strong baseline, we conduct a set of experiments to tune the parameter b and we set it equals 0.75.

4.2.2 Concept Based Image Retrieval

As a concept based model, we use a simple but effective concept based image retrieval model. First, we extract the candidate concepts using METAMAP and UMLS; second, a concept based retrieval process is applied. Several works show the efficiency of the MetaMap tool with UMLS [12]. For this reason, we propose to map textual representation of images into concepts by applying the MetaMap tool. Extracted concepts are identified by a CUI (Concept Unique Identifier). Typically each term will relate to several possible concepts, whence, for each term, several concepts could be extracted. These concepts are called candidate concepts. Taking the phrase "Ocular complications" as an example, 6 UMLS concept candidates are identified by MetaMap and used for the conceptual representation of the text "Ocular complications". They are "{C0009566, C1171258, C0231242, C1522701, C0015392, C1555959}". After this processing, the dataset considered in the retrieval process is a set of medical concepts.

The retrieval process is presented in three main steps: first, we compute the relevance score that measures the similarity between a document and a query. This is the baseline score which represents the correspondence degree between document and query based on terms; second, we measure the relevance score of query and document representations through medical concepts by using the same baseline model; finally, in order to take advantages of both datasets (concept, text) we combine the medical concept (MC) score with the baseline (BM) score to form the new retrieval score (MC-BM), and thus by using a linear combination after a normalization step. In order to obtain the best linear combination, we conduct a set of experiments to tune the parameter α and we set it equals 0.4.

5 Experimental Results

5.1 Results of the Proposed Models

In these experiments, we evaluate the impact of MDF-BM, MC-BM, BM25 model using terms, according to the MAP. Figure 1 presents a comparison according to MAP values between the MDF-BM model results, the MC-BM model results and BM25 using the terms results for all datasets. Based on those barplots, we observe that the MAP values depend on the used model (BM25, MDF, MDF-BM). For both datatsets, we can clearly see that the MAP values of MDFBM and MC-BM are comparable. For example, the MAP value of 2009 dataset when using MDF model equals to 0.148 and achieved 0.39 by MDF-BM model. In addition, it equals to 0.216 when using only concepts (MC) for research and achieved to 0.393 when using combination (concept + term) MC-BM for retrieval. We have the same observation for 2010 collections. These results confirm that MDFs and concepts are good additional sources of evidence to enhance medical image retrieval. Using only

Fig. 1 Comparison based on the MAP values

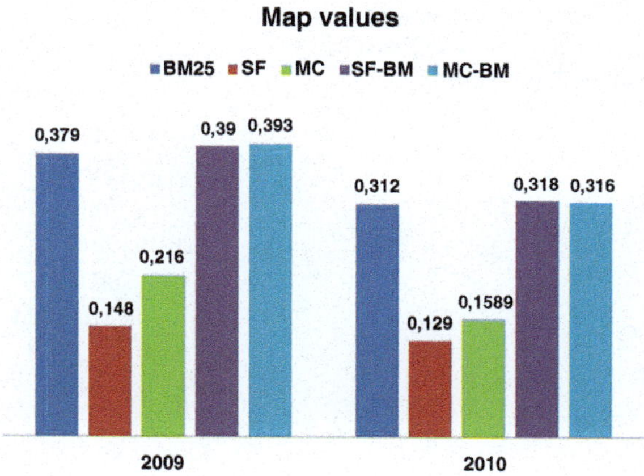

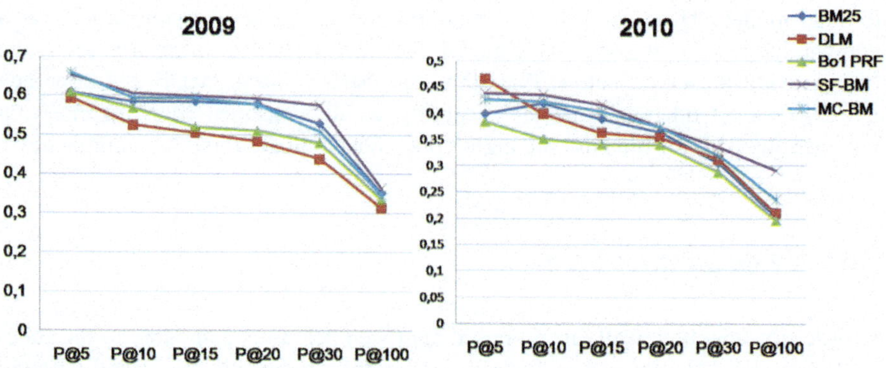

Fig. 2 Comparison of the precision at top ranks

features is not sufficient, and it is not surprising given the following explanation: A query cannot contain a large number of features, so it will be hard to find relevant images by using only features. Moreover, the decreasing MC results compared to BM25 may be explained by the fact that some UMLS concepts extracted based on image text are not correct. Consequently, it can negatively affect the obtained results. However, we can clearly see the improvement of results when combing feature/concept scores with BM25 scores.

5.2 *Further Analysis and Discussion*

In this experiment, we compare the precision at top ranks obtained by MDF-BM and MC-BM models to the state-of-the art models namely BM25, Dirichlet Language and Bo1 pseudo relevance feedback models. We use the same parameters for all datasets. Figure 2 presents the precision values for the different models.

Table 2 Comparison with the official imageCLEFmed approaches results

	Team	Rank	MAP	P@10	Bpref
2009	Liris	**1**	**0.43**	**0.66**	**0.46**
	MDF-BM	–	0.39	0.651	0.415
	MC-BM	–	0.393	0.623	0.41
	SINAI	2	0.38	0.62	0.39
	York	3	0.37	0.60	0.38
2010	Xrce	**1**	**0.338**	**0.506**	**0.382**
	AUEB	2	0.323	0.468	0.31
	MDF-BM	–	0.318	0.438	0.338
	MC-BM	–	0.316	0.427	0.34
	OHSU	3	0.302	0.431	0.34

According to the results, the MDF-BM model gives the best precision compared to other models. However, it is important to note that MC-BM results model has a comparable result with MDF-BM model. Our interpretations in regards to results of Fig. 2 are presented below. For 2009 and 2010 datasets, MDF-BM approach outperforms all other approaches according to all measures. More precisely, it outperforms BM25 which has the higher precision compared to other approaches.

5.3 A Comparative Study

In order to show how well our proposed approach performs compared to the state-of-the-art [10, 11] approaches, further comparative studies are conducted with the top three teams that achieved the best MAP using textual runs on the medical image retrieval task. Table 2 presents a comparison based on the MAP, P@10, and Bpref between the MDF-BM, the MC-BM model results, and the official imageCLEFmed approaches results. The results of the models (MDF-BM and MC-BM) are comparable to the results of the state of the art approaches, as shown in Table 2. For 2009 and 2010 datasets, our models do not outperform the highest values (MAP, p@10 and Bpref) founded by existing approaches. This can be explained by the fact that these models are highly dependent on the baseline results. However, for both datatsets, our models outperform the third highest values founded by existing approaches. This validates our assumption that our model has a positive impact on the retrieval performance.

5.4 Time and Space Complexity

In this paper, we used three datasets types (concept based, MDF based and text based) for retrieval approach. In this section, we present the indexing time and the

Table 3 Comparison of time/space occupancy

	2009			2010		
Index	Term	Concept	MDF	Term	Concept	MDF
Size(MB)	38.6	34.3	15.2	40.2	21.3	15.7
Time(s)	155.2	Few days	102.3	103.3	Few days	89.1

memory consumption using the three models: text-based, concept-based, and MDF-based. The experiment was conducted on a Pentium Dual Core 2.2 GHz machine with 2 GB DDR3 of RAM running ubuntu 12.04. As shown in Table 3, the size occupancy of MDFs, for the 2009 dataset, equals to 15.2 MB, while, for concept based indexing it is 34.3 MB and the term-based indexing, the size is 38.6 MB. The indexing time taken by MDFs approach is faster than the indexing time taken by term based and concept based indexing time. Based on result shown in Table 3, the indexing time is reduced from few days and 155.2–102.3 s by using MDFs. This reduction in indexing time as well as the size occupancy is due to the restriction of indexing on MDFs and thoughtlessness of all keywords of documents. This proves that these features are critical terms in the search process.

6 Conclusions and Future Work

In this paper, we studied the performance of medical-dependent-feature-based medical image indexing and retrieval according to both criteria: efficiency and effectiveness. MDFs are used to represent medical imageCLEF datasets as feature based representation. In addition, a classic retrieval method for computing the feature based score is used. We combined the feature based score with the baseline (BM25) score to form the new retrieval score. Using two medical imageCLEF collections (2009 and 2010), we compare the performance of MDF retrieval with approaches from the literature and analyze where it is effective. Results show that using that the MDF based approach gives accuracy results comparable to those found by concept based approach. In addition, the MDF approach has several strengths compared to literature indexing approaches, especially as regards space-time occupancy. In future work, we plan to include more MDFs that could cover more characteristics of any user information need in the context of image retrieval. Moreover, we plan to evaluate the performance of our model on other standard dataset collections.

References

1. Ayadi, H., Khemakhem, M.T., Daoud, M., Huang, J.X., Jemaa, M.B.: Mf-re-rank: a modality feature-based re-ranking model for medical image retrieval. JASIST **69**(9), 1095–1108 (2018)

2. Bouslimi, R., Messaoudi, A., Akaichi, J.: Using a bag of words for automatic medical image annotation with a latent semantic. CoRR abs/1306.0178 (2013)
3. Cao, Y., Steffey, S., He, J., Xiao, D., Tao, C., Chen, P., Müller, H.: Medical image retrieval: a multimodal approach. Cancer Informat. **2014**, 125–136 (2015)
4. Díaz-Galiano, M.C., García-Cumbreras, M.A., Martín-Valdivia, M.T., Ureña-López, L.A., Montejo-Ráez, A.: Query Expansion on Medical Image Retrieval: MeSH vs. UMLS, pp. 732–735. Springer, Berlin/Heidelberg (2009)
5. Gasmi, K., Khemakhem, M.T., Jemaa, M.B.: A conceptual model for word sense disambiguation in medical image retrieval. In: Information Retrieval Technology – 9th Asia Information Retrieval Societies Conference, AIRS 2013, Singapore, 9–11 Dec 2013. Proceedings, pp. 296–307 (2013)
6. He, B., Ounis, I.: Inferring query performance using pre-retrieval predictors. In: Proceedings of SPIRE, pp. 43–54 (2004)
7. Lu, Z., Kim, W., Wilbur, W.: Evaluation of query expansion using MeSH in PubMed. Inf. Retr. **12**(1), 69–80 (2009). https://doi.org/10.1007/s10791-008-9074-8
8. Maisonnasse, L., Gaussier, E., Chevallet, J.P.: Model Fusion in Conceptual Language Modeling, pp. 240–251 (2009)
9. Miller, D.R.H., Leek, T., Schwartz, R.M.: A hidden Markov model information retrieval system. In: Proceedings of the 22nd ACM SIGIR, pp. 214–221 (1999)
10. Muller, H., Kalpathy-Cramer, J., Eggel, I., Bedrick, S., Radhouani, S., Bakke, B., Khan, C.E., Jr., Hersh, W.R.: Overview of the CLEF 2009 medical image retrieval track. In: Proceedings of CLEF, pp. 72–84 (2009)
11. Müller, H., Kalpathy-Cramer, J., Eggel, I., Bedrick, S., Reisetter, J., Khan, C.E., Jr., Hersh, W.R.: Overview of the CLEF 2010 medical image retrieval track. In: CLEF (Notebook Papers/LABs/Workshops) (2010)
12. Pratt, W., Yetisgen-Yildiz, M.: A study of biomedical concept identification: Metamap vs. people. AMIA ... Annual Symposium Proceedings. AMIA Symposium, pp. 529–33 (2003)
13. Quellec, G., Lamard, M., Bekri, L., Cazuguel, G., Roux, C., Cochener, B.: Medical case retrieval from a committee of decision trees. Trans. Info. Tech. Biomed. **14**(5), 1227–1235 (2010)
14. Robertson, S.E., Walker, S.: Some simple effective approximations to the 2-poisson model for probabilistic weighted retrieval. In: Proceedings of SIGIR, pp. 232–241 (1994)
15. Souissi, N., Ayadi, H., Khemakhem, M.T.: Text-based medical image retrieval using convolutional neural network and specific medical features. In: Proceedings of the 12th International Joint Conference on Biomedical Engineering Systems and Technologies (BIOSTEC 2019) – Volume 5: HEALTHINF, Prague, 22–24 Feb 2019, pp. 78–87 (2019)
16. Wu, H., Sun, K., Deng, X., Zhang, Y., Che, B.: UESTC at imageCLEF 2012 medical tasks. In: Proceedings of CLEF, pp. 1–1 (2012)

Brain Image Processing Using Deep Learning: An Overview

Rahma Kadri, Mohamed Tmar, and Bassem Bouaziz

1 Introduction

Lately with the availability of smart technologies such as wearable technologies and the brain imaging tools, there have been great leaps forward the brain imaging processing and neuroscience. This discipline allows to better understand the mechanisms of the brain and the way we process and record information. One of the most challenging questions regarding this context is the automatic brain diseases and disorders diagnosis. Toward this end neuroscientists around the world collect data about brain function, structure and behavior using various neuroimaging tools at an ever-increasing rate. This data is the lifeblood of the brain behavior analysis. However the neuroimaging data are collected in various formats (text, image, video, sound..). The overarching challenge is how we can extract insights from it. Extracting knowledge is a tedious task that necessitates integration of well validated data described in a common standard and format. One interesting way to enable such process is to deal with a common international platform to collect, store, validate, analyze and publish neuroimaging data. The breakthrough in neuroimaging or brain imagining is the availability of powerful and advanced imaging modalities to understand the brain function. Brain imaging analysis encompasses many tasks such as the brain activity analysis, brain image segmentation, brain disease analysis and prediction. For this end, there are processing brain image modalities used to uncover and image the brain structure, behavior and activity.

R. Kadri (✉) · M. Tmar · B. Bouaziz
Higher Institute of Computer Science and Multimedia, University of Sfax, Sfax, Tunisia

L. Chaari (ed.), *Digital Health in Focus of Predictive, Preventive and Personalised Medicine*, Advances in Predictive, Preventive and Personalised Medicine 12,
https://doi.org/10.1007/978-3-030-49815-3_10

1.1 Brain Image Modalities

Typically brain imagining falls into two classes: the structural and the functional imaging.

Structural imaging which enables to illustrate the brain structure. Under this category there are the Computed Tomography (CT) and Magnetic Resonance Imaging (MRI) techniques.

- **CT** is a computerized x-ray imaging technique which provides axial images called slices.
- **MRI** is an advanced technique that produce detailed brain image structure. It allows to examine the brain anatomy in all three planes: axial, sagittal and coronal. the most commonly used MRI images are T1-weighted and T2-weighted.

Functional imaging is devoted to study the brain function. This technique uncovers the brain's information processing. It is based on well known scan techniques such as the Electroencephalography (EEG), functional Magnetic Resonance Imaging (fMRI), Positron Emission Tomography (PET) and the Magnetoencephalography (MEG).

- **fMRI**: is extremely used to detect the brain's functional anatomy by measuring the brain activity. It also examines the main changes in the brain.
- **(EEG)**: visualizes the electrical activity in the brain neurons. It also uncover the state of the brain.
- **(PET)**: uses a radioactive substance also known as tracer to illustrate the brain activity. This technique detects such injury on the brain.
- **(MEG)**: measures the magnetic fields relating to such electrical activity in the brain.

The automatic diagnosis and knowledge extraction from these tools became a hard question to meet. The tremendous success of deep learning meet the need of an efficient neuroimaging data analysis approaches. We investigate the recent application of deep learning regarding the neuroimaging data collection and analysis. Hence we define a set of research questions:

- RQ1: What are the most used datasets for each image brain analysis methods using deep learning. This question highlights the most used dataset sources for image brain analysis. The main motivation underlying this question is the need of data collection for the brain image analysis.
- RQ2: What are the most relevant contributions of deep learning regarding the brain image analysis. The underlying purpose of this question is to overview the current brain image processing methods and explore the recent publications and approaches within this context.

- RQ3: What are the preprocessing steps for an effective brain image analysis. The main motivation of this question is to figure out the main key preprocessing steps for the brain image analysis.
- RQ4: What are the main current challenges today regarding the brain image analysis.

We conducted a Systematic Literature Review (SLR) to investigate the recent existing publications in order to meet these research questions.

2 Brain Image Processing Using Deep Learning

Deep learning was widely used for different brain image analysis tasks:

Brain image reconstruction: is an active area that aims to create two or three-dimensional image from scattered or incomplete data. Brain image reconstruction is the key step for many tasks such as disease, classification and recognition. Further, this task is extremely applied for the reconstruction of the image from the brain activity.

Brain image super-resolution: medical image with high resolution is very expensive. For this end, the brain image super-resolution incorporates a set of techniques that aim to reconstruct a high-resolution MRI images from low-resolution image. This task is vital to ensure the relevant quantitative analysis.

Brain Image Segmentation: this task is critical for image brain analysis and understanding. It simplifies the representation of the image in order to make it easier to analyse.

Automated Brain Disorders Diagnosis: a lot of attention today is accorded to the brain disease classification. Examples include Alzheimer's disease, brain cancer, migraine disease and dementia.

Brain image generation and synthesis: data collection within the neuroimaging is challenging and difficult task. Brain image analysis using deep learning is relying on a huge amount of training data. Significant effort has been invested on this task such as the data augmentation and the synthetic image generation.

2.1 Data Preparation and Collection

Data preparation is a key pre-processing process consisting of data gathering, cleaning, structuring, organizing, augmentation, fusion and transforming into suitable data from for analysis task. Researchers adopt many methods to collect and prepare their data. The key challenge today within the brain image analysis is the lack of annotated brain images. There is an effective effort to ensure centralized access and data availability by creating tools for neuroimaging data exchange examples includes (OpenfMR,[1] ADNI,[2] OASIS[3]). The data preparation and collection here depends on the target task such as brain image segmentation, reconstruction, super-resolution and brain disease detection. Within the context of the brain disease detection and analysis many researchers collect different brain image modalities. Jain et al. [1] collect T1-weighted MRI data of 150 subject 50 Alzheimer's Disease (AD) 50 Normal Control (CN), 50 Mild Cognitive Impairment (MCI) from the Alzheimer's Disease Neuroimaging Initiative (ADNI) for alzheimer's disease classification. The feature selection involves demographic characteristics of the selected subjects such as age, gender and Mind Mental State Examination (MMSE). They select the most informative RMI slices using an entropy function. They used a FreeSurfer software for the pre-processing. They adopt different preprocessing methods such as motion correction, non-uniform intensity normalization and skull stripping. Another intelligent selection of the most informative MRI slices from the ADNI dataset also was proposed by [2] for the prediction of Alzheimer's disease. An intelligent data augmentation process with balancing method is proposed by [3] using the same dataset also for the Alzheimer's disease. Here data selection involves 214 patients: 48 AD patients, 108 MCI and 58 NC. The input used images are T1-weighted Structural magnetic resonance imaging (sMRI) image and a Diffusion Tensor Imaging (DTI) image. They also adopt the age, gender and (MMSE) score as the demographic characteristics. For the preprocessing steps they applied a correction of eddy currents and head motion, skull stripping using the Brain Extraction Tool (BET) on the DTI brain images. For the same task [4] collect 18F-FDG PET images about 1002 patients with various scans. Here the dataset is from different sources such as (ADNI)-1, ADNI2 and ADNI-GO studies. To prepare data for analysis, they adopt a grid method based on the input images resampling to 2-mm isotropic voxels. Here the feature selection consists of extracting the caudal-most sections that represent more than $100 \times 100\,\text{mm}^2$ of brain parenchyma. For the brain voxels selection they utilize an Otsu threshold function. They also use a connected component analysis to extract the relevant imaging volume. For this end they find a use for Python Software Foundation.

Feng et al. [5] adopt 2 different brain image modalities MRI and PET also from the ADNI dataset for the diagnosis of Alzheimer disease. They applied different methods for the MRI preprocessing such as the image resampling, Anterior Commissure (AC), posterior commissure reorientation, skull striping and segmentation using Field Service Lightning(FSL) package. Here they applied different algorithms for elastic image registration using the hierarchical attribute matching method. Whereas [6] use a 3D FDG-PET images from the ADNI dataset about 339 patients: 93 AD patients, 146 MCI and 100 NC acquired by 30–60 min post-injection for the Alzheimer's disease classification. They use the same demographic characteristics of the previous contributions (age, gender, education..). Data preprocessing here

[1] openfmri.org

[2] adni.loni.usc.edu

[3] www.oasis-brains.org

includes the intensity normalization, the conversion to a uniform isotropic resolution of 8 mm FWHM, the image decomposition into 2D slices and the image size reduction. Yang et al. [7] use a small custom dataset for migraine classification including 21 migraine patients without aura, 15 migraineurs with aura, and 28 healthy controls. For the data acquisition they utilize a 3.0 Tesla MRI system and Echo-Planar Imaging (EPI). During this acquisition, patients were rest with their eyes closed and not to fall asleep. The key feature here is the feature mapping method in order to illustrate the brain activity and state. They calculated three functional maps for each subject the amplitude of low frequency fluctuations, the regional homogeneity and the brain functional connectivity state. Within the context of brain image segmentation [8] collect 2 medical datasets: the BraTS2016 and the LiTS2017 benchmark for brain tumor segmentation including MRI and CT images. They applied different preprocessing steps on the MRI images for example the intensity non-uniformity and the histogram matching. Further they perform a slice-wise fashion on the CT images. To remove the irrelevant object on the CT images, they calculated the Hounsfield Unit (HU) values. Finally they adopt the histogram equalization to improve the contrast. They introduce a patient-wise mini-batch normalization as preprocessing step to enhance the segmentation task. Ang et al. [9] collect an fMRI data about specific brain tissue such as gray matter, white matter, blood vessel, non-brain and cerebrospinal fluid also for brain tissue and tumor classification. For the preprocessing they adopt a motion correction, slice scan time correction and intensity normalization. Whereas for this task [10] use the Brats2017 training dataset. Here a few preprocessing steps are performed such as intensity normalization. Chen et al. [11] also collect data within the context of brain image segmentation from the MRBrainS challenge. They adopt different brain image modalities including the T1, T1-IR, and T2-FLAIR of patients with diabetes.

2.2 *Training Process and Classification*

The training and the learning process involves the main architectures used to meet such tasks on the brain image processing. The methods are based on different learning process algorithms. Examples include supervised learning methods based on the transfer learning, unsupervised learning and fusion methods.

2.2.1 Transfer Learning

The transfer learning is a machine learning method based on the reuse of a model which is created for solving specific task as a starting point for another task. Within the context of brain disease detection the transfer learning is widely used. Within the context of brain disease diagnosis and detection such as the Alzheimer's disease [1] adopt the transfer learning using a pretrained VGG16 for Alzheimer's disease classification. Whereas [2] use the VGG19 for Alzheimer's disease prediction. The transfer learning meet the need of the huge amount of data for training. However the VGG network used in this works is slow to train due to the huge number of the network parameters. Another transfer learning based on the inception model was proposed by [4] with the same training dataset to predict a diagnosis of Alzheimer disease using 18F-FDG PET of the brain data. The network consists of 11 inception modules. Each module incorporates a convolution layers, pooling layers and convolutional filters with rectified linear units. The main advantage of this work over the previous methods is the multi-level feature extraction. Khvostikov et al. [3] present a 3D Convolution Neural Network (CNN) architecture which consists of a set of convolutions blocks using a sMRI and DTI images as inputs for alzheimer disease classification. Each block is composed by a 3D convolution, batch normalization, rectifier linear unit and 3D pooling. The discriminate feature of this work is the fusion method of 2 different image modalities(sMRI and MD-DT) using a hippocampal Region of interest pooling (ROI). Here the inception model allows the extraction of the local and global features at the same time. However this work just handles 2D images. A recent work [12] of the same researchers consists of using a 3D inception model. Compared with their previous work the inception model decreases the number of network parameters and enhances the feature extraction process. Yang et al. [7] address the problem of the migraine classification and compare the inception model with the Alexnet to classify healthy brains, brains affected by Migraines with aura (MWA) and brains affected by Migraines without aura (MWoA). Within the context of brain image segmentation, [8] propose a multitask convolutional neural network for tumor brain instance segmentation. The learning process involves 2 stages. The first stage is a tumor detection using a region proposal network correlated with the though transform technique. The second stage is the tumor segmentation using the VGG19 network. Chen et al. [11] present a new deep residual learning namely deep voxelwise residual networks for brain segmentation also from 3D MR images. They propose a stacked of residual module(25 volumetric convolutional/deconvolutional). The main advantage here is the multi-modality and auto-context information fusion to enhance the segmentation task. Their method holds different image sizes.

2.2.2 Fusion Methods

In order to enable an effective feature extraction from brain images. Researches adopt fusion methods that extract special and temporal features using the Recurrent Neural Network (RNN) such as the Long short-term memory (LSTM) and the Bidirectional gated recurrent unit (BGRU) combined with the convolution neural network. The application of CNNs for 3D volumetric classification is difficult to optimize. To improve the CNN performance regarding the Alzheimer's diagnosis, [5] combine a 3D-CNN and fully stacked bidirectional (FSBi-LSTM) using a RMI and PET images. They compare different fusion methods such as FSBi-RNN,

FSBi-GRU. They point out that FSBi-LSTM is the best fusion method. The key contribution of this method is the multi-modal fusion which yields good results of diagnosis than a single modality methods. Another fusion method on the same the context demonstrated by [6] consists of a convolutional and bidirectional gated recurrent neural network using FDG-PET images. The 2D CNN is trained to capture the intra-slice features and the BGRU for the inter-slice feature extraction. Different from the previous work, they adopt 2 activation functions Tanh for the BGRU and the Rectified Linear Activation Function (ReLU) for the CNN. To improve the segmentation task, [9] combine the CNN with the LSTM for automatic brain tissue tumor segmentation for fmri voxel classification into 5 classes gray matter, white matter, blood vessel, non-brain (NB) and cerebrospinal fluid. The training encompasses spatial and temporal feature extraction.

2.2.3 Unsupervised Learning

The unsupervised leaning overcome the lack of labeled data within the context of the neuroimaging. Regarding the context of brain disease detection, [13] introduce a method to model the progression of Alzheimer's disease in the MRI brain images. They modify the Wasserstein training process by a AdaBoost learning in order to extract the more extreme cases of AD on the ADNI training dataset. Mallick et al. [14] also propose an unsupervised learning using a combination of the deep wavelet autoencoder and the deep neural network for brain cancer detection. The main contribution here over the existing methods is the feature reduction and the image decomposition using an autoencoder and the wavelet transformation. Authors compare their proposed network with other methods such as Autoencoder-DNN and Deep Neural Network (DNN). Within the context of brain image segmentation [10] notice that it is vital to improve the spatial contiguity of the network output by using unsupervised learning. Toward this end, they adopt an adversarial network using tow different CNN networks. This adversarial learning consists of a generator that generates synthetic labels and the discriminator tries to distinguish between the truth and the synthetic labels produced by the generator. Data augmentation and brain image generation is another challenging task. The generative adversarial network is extremely used to meed this task. Han et al. [15] propose to generate synthetic brain MR images using a deep generative adversarial network. They adopt unsupervised learning basing on a generator and discriminator network. The generator used up-convolutions layers with a non-linearity and batch-normalization in order to create synthetic images. The discriminator is another network that distinguish between the real and the generated images. Han et al. [16] use a progressive Generative Adversarial Network (pGAN) for brain MRI augmentation. Han et al. [17] improve the data augmentation by a cascade method that combines different GAN architectures to generate brain MR images without and with tumors separately. For this end they combine the noise-to-image GANs and image-to-image GANs. They also adopt a pGAN to generate brain images. Dar et al. [18] propose a method for a multi-contrast MRI synthesis using the conditional generative adversarial network. For the registered images they use a pGAN to learn the function map between the source and the target image. They use a cGAN for the unregistered images. Yang et al. [19] adopt a cycleGAN with structure-constrained for synthesizing CT images from brain MR images.

For the classification both methods are based on the softmax classifier.

2.3 Results

The transfer learning based on the convolution neural network was widely used for the context of brain disease detection such as the Alzheimer's disease. Jain et al. [1] achieve accuracy of 95.73% using the VGG 16 to classify brain sMRI 2D slices into 3 different classes: AD, NC and MCI. Over the CNN architecture the inception model yields the best accurate results. This is illustrated by many researchers such as [3]. Here authors reach 0.933% for AD/NC binary, 0.867% for AD/MCI, 0.733% for MCI/NC and 0.68% ternary for AD/MCI/NC classification problem. Ding et al. [4] reaches a good results using an inception model for Alzheimer's early prediction about 75.8 months before the final diagnosis. Fusion method based on the combination of the CNN and RNN architectures also shows an accurate results on this context such as [5]. Regarding the unsupervised learning the GAN and the autoencoder are widely used by researchers for the brain disease diagnosis. Bowles et al. [13] return relevant results regarding the illustration of the Alzheimer's disease progression using the GAN. Mallick et al. [14] with the combination of the deep network and the autoencoder obtain an accuracy of 93% to detect brain cancer. The convolution neural network is also used extremely for the brain image segmentation and tumor classification. A cascade method proposed by [9] reach a classification accuracy of 84.04% to classify brain tumor and segmentation. Chen et al. [11] achieve the first place in a challenge including 37 contributions on brain image segmentation. Rezaei et al. [8] present a prominent result regarding the brain tumor instance segmentation using a multitask convolution neural network basing on VGG19. Whereas [10] with the GAN architecture obtain more reliable results on the brain tumor segmentation. Regarding the context of the brain image synthesis and generation, the GAN architectures are the first choice of many researchers. Kazuhiro et al. [20] shows a good results using a deep GAN on the MRI image generation. Whereas the fusion method [17, 21] that based on the combination of the different architectures of the GAN such as pGAN, cGAN provide more accurate results.

3 Conclusion and Current Challenges

Neuroimaging is an interdisciplinary filed devoted to the study of the brain structure, function, behavior and activity. This domain brings different fields such as medicine, statistics, biology and computer science. The advancement of the brain imaging technique enhances the brain analysis. However it is critical to extract the meaningful information within these techniques. Deep learning fill this need. In the present paper, we highlight the main techniques used on the deep learning networks for brain image processing such as the data preparation, augmentation and the training process. For the data preparation and collection, there is a hardest question to meet which is the lack of annotated datasets for the supervised learning.

The preprocessing and feature extraction are another key steps for an effective brain image analysis. Significant efforts have been made to handle different preprocessing for various brain image modalities. It is crucial today to ensure an analysis methods that handle different image brain modalities in order to exploit the information within these images.

The generative adversarial networks were extremely used for the data augmentation on the brain images analysis to enhance the training process. This network was also widely used for the brain image super-resolution and synthesis. The Convolution neural network was applied for the brain images classification and brain diseases classification. The inception model is the most used among the CNN architectures. To improve the CNN performance on the image brain analysis researches combine it with the RNN networks such as the LSTM and the BGRU. To enhance the training process and optimize the network, researchers utilize different regulations methods such as dropout layer, batch normalization and data augmentation. The brain image processing includes different tasks such as brain image segmentation, generation, brain disease prediction and brain image enhancement.

However there is a need today for the image to text within the context of neuroscience to enhance the brain image understanding which is not found on the recent deep learning application regarding this context. There are many challenges regarding the brain image analysis today such as the early prediction of the brain disease before years. However this needs a huge amount of medical data. Another challenge is ensuring a unified infrastructure to share neuroimaging data. The data augmentation and synthetic data generation is trending today due to the lack of the annotated datasets. The brain activity analysis is another key challenge.

References

1. Jain, R., Jain, N., Aggarwal, A., Jude Hemanth, D.: Convolutional neural network based Alzheimer's disease classification from magnetic resonance brain images. Cogn. Syst. Res. **57**, 147–159 (2019)
2. Khan, N.M., Abraham, N., Hon, M.: Transfer learning with intelligent training data selection for prediction of Alzheimer's disease. IEEE Access **7**, 72726–72735 (2019)
3. Khvostikov, A., Aderghal, K., Benois-Pineau, J., Krylov, A., Catheline, G.: 3D CNN-based classification using SMRI and MD-DTI images for Alzheimer disease studies, Jan (2018)
4. Ding, Y., Sohn, J.H., Kawczynski, M.G., Trivedi, H., Harnish, R., Jenkins, N.W., Lituiev, D., Timothy, P.: A deep learning model to predict a diagnosis of Alzheimer disease by using 18f-FDG PET of the brain. Radiology **290**(2), 456–464 (2019)

5. Feng, C., Elazab, A., Yang, P., Wang, T., Zhou, F., Hu, H., Xiao, X., Lei, B.: Deep learning framework for Alzheimer's disease diagnosis via 3D-CNN and FSBi-LSTM. IEEE Access **7**, 63605–63618 (2019)
6. Liu, M., Cheng, D., Yan, W.: Classification of Alzheimer's disease by combination of convolutional and recurrent neural networks using FDG-PET images. Front. Neuroinform. **12**, 35 (2018)
7. Yang, H., Zhang, J., Liu, Q., Wang, Y.: Multimodal MRI-based classification of migraine: using deep learning convolutional neural network. BioMed. Eng. Online **17**(1):138 (2018)
8. Rezaei, M., Yang, H., Meinel, C.: Instance tumor segmentation using multitask convolutional neural network. In: 2018 International Joint Conference on Neural Networks (IJCNN). IEEE, July 2018
9. Ang, S.P., Phung, S.L., Schira, M.M., Bouzerdoum, A., Duong, S.T.M.: Human brain tissue segmentation in fMRI using deep long-term recurrent convolutional network. In: 2018 Digital Image Computing: Techniques and Applications (DICTA). IEEE, Dec (2018)
10. Li, Z., Wang, Y., Yu, J.: Brain tumor segmentation using an adversarial network. In: Brainlesion: Glioma, Multiple Sclerosis, Stroke and Traumatic Brain Injuries, pp. 123–132. Springer International Publishing (2018)
11. Chen, H., Dou, Q., Yu, L., Qin, J., Heng, P.-A.: VoxResNet: Deep voxelwise residual networks for brain segmentation from 3D MR images. NeuroImage **170**, 446–455 (2018)
12. Khvostikov, A., Aderghal, K., Krylov, A., Catheline, G., Benois-Pineau, J.: 3D inception-based CNN with SMRI and MD-DTI data fusion for Alzheimer's disease diagnostics. arXiv preprint arXiv:1809.03972 (2018)
13. Bowles, C., Gunn, R., Hammers, A., Rueckert, D.: Modelling the progression of Alzheimer's disease in MRI using generative adversarial networks. In: Angelini, E.D., Landman, B.A. (eds.) Medical Imaging 2018: Image Processing. SPIE, Bellingham, Mar (2018)
14. Mallick, P.K., Ryu, S.H., Satapathy, S.K., Mishra, S., Nguyen, G.N., Tiwari, P.: Brain MRI image classification for cancer detection using deep wavelet autoencoder-based deep neural network. IEEE Access **7**, 46278–46287 (2019)
15. Han, C., Hayashi, H., Rundo, L., Araki, R., Shimoda, W., Muramatsu, S., Furukawa, Y., Mauri, G., Nakayama, H.: Gan-based synthetic brain MR image generation. In: 2018 IEEE 15th International Symposium on Biomedical Imaging (ISBI 2018), pp. 734–738. IEEE (2018)
16. Han, C., Rundo, L., Araki, R., Furukawa, Y., Mauri, G., Nakayama, H., Hayashi, H.: Infinite brain MR images: PGGAN-based data augmentation for tumor detection. arXiv preprint arXiv:1903.12564 (2019)
17. Han, C., Rundo, L., Araki, R., Nagano, Y., Furukawa, Y., Mauri, G., Nakayama, H., Hayashi, H.: Combining noise-to-image and image-to-image gans: brain MR image augmentation for tumor detection. arXiv preprint arXiv:1905.13456 (2019)
18. Dar, S.U.H., Yurt, M., Karacan, L., Erdem, A., Erdem, E., Çukur, T.: Image synthesis in multi-contrast MRI with conditional generative adversarial networks. IEEE Trans. Med. Imaging **38**, 2375–2388 (2019)
19. Yang, H., Sun, J., Carass, A., Zhao, C., Lee, J., Xu, Z., Prince, J.: Unpaired brain MR-to-CT synthesis using a structure-constrained cyclegan. In: Deep Learning in Medical Image Analysis and Multimodal Learning for Clinical Decision Support, pp. 174–182. Springer (2018)
20. Kazuhiro, K., Werner, R.A., Toriumi, F., Javadi, M.S., Pomper, M.G., Solnes, L.B., Verde, F., Higuchi, T., Rowe, S.P.: Generative adversarial networks for the creation of realistic artificial brain magnetic resonance images. Tomography **4**(4), 159–163 (2018)
21. Gu, J., Li, Z., Wang, Y., Yang, H., Qiao, Z., Yu, J.: Deep generative adversarial networks for thinsection infant MR image reconstruction. IEEE Access **7**, 68290–68304 (2019)

Discrete Optimization Model of Free-Fall-Flow-Rack Based Automated Drug Dispensing System

Dhiyaeddine Metahri and Khalid Hachemi

1 Introduction

Medicine is changing paradigm; it is switching from diagnosis and treatment to prediction and prevention. This is encompassed in the new concept of Predictive, Preventive and Personalized Medicine (PPPM). "True personalised medicine" is based on the "individual patient profile" directing to a tailored therapy that maximises the efficacy for that one patient in particular [12].

Going from a reactive medicine to a proactive medicine has multiple consequences for the management of the medication-use process within a healthcare structure, including an increase in the number of drug references underlying the individualization of treatments. In this context, automated dispensing systems are a key choice to meet the demands of speed and accuracy of patient service.

Materials handling technologies have enabled companies to control and manage their inventory. This can be achieved through an automated storage and retrieval system (AS / RS). AS / RSs are used in multiple industries and advanced manufacturing systems [30]. The main advantages of these systems are the saving of labor and floor space costs, the ease and speed of handling items and enhance throughput [21].

The main components of an AS/RS are storage racks, aisles, storage and retrieval (S/R) machines, Input/output stations (I/O) stations and the control system. Racks consist of several bins that can store items. The racks are separated by aisles, which allow the movement of storage and retrieval machines to pick up and drop off loads.

D. Metahri · K. Hachemi (✉)
Institute of Maintenance and Industrial Safety, Oran 2 Mohamed Ben Ahmed University, Oran, Algeria
e-mail: hachemi.khalid@univ-oran2.dz

L. Chaari (ed.), *Digital Health in Focus of Predictive, Preventive and Personalised Medicine*, Advances in Predictive, Preventive and Personalised Medicine 12,
https://doi.org/10.1007/978-3-030-49815-3_11

The Input/output stations (I/O) receive incoming and outgoing products. The control system is used for managing storage and retrieval operations.

There are different types of ASRS, namely, unit-load AS/RS, mini-load AS/RS, man-on-board AS/RS, carousel AS/RS, multi aisles AS/RS, Mobil-racks AS/RS, and flow-rack AS/RS (deep-lane AS/RS).

A new kind of flow-rack AS/RS has been introduced by MEKAPHARM [23], this system is served by a human operator or a single machine for storage operations, and combines the free-fall movement and a transport conveyor for retrieval operations. It can operate without any storage/retrieval machines, compared to the classic flow-rack AS/RS, where the system uses a (S/R) machine.

Since AS/RS require a very high investment, the design of AS/RS represents a crucial step during the feasibility conception study. In fact, once the AS/RS is implemented, it is very difficult to modify the rack layout and storage capacity. For this, the purpose of this paper is to find the optimal dimensions (length, height and depth) of the rack, which minimize the retrieval-travel-time. We formulate the optimization problem as a non-linear discrete model instead of a continuous model, which does not reflect the discrete nature of the rack. The aim of this study is to give a practical support to the AS/RS designer.

The structure of the paper is as follows. Section 2 gives an overview of the previous research. The FF-flow-rack AS/RS operation and structure are presented in Sect. 3. The optimization model and the obtained results are provided and discussed in Sect. 4. Section 5 draw conclusion and further research.

2 Literature Review

Different approaches have been proposed to increase the AS/RS performance by the means of request sequencing, storage assignment policy, and system configuration. The expected travel time was the main indicator used to assess the AS/RS performance.

Several studies exist on the modelling of the expected travel time. The most interesting approach to this issue has been proposed by Bozer and White [5]. They developed the expected single and dual travel time models of a rectangular rack under a random storage and for different positions of input/output point. Additionally, various dwell-point strategies for the storage/retrieval machine were examined. This model was used by Sari et al. [28], where they presented two mathematical models for the expected travel-time for a flow-rack AS/RS, which use two (S/R) machines. The first model is developed by using a continuous approach and compared with a second discrete model for accuracy via simulation. The authors conclude that the expressions based on continuous approach are extremely practical due to the difference in computation time.

For other flow-rack AS/RS variations, Sari and Bessnouci [27] have proposed a new kind of flow-rack AS/RS that using a single machine for both storage and retrieval operations instead of two machines. They developed analytical-travel-time models of the storage and retrieval machine, under randomized storage assignment. Two dwell point positions were considered. Otherwise, De Koster et al. [10] used a lifting mechanism in the opposite face of the S/R machine for a flow-rack AS/RS. They presented a closed-form expression of expected retrieval travel-time for single-command cycles, and derived an approximate travel-time expression for dual command cycles of the system. Also, Chen et al. [7] designed a bi-directional flow-rack (BFR) in which bins in adjacent columns slope to opposite directions. They develop a travel-time model for BFR systems.

Various methods have been proposed to deal with reducing the travel time for the flow-rack AS/RS. Sari et al. [29] Studied the impact of P/D stations and restoring conveyor locations on expected retrieval-time and classified their optimal positions. Meghelli-Gaouar and Sari [22] used a two class-based storage policy for the flow-rack AS/RS, where each item is assigned to the same bin as closely as possible to the P/D point. This work was extended by Bessenouci et al. [4] by developing two metaheuristic algorithms (tabu search and simulated annealing) applied to the control of the S/R machine. Hachemi and Alla [13] presented an optimization method of retrieval sequencing where the AS/RS was represented by a colored Petri net model. In a recent paper, Hachemi and Besombes [14], extended the problem of retrieval sequencing for flow-rack AS/RS by integrating the product expiry date. They introduced an optimization method as a decision process which performs a real-time optimization into two phases and formulated as an integer program. Kota et al. [16] Developed analytical expressions for retrieval times and heuristic algorithms to determine optimal or near-optimal movement of objects in a high-density, puzzle-based storage system.

Various researchers study the sequencing problem for different type of AS/RS. Chung and Lee [8] introduced heuristic methods to solve a generalized sequencing problem for unit-load AS/RS. These methods determine both specific bin locations for the retrieval requests and sequencing with the chosen bin locations. From a series of realistic case problems Kuo et al. [18] proposed a cycle-time model for class-based storage policies for automated unit load AS/RS that use autonomous vehicle technology. The model was designed specifically for the practice of AVS/RS design conceptualization by utilizing a network queuing approach. In order to minimize the distance travelled by the Storage and Retrieval (S/R) machine. Asokan et al. [3] implemented non-traditional optimization techniques (Adaptive Genetic Algorithm (AGA) and Particle Swarm Optimization (PSO)). In order to optimize the performance of man on board AS/RS, Dallari et al. [9] compares different storage policies with two tour construction heuristic. Authors conclude that the introduction of BI heuristic and class based storage policy provide substantial travel time reduction. According to (Fohn et al. [11]; Robert terry et al. [26]), AS/RS designs are difficult because these systems evolve in highly dynamic environments. For this, an optimal design procedure should be combined with control policies.

AS/RS design has received some attention in the literature. Ashayeri et al. [2] proposed a microcomputer-based optimization model to calculate the optimum number of racks and the optimum width and length of automated warehouses. Malmborg [20] studied the design and modelling of double-shuttle AS/RS.

Kuo et al. [17] proposed effective design calculation models for unit load AS/RS using autonomous vehicle technology. Yang et al. [32] deals with the optimization of 3D multi-deep AS/RS with a full turnover-based storage policy by considering the operating characteristics of the S/R machine, to close to the real operation of the compact warehouse.

De Koster et al. [10] derived the expressions of the expected travel time for single and dual command cycle of flow-rack AS/RS that used a lifting mechanism. They used these expressions to optimize the systems dimensions. The authors found that the cubic-in-time system (i.e. all dimensions are equal in time) is not the optimal configuration. This work was extended by Yang et al. [31], who considered the real operating characteristics of the S/R machine to obtain the optimal rack dimensions. Concerning the AS/RS introduced by Sari and Bessnouci [27]. Hamzaoui and Sari [15] determined the optimal dimensions of this AS/RS by using an enumeration technique. These dimensions minimize the expected travel times of the S/R machine.

An interesting study that was presented by Meneghetti et al. [24]. The authors proposed the adoption of a two-stage design approach of unit-load AS/RS by taking into account the economical and environmental perspectives (energy consumption, costs and carbon dioxide emissions). Based on discrete events simulation Caputo and Pelagagge [6] check and identify correct design choices for capacity upgrade of large-intensive material handling and storage systems. Asef-Vaziri et al. [1] designed and analyzed an automated container handling and storage system, which integrates AS/RS and Automated Guided Vehicle Systems (AGVS) for use at seaport terminals. They performed a computer simulation study to show the impact of such automation on the system performance (throughput, space utilization, and equipment utilization). Lättilä et al. [19] developed a decision-making tool based on the combination between static spreadsheet modelling and Monte Carlo simulation. This tool was used to compare warehouse design, calculate investment payback time of two suggested AS/RS investments, and to identify the main factors affecting their economic feasibility.

3 FF-Flow-Rack AS/RS

3.1 System Description and Structure

Mekapharm company® has launched a new type of flow-rack AS / RS, known under the trade name "APOTEKA" [23]. It is mainly used in all areas handling products resistant to free fall impact, and in particular for the automation of drug distribution in pharmacies. We are referring to the new type of AS / RS: the Free-Fall-flow rack AS/RS, or FF-Flow-rack AS/RS. The most important divergence between the FF-flow-rack AS/RS and the other types of flow-rack AS/RS presented by (Sari et al. [28]; De Koster et al. [10]; Sari and Bessnouci [27]) is that the picking operations

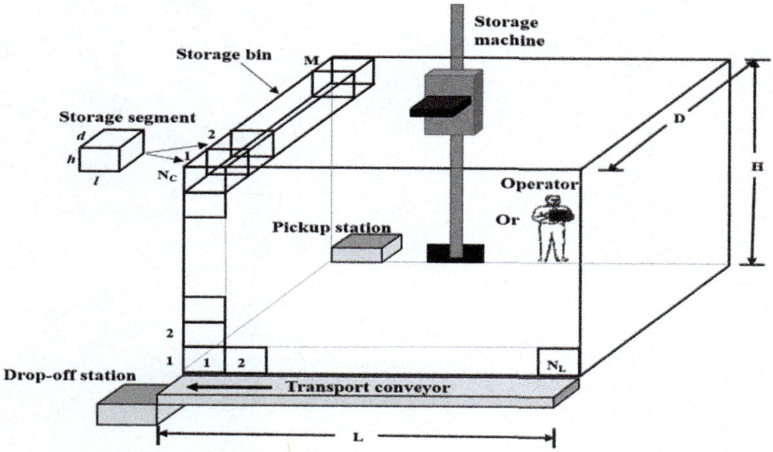

Fig. 1 Typical configuration of FF-flow-rack AS/RS

are realized by combining the free-fall movement and transport conveyor to replace the retrieval machine.

The use of FF-flow-rack AS/RS has several advantages like: saving the floor space, better inventory management, throughput increasing, and removal of the S/R machines. Especially, in the pharmaceutical distribution, this system offers the possibility of simultaneous retrieval of several drugs, reduces customer wait time, reduces queue sizes leading more time for advising customers, and reduces the dispensing error.

As shown in Fig. 1, the FF-flow-rack AS/RS structure is built of: a deep rack with a multitude of sloping bins, equipped with rolling wheels to allow the sliding of products by gravity from the storage to the picking side. Each bin is made of a set of segments (locations) that contains multiple identical products (the same SKU: Stock Keeping Unit) placed according to a FIFO file. A pickup station is located on the storage side, and a drop-off station is located on the retrieval side. A transport conveyor used to make the connection between the rack and the drop-off station. An operator or a storage crane performs the storage of items. The Fig. 2 shows a real view of the Apoteka© system.

As illustrated in Fig. 1, the rack dimensions are: length (L), height (H) and depth (D). The rack has (N_L) bins in each tier and (N_c) bins in each column. Each bin has (M) storage segments. Since the use of a person for the storage operation, the maximum height of the rack should be less than 3 m, in regard to practical and ergonomic considerations.

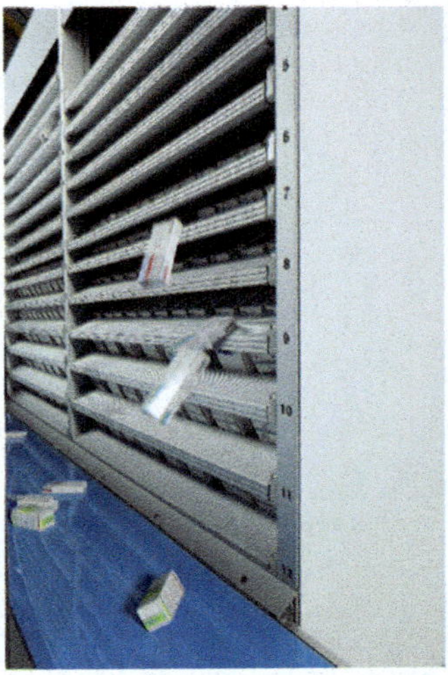

Fig. 2 Real view of the Apoteka system

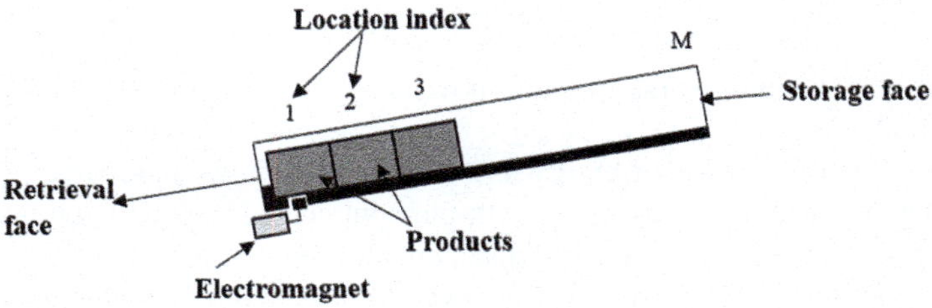

Fig. 3 Product layout inside a storage bin

3.2 System Operation

The FF-flow-rack AS/RS operating is as follows:

(a) The storage operation is fulfilled by a storage machine or an operator, where the products are moved from the pickup station to store them in the corresponding bins.
(b) The retrieval operation is done in two steps: The first one is the ejection of the item, where it is accomplished by the excitement of the electromagnet of the bin containing the desired product. This induces the free fall of the product on the transport conveyor. The second step is the product transport by the conveyor until the drop-off station.

The ejection of a product causes the progressive sliding by the gravity of all other products in the bin, as shown in Fig. 3 that highlight the layout of products inside a bin.

3.3 *Retrieval Travel Time Model*

Eq (1) gives expected retrieval-travel-time models that have been developed by Metahri and Hachemi [25].

$$E\left(T_g'\right) = \frac{1}{2\,V_c}L + \frac{2}{3}\sqrt{2H/g} \tag{1}$$

Where:

L, H the length and height of the rack
V_c the speed of the transport conveyor
g the acceleration due to gravity
$E\left(T_g'\right)$ the expected retrieval travel-time

4 Rack Dimensions Optimization

4.1 *Problem Statement*

The rack dimensions are a key of AS/RS performance improvement.

However, space constraints require that rack dimensions must not exceed the admissible values (L_A, H_A, D_A), the storage capacity is fixed into N storage segments, and the segment dimensions (l, h, d) are predefined. Consequently, there are several possible configurations to design this system (See Fig. 4), so what are the optimal rack-dimensions that lead to the minimum retrieval travel time? In order to solve this problem, we built an optimization model where the objective function to be minimized is the non-linear function of the retrieval travel time $E\left(T_g'\right)$.

To purchase this aim, we have developed a discrete optimization model which matches more accurately the real nature of the rack. Indeed, the enumeration technique is not practical because it leads to a combinatorial explosion, while a continuous model does not reflect the nature of the rack. In the continuous approach, approximating a solution to the nearest integer does not necessarily correspond to the optimal solution.

4.2 *Optimization Model Formulation*

Let us first introduce the following notations.

Parameters:

L_A, H_A, D_A the admissible length, height and depth of the rack
l, h, d the length, height and depth of a storage segment.

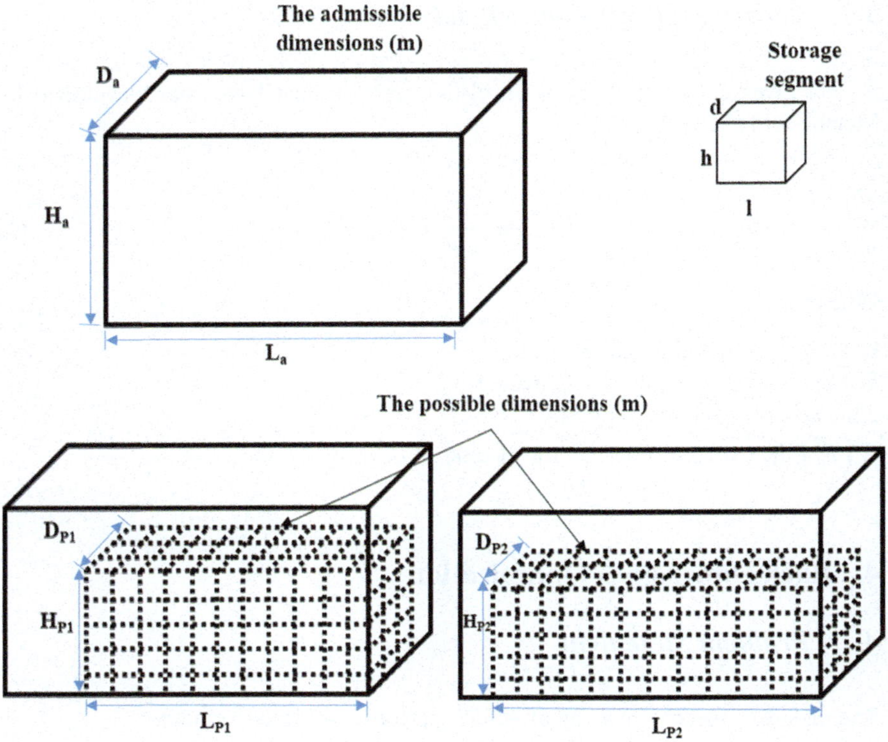

Fig. 4 Depiction of the admissible and possible rack dimensions

N_{LA}, N_{CA}, M_A the admissible number of bins per line, column and segments in each bin. Where: $N_{LA} = L_A/l$, $N_{CA} = H_A/h$, $M_A = D_A/d$.

V_c the speed of the transport conveyor

N the storage capacity (total number of bins)

N_A the admissible storage capacity

Variables:

m the number of bins per line

n the number of bins per column

q the number of segments in each bin

Recall that $E\left(T'_g\right) = \frac{1}{2\,V_c}L + \frac{2}{3}C\sqrt{H}$

$m = L/l$, $n = H/h$, $q = D/d$

So, the optimization problem can be formulated as follows:

$$\min \frac{1}{2\,V_c}m + \frac{2}{3}C\sqrt{n} \tag{2}$$

Subject to the following constraints:

$$m \leq N_{LA} \tag{3}$$

$$n \leq N_{CA} \tag{4}$$

$$q \leq M_A \tag{5}$$

$$m * n * q \geq N \tag{6}$$

$$m, n \text{ and } q \text{ are integer} \tag{7}$$

Where:

- The objective (2) minimizes the retrieval time,
- The constraints (3, 4 and 5) ensure that the dimensions of the rack are limited to the admissible values.
- The constraint (6) allows the rack storage capacity to be greater or equal to the admissible storage capacity.
- The constraint (7) ensures that decision variables are integers.

We propose a flow chart that effectively shows the different part of the discrete optimization model. As outlined in Fig. 5, the model evolves the following phases:

- Initialization of system parameters such as the storage capacity *N*, the admissible dimensions of the rack (L_A, H_A, D_A), the storage segment dimensions (*l*, *h*, *d*), and the transport conveyor velocity V_c.
- Determination of the resulted optimal dimensions of *m*, *n*, and *q* which are noted N_{Lo}, N_{Co}, M_o, respectively. Where: $N_{Lo} = L_o/l$, $N_{Co} = H_o/h$, $M_o = D_o/d$.

4.3 Optimization Results and Discussion

In order to show the effectiveness of the optimization method, we consider different configurations of industrial-sized problems with a storage capacity ranging from 400 to 27,000 segments. For each storage capacity, we assumed that the dimensions of storage segment are $(l, h, d) = (0.15; 0.10; 0.10)(m)$, and the transport conveyor velocity is: $V_C = 3m/s$.

Moreover, the optimization problem is solved using Generalized Reduced Gradient (GRG) solver, and executed on a PC with 2.17 GHz CPU and 2 GB RAM. In our study, we used the GRG solver because the optimized model is a discrete nonlinear problem.

To illustrate the optimization procedure, Table 1 presents the optimization results of 20 storage capacities. Columns 2, 3 and 4 of this table represent the studied storage capacity (*N*), the admissible dimensions (L_A, H_A, D_A) and the optimal

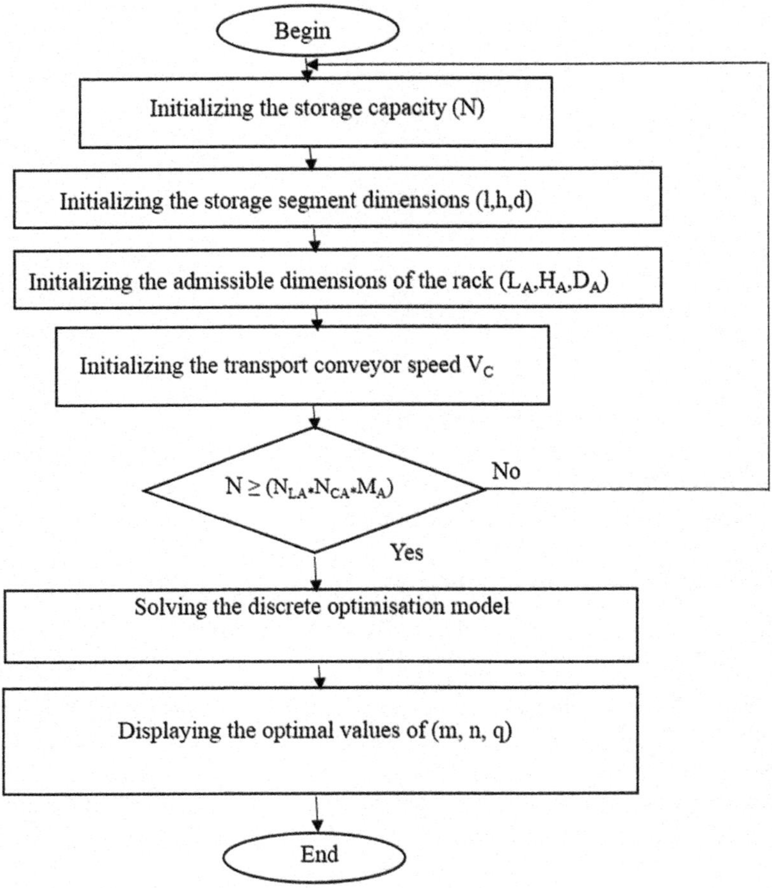

Fig. 5 Flow chart of the discrete optimization model

configuration (N_{Lo}, N_{Co}, M_o), respectively. While, Columns 5 and Column 6 represent the optimal dimensions (L_o, H_o, D_o) and their corresponding retrieval travel time $E\left(T'_g\right)$, respectively.

The analysis of the results allowed us to make the following insights:

- The optimal rack is not cubic-in-time (i.e. travel time along length, high, and depth are not equal).
- The optimization model tends generally to choose the maximum possible depth, and prevails rather the height to the length.
- The computing time is very short (few seconds).

Table 1 Optimal rack configuration for a different storage rack capacity

	N	The admissible dimensions (m)			The optimal configuration			The optimal dimensions (m)			$E\left(T_g'\right)$
		L_A	H_A	D_A	N_{Lo}	N_{Co}	M_o	L_O	H_O	D_O	
1	400	2	1	0.6	8	10	5	1.2	1	0.5	0.501016
2	500				10	10	5	1.5	1	0.5	0.551016
3	600				10	10	6	1.5	1	0.6	0.551016
4	900	4	1.5	0.8	10	15	6	1.5	1.5	0.6	0.618668
5	1000				20	10	5	3	1	0.5	0.801016
6	1200				10	15	8	1.5	1.5	0.8	0.618668
7	1400				20	10	7	3	1	0.7	0.801016
8	1800	6	2	1	9	20	10	1.35	2	1	0.650701
9	2000				10	20	10	1.5	2	1	0.675701
10	2500				25	10	10	3.75	1	1	0.926016
11	3000				15	20	10	2.25	2	1	0.800701
12	4000				20	20	10	3	2	1	0.925701
13	5000	8	2.5	1.2	20	25	10	3	2.5	1	0.975948
14	6000				20	25	12	3	2.5	1.2	0.975948
15	7000				28	25	10	4.2	2.5	1	1.175948
16	8000				32	25	10	4.8	2.5	1	1.275948
17	10,000	15	3	1.5	40	25	10	6	2.5	1	1.475948
18	21,000				50	28	15	7.5	2.8	1.5	1.753696
19	24,000				64	25	15	9.6	2.5	1.5	2.075948
20	27,000				60	30	15	9	3	1.5	2.021375

5 Conclusion

According to the fact that automated drug dispensing systems better meet the requirements of the PPP medicine, we are interested, in this paper, in the determination of the optimal configuration of an automated dispensing system based on a free-fall-flow-rack AS/RS. A useful way to do this is to determine the expression of the expected retrieval travel time and minimize it through an optimization model. We first presented an overview of the FF flow-rack AS/RS structure and then we presented its analytical retrieval time. Subsequently, we formulate this problem as a discrete nonlinear optimization model, which is solved by using Generalized Reduced Gradient (GRG) solver.

To show the power of the optimization method we applied the proposed model on different rack configurations under the constraints on the admissible dimensions and storage capacity. The results show that rack configuration has a significant effect on the expected retrieval time, and the optimal rack is not cubic-in-time (i.e. travel time along length, high, and depth are not equal). In addition, we find that the optimization model generally favors longer depth over the other two dimensions in retrieval time optimization. Note that the solving time for industrial sized rack configurations is very short (few seconds). This optimization method could be very useful for the AS/RS designer. Subsequently, according to numerical study the optimization model tends generally to choose the maximum possible depth then it prevails rather the height to the length. This optimization method could be used to give a decision support to the AS/RS designer.

In our future research, we will perform a comparison study in order to evaluate the gap between this approach and the continuous optimization approach, and investigate the optimal location of the drop-off station that minimize the retrieval travel time of the FF-flow-rack AS/RS.

References

1. Asef-Vaziri, A., Khoshnevis, B., Rahimi, M.: Design and analysis of an automated container handling system in seaports. Int. J. Agile Syst. Manag. **3**(1–2), 112–126 (2008)
2. Ashayeri, J., Gelders, L., Wassenhove, L.V.: A microcomputer-based optimization model for the design of automated warehouses. Int. J. Prod. Res. **23**(4), 825–839 (1985)
3. Asokan, P., Jerald, J., Arunachalam, S., Page, T.: Application of adaptive genetic algorithm and particle swarm optimisation in scheduling of jobs and AS/RS in FMS. Int. J. Manuf. Res. **3**(4), 393–405 (2008)
4. Bessenouci, H.N., Sari, Z., Ghomri, L.: Metaheuristic based control of a flow rack automated storage retrieval system. J. Intell. Manuf. **23**(4), 1157–1166 (2012)
5. Bozer, Y.A., White, J.A.: Travel-time models for automated storage/retrieval systems. IIE Trans. **16**(4), 329–338 (1984)
6. Caputo, A.C., Pelagagge, P.M.: Capacity upgrade criteria of large-intensive material handling and storage systems: a case study. J. Manuf. Technol. Manag. **19**(8), 953–978 (2008)
7. Chen, Z., Li, X., Gupta, J.N.: A bi-directional flow-rack automated storage and retrieval system for unit-load warehouses. Int. J. Prod. Res. **53**(14), 4176–4188 (2015)

8. Chung, E., Lee, H.F.: A generalised sequencing problem for unit-load automated storage and retrieval systems. Int. J. Ind. Syst. Eng. **2**(4), 393–412 (2007)
9. Dallari, F., Marchet, G., Ruggeri, R.: Optimisation of man-on-board automated storage/retrieval systems. Integr. Manuf. Syst. **11**(2), 87–93 (2000)
10. De Koster, R.M.B., Le-Duc, T., Yugang, Y.: Optimal storage rack design for a 3-dimensional compact AS/RS. Int. J. Prod. Res. **46**(6), 1495–1514 (2008)
11. Fohn, S.M., Greef, A.R., Young, R.E., O'Grady, P.J.: A constraint-system shell to support concurrent engineering approaches to design. Artif. Intell. Eng. **9**(1), 1–17 (1994)
12. Golubnitschaja, O., Baban, B., Boniolo, G., Wang, W., Bubnov, R., Kapalla, M., et al.: Medicine in the early twenty-first century: paradigm and anticipation-EPMA position paper 2016. EPMA J. **7**(1), 23 (2016)
13. Hachemi, K., & Alla, H. (2008). Pilotage dynamique d'un système automatisé de stockage/déstockage à convoyeur gravitationnel. J. Eur. Syst. Automatisés (JESA), 42(5/2008), 487–508
14. Hachemi, K., Besombes, B.: Integration of products expiry dates in optimal scheduling of storage/retrieval operations for a flow-rack AS/RS. Int. J. Ind. Syst. Eng. **15**(2), 216–233 (2013)
15. Hamzaoui, M.A., Sari, Z.: Optimal dimensions minimizing expected travel time of a single machine flow rack AS/RS. Mechatronics. **31**, 158–168 (2015)
16. Kota, V.R., Taylor, D., Gue, K.R.: Retrieval time performance in puzzle-based storage systems. J. Manuf. Technol. Manag. **26**(4), 582–602 (2015)
17. Kuo, P.H., Krishnamurthy, A., Malmborg, C.J.: Design models for unit load storage and retrieval systems using autonomous vehicle technology and resource conserving storage and dwell point policies. Appl. Math. Model. **31**(10), 2332–2346 (2007)
18. Kuo, P.H., Krishnamurthy, A., Malmborg, C.J.: Performance modelling of autonomous vehicle storage and retrieval systems using class-based storage policies. Int. J. Comput. Appl. Technol. **31**(3–4), 238–248 (2008)
19. Lättilä, L., Saranen, J., Hilmola, O.P.: Decision support system for AS/RS investments: real benefits out of Monte Carlo simulation. Int. J. Technol. Intell. Plan. **9**(2), 108–125 (2013)
20. Malmborg, C.J.: Interleaving models for the analysis of twin shuttle automated storage and retrieval systems. Int. J. Prod. Res. **38**(18), 4599–4610 (2000)
21. Mathisen, K.: From traditional stacks to an automated storage and retrieval system. Libr. Manag. **26**(1/2), 97–101 (2005)
22. Meghelli-Gaouar, N., Sari, Z.: Assessment of performance of a class-based storage in a flow-rack AS/RS. J. Stud. Manuf. **1**(2–3), 100–107 (2010)
23. MEKAPHARM: C. Fiche caractristiques de l'automate APOTEKA (2016). http://mekapharm.com/apoteka/.1999. Accessed 22 Oct 2016
24. Meneghetti, A., Borgo, E.D., Monti, L.: Decision support optimisation models for design of sustainable automated warehouses. Int. J. Shipp. Transport. Logist. **7**(3), 266–294 (2015)
25. Metahri, D., Hachemi, K.: Retrieval–travel-time model for free-fall-flow-rack automated storage and retrieval system. J. Ind. Eng. Int. **14**(4), 807–820 (2018)
26. Robert Terry, W., RAO, H.G., SON, J.Y.: Application of a computer-based approach to designing real-time control software for an integrated robotic assembly and automated storage/retrieval system. Int. J. Prod. Res. **26**(10), 1593–1604 (1988)
27. Sari, Z., Bessnouci, N. H.: Design & modeling of a single machine flow rack AS. RS, proceeding of IMHRC2012, Gardanne, France (2012)
28. Sari, Z., Saygin, C., Ghouali, N.: Travel-time models for flow-rack automated storage and retrieval systems. Int. J. Adv. Manuf. Technol. **25**(9), 979–987 (2005)
29. Sari, Z., Grasman, S.E., Ghouali, N.: Impact of pickup/delivery stations and restoring conveyor locations on retrieval time models of flow-rack automated storage and retrieval systems. Prod. Plan. Control. **18**(2), 105–116 (2007)
30. Van Den Berg, J.P., Gademann, A.J.R.M.: Simulation study of an automated storage/retrieval system. Int. J. Prod. Res. **38**(6), 1339–1356 (2000)

31. Yang, P., Miao, L., Xue, Z., Qin, L.: Optimal storage rack design for a multi-deep compact AS/RS considering the acceleration/deceleration of the storage and retrieval machine. Int. J. Prod. Res. **53**(3), 929–943 (2015)
32. Yang, P., Yang, K., Qi, M., Miao, L., Ye, B.: Designing the optimal multi-deep AS/RS storage rack under full turnover-based storage policy based on non-approximate speed model of S/R machine. Transport. Res. Part E Logist. Transport. Rev. **104**, 113–130 (2017)

Intuitive and Intelligent Solutions for Elderly Care

Neja Samar Brenčič, Marius Dragoi, Irina Mocanu, and Tomasz Winiarski

1 Introduction

Vast demand for some particular, advanced and seamless solutions is spurring from current demographic realities, aging population, and burden of chronic diseases. Changing life-style related illnesses, increased demands of people for new, more sophisticated therapeutic and care methods are stretching the limits of innovations, specifically for the respected field considered in this article, the increase of symp-

This work was supported by a grant of the Romanian National Authority for Scientific Research and Innovation, the AAL Program with co-funding from the Horizon 2020 program projects "IONIS – Improving the quality of life of people with dementia and disabled persons" – AAL2017-AAL-2016-074-IONIS-1 and AAL-2016-074-IONIS-2 and – INCARE – Integrated Solution for Innovative Elderly Care", project number AAL-2017-059-INCARE, by the Slovenia Ministry of Public Administration and by the subsidiary contract "CoRSAr" no. 1226/22.01.2018 for the grant 53/05.09.2016, ID 40270, cod MySMIS: 105976.

N. S. Brenčič (✉)
IZRIIS Institute, Ljubljana, Slovenia
e-mail: neja.samar-brencic@izriis.si

M. Dragoi
IT Center for Science and Technology, Bucharest, Romania

I. Mocanu
Computer Science Department, University Politehnica of Bucharest, Bucharest, Romania
e-mail: irina.mocanu@upb.ro

T. Winiarski
Institute of Control and Computation Engineering, Warsaw University of Technology, Warszawa, Poland
e-mail: tomasz.winiarski@pw.edu.pl

L. Chaari (ed.), *Digital Health in Focus of Predictive, Preventive and Personalised Medicine*, Advances in Predictive, Preventive and Personalised Medicine 12,
https://doi.org/10.1007/978-3-030-49815-3_12

toms and consequences related to older age, (like Alzheimer's disease, Dementia and Cognitive impairment). The European Commission in light of the challenge that also concerns stakeholders worldwide is encouraging many streams of endeavors. One of them being innovation in introducing solutions based on new models of services and state-of-the-art technology. Health services and home care services at a distance are the future for the aging population in many countries of the world. They present the possibility for building a sustainable health care system and contribution to a better life for older adults.

In this context, the current work is focusing on two Active and Assisted Living (AAL) projects which are developing information and communications technology (ICT) based platforms to support elderly persons and their caregivers. Both AAL IONIS [12] and AAL INCARE [11] projects originate from the very successful NITICS project [13, 17, 18]. In addition, contributions from the CoRSAr project (Platforma de Programare si Configurare a Robotilor Sociali si Asistivi) which is focusing on robotic based functionalities are also included in this research. IONIS exploits the innovation in NITICS and extends the platform with new technologies and upgraded services dedicated to persons suffering from mild cognitive impairment or incipient dementia and to their caregivers. It offers a fully integrated and validated solution at an affordable cost and with a high degree of personalization. IONIS is developed by exploiting location based services, sleep quality monitoring, communication services and the NITICS functionalities in order to offer continuous support at home (indoor area) and outside (outdoor area). A user-centered design involves extensive trials and piloting employed to both develop and validate the IONIS solution. The INCARE platform is extending NITICS with robotic features following a similar path as the CoRSAr project which can offer active support to the end-users, as exemplified further in this work. All presented projects implement functionalities specific for predictive (health, mobility and sleep patterns), preventive (medication compliance, hazard detection and enhanced activity) and personalized (e.g. robotic platforms).

2 Results and Discussions

2.1 End-User Involvement

A user-centered design was implemented in both IONIS and INCARE by involving elderly and caregivers during the whole development process. User input was also gathered in CoRSAr focusing on the perception of robotic platfomrs. Some important findings of the IONIS multinational survey and conjoint analysis are presented next.

A multinational survey The survey was carried out in four countries: Hungary, Poland, Romania and Slovenia. A total number of 121 primary (elderly) and 103 secondary (caregivers) users filled the dedicated questionnaires. The primary users

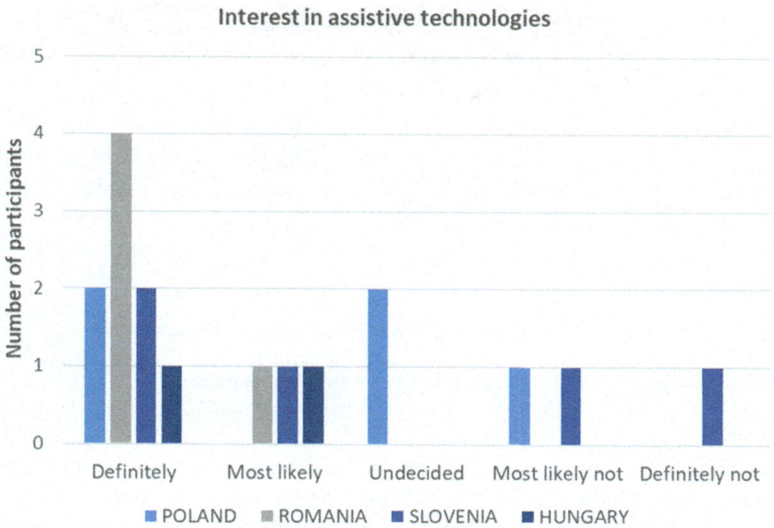

Fig. 1 Interest in using Assistive Technologies among the survey participants

were selected based on their score in the Mini-Mental State Examination (MMSE) test, the eligibility criterion being the presence of mild cognitive impairment or mild dementia signs (MMSE score 19–27 points).

The questionnaires focused on data useful for services design, implementation and testing, such as the living conditions, caregiving status and technology experience. Additional data covered the socialization activities of the primary users, their health status and acceptance [15] of the proposed IONIS services and their financial costs, memory impairment, sleep problems and independence in everyday tasks performed home and outdoors. The processed data was exploited in order to elaborate the Persona Cards and to generate reliable and realistic representations of potential elderly users. The survey results have shown that, although the primary users are generally not acquainted with the ICT solutions, the majority of them perceives the proposed services as useful (see Fig. 1). Most of the participants (70%) would definitely or most likely use Assistive Technology to help them in the activities of daily living. 15% of participants are not interested in Assistive Technologies and would most likely or definitely not use it. About 53% of included participants would definitely use Assistive Technology, 17.6% would most likely use it, about 16% of included participants would most likely or definitely not use it and 11.8% are undecided.

Conjoint analysis The goal of performing a conjoint analysis was to order the users' preferences towards the IONIS functionalities and their possible implementation. A thorough conjoint user preference analysis was designed and implemented at this stage involving 61 total end-users (representing assisted persons and caregivers) from the same four end-user countries. Elderly and their informal caregivers expressed almost similar preferences, with a very small difference for the reminders

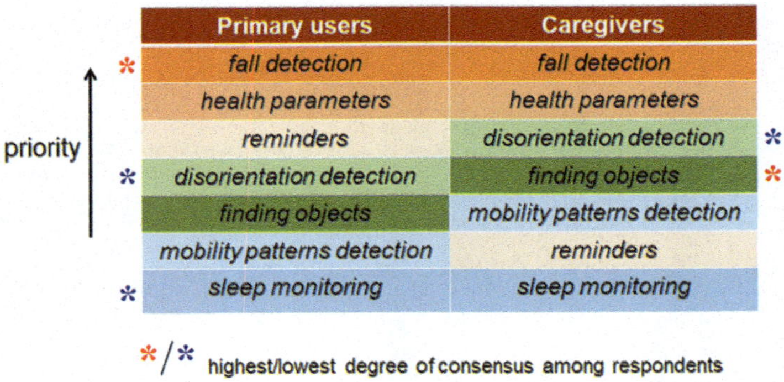

Fig. 2 End-user preferences for the identified services/functionalities

functionality. This scored much higher (3rd) for the elderly than for the caregivers (5th), trumping both the disorientation detection and finding objects (see Fig. 2). The main conclusion regarding the reminders functionality is that both the elderly and the caregivers appraised the email alternative as the least useful with almost the same levels of consensus. Also, both groups valued visual messages with approximately the same 'strength', but the persons in need found the voice messages as being the most useful.

2.2 *Novel ICT Approaches in IONIS and INCARE*

Both IONIS and INCARE projects follow an intelligent and innovative approach regarding the technologies considered in their integration. Particularly, INCARE aims to integrate robotic platforms as service robots. Additionally, distributed AI approaches are considered for privacy compliance purposes. In this section, we present an overview the end-user needs identified in elderly-robot interaction experiments, a laboratory environment example to be tested within INCARE and recent trends in federated learning.

Elderly-robot interaction For a successful integration in elderly care environments, robots must be carefully designed such that their appearance and functionality match the needs and expectations of both elderly and caregivers [8, 16]. The human necessities and reception of robots within an elderly care environment are usually identified through the use of questionnaires, focus groups and live sessions. The quality evaluation of human-robot interaction in the context of elderly care is focused on the quality of life impact for the caregivers and caretakers [8], but also on psychological and behavioral effects on the elderly, such as decreases in their level of stress and loneliness and improvements in their predisposition to engage in communication activities and overall mood [4]. A review on the robot acceptance identifies age, gender, experience with technology and cultural background as human factors, while appearance, human resemblance and dimensions, gender and personality are the robot characteristics of high importance [3]. Concern is also directed towards personal data confidentiality and the assessment of the risks and benefits [1]. According to multiple studies, robots resembling human beings usually receive a negative feedback, the robots with a more machine-like appearance being preferred [1, 3, 16, 24].

In general, the preexisting attitudes towards robots proved to be a major factor in their acceptance [20]. In [2], the previous perception of robots and the quality of experience in a setup examining the feelings of the patients during blood pressure and heart rate readings performed by a robot assistant and by a medical student showed a high correlation. The patients were able to identify multiple benefits of the healthcare robots, such as workload balancing for the caregivers, daily routine scheduling and compensating for staff shortages, indicating that low human comfort around robots due to lack of exposure might be a principal negative factor in their acceptance. Several areas of improvement for elderly-robot interaction include empathy emulation, behavior adaptability [21] and unpredictability, as the capacity to generate actions that are not necessarily reactions to user input [10].

Scenario in laboratory environment Various scenarios are intended to be tested within INCARE and CoRSAr, where a robot interacts with elderly and their formal and informal caregivers. The development of cloud services [6] and map creation methods [22] substantially support the effectiveness of not only robot navigation, but also both speech recognition and speech synthesis. Hence, this type of communication was chosen for being both effective and intuitive.

The first scenario covers the need for delivery of small items (e.g. drinks) ordered by the elderly, where the robot substitutes the staff of e.g. elderly facility and the staff can concentrate on more complicated activities. It is assumed that the older person stays in one room, while the staff operates in the other room – i.e. kitchen. The robot will perform its delivery task while also detecting hazards [5, 7] and informing about them. The robot considered for the scenarios is the TIAGo [14, 23] by PAL robotics. The scenario consists of the following, subsequent steps: (1) An elderly person calls for a robot; (2) The robot approaches the elderly person; (3) The robot asks for orders; (4) The elderly person requests for a drink, e.g. tea; (5) The robot confirms an order; (6) The robot goes to the kitchen; (7) The robot approaches the staff in the kitchen and asks for the particular drink to be put on it; (8) The staff confirms that the delivery is ready and placed on the robot; (9) The robot informs that it starts to go back to deliver the order; (10) The robot approaches the elderly person and informs that it has the delivery; (11) The robot asks the elderly person to take the drink; (12) The older person takes the drink and confirms the action.

Federated learning in AI In the past few years, machine learning has led to major breakthroughs in various areas, such as computer vision. Much of this success has been based on collecting huge amounts of data. Machine learning applications need to collect data that are privacy-invasive.

Federated Learning is a distributed form of machine learning approach where the training process is distributed among many users using a training data set composed of decentralized data. A server has the role of coordinating everything and most of the work is performed by each device. Steps involved in the federated learning are: (1) the server initializes the model and each device/client downloads the global model; (2) the model is updated using its own data; (3) each personalised trained model is sent to the server; (4) on the server a federated average function is used to generate a much improved version of the model than the previous one; and (5) the improved version is sent to all the devices.

Federated learning looks similar with distributed machine learning on a technical level. But there are some major differences: (1) huge number of clients; (2) learning data for each user is obtained from different distribution – two similar users might have similar training data, but two randomly users can obtain totally different data; (3) unbalanced number of examples per device and (4) slow and unstable communication.

In 2018, Intel began a collaboration with the Center for Biomedical Image Computing and Analytics at the University of Pennsylvania showing the first proof concept for federated learning applied for real medical images used for semantic segmentation of brain tumors from images. The study demonstrated training of a convolutional neural network (U-Net model) using federated learning with an accuracy of 99% as the same model trained with the traditional methods [19]. Paper [9] uses electronic medical records together with federated learning to predict disease incidence, patient response to treatment, and other healthcare events. A community-based federated machine learning method was proposed. The method clusters patients into similar clinically communities that has similar diagnoses and geographical locations, learning one model for each community. Also, the learning process keeps data locally at hospitals. Evaluation was performed on 50 hospitals, each with 560 patients. Results show that the proposed method outperforms the baseline federated machine learning method.

3 Conclusions

Many professional teams, companies, policy makers and individuals are working in the field of the challenges posed by AAL. All efforts are necessary to make worthwhile changes providing technological and procedural solutions and to bring them closer to the end-users. Understanding their needs and experiences and enhancing the acceptance of solutions being developed are crucial to make AAL solutions widely and fairly available and bring about significant structural change. For this purpose, the presented projects offer predictive, preventive and personalized support through their design and implemented functionalities.

References

1. Broadbent, E., Jayawardena, C., Kerse, N., Stafford, R.Q., MacDonald, B.A.: Human-robot interaction research to improve quality of life in elder care – an approach and issues. In: Workshops at the Twenty-Fifth AAAI Conference on Artificial Intelligence (2011)

2. Broadbent, E., Kuo, I.H., Lee, Y.I., Rabindran, J., Kerse, N., Stafford, R., MacDonald, B.A.: Attitudes and reactions to a healthcare robot. Telemed. e-Health **16**(5), 608–613 (2010)
3. Broadbent, E., Stafford, R., MacDonald, B.: Acceptance of healthcare robots for the older population: review and future directions. Int. J. Soc. Robot. **1**(4), 319 (2009)
4. Broekens, J., Heerink, M., Rosendal, H., et al.: Assistive social robots in elderly care: a review. Gerontechnology **8**(2), 94–103 (2009)
5. Dudek, W., Banachowicz, K., Szynkiewicz, W., Winiarski, T.: Distributed nao robot navigation system in the hazard detection application. In: 2016 21st International Conference on Methods and Models in Automation and Robotics (MMAR), pp. 942–947. IEEE (2016)
6. Dudek, W., Szynkiewicz, W., Winiarski, T.: Cloud computing support for the multi-agent robot navigation system. J. Autom. Mob. Robot. Intell. Syst. **11**, 67–74 (2017)
7. Dudek, W., Wegierek, M., Karwowski, J., Szynkiewicz, W., Winiarski, T.: Task harmonisation for a single–task robot controller. In: Kozłowski, K. (ed.) 12th International Workshop on Robot Motion and Control, pp. 86–91. IEEE (2019)
8. Feil-Seifer, D., Skinner, K., Matarić, M.J.: Benchmarks for evaluating socially assistive robotics. Interact. Stud. **8**(3), 423–439 (2007)
9. Huang, L., Shea, A.L., Qian, H., Masurkar, A., Deng, H., Liu, D.: Patient clustering improves efficiency of federated machine learning to predict mortality and hospital stay time using distributed electronic medical records. J. Biomed. Inform. **99**, 103291 (2019)
10. Hutson, S., Lim, S.L., Bentley, P.J., Bianchi-Berthouze, N., Bowling, A.: Investigating the suitability of social robots for the wellbeing of the elderly. In: International Conference on Affective Computing and Intelligent Interaction, pp. 578–587. Springer (2011)
11. Integrated solution for innovative elderly care (INCARE). http://www.aal-europe.eu/projects/incare/
12. Indoor and outdoor niticsplus solution for dementia challenges (IONIS). http://www.aal-europe.eu/projects/ionis/
13. Networked infrastructure for innovative home care solutions (NITICS). http://www.aal-europe.eu/projects/nitics/
14. Pages, J., Marchionni, L., Ferro, F.: Tiago: the modular robot that adapts to different research needs. In: International Workshop on Robot Modularity (2016)
15. Paraciani, N., Tabozzi, S., Di Pasquale, D., Padula, M., Biocca, L., Lafortuna, C., Maiuri, F., Rudel, D., Fisk, M.: The telescope code. quality standards for telehealth practice across Europe. In: 2017 E-Health and Bioengineering Conference (EHB), pp. 297–300. IEEE (2017)
16. Pino, M., Boulay, M., Jouen, F., Rigaud, A.S.: "Are we ready for robots that care for us?" Attitudes and opinions of older adults toward socially assistive robots. Front. Aging Neurosci. **7**, 141 (2015)
17. Samar-Brencic, N.: Service requirements for supporting daily activities of elderly people living at home – multi-national survey within aal project nitics. In: Information Society IS 2014, Proceedings of the 17th International Multiconference. IJS, Ljubljana (2014)
18. Samar-Brencic, N.: System elements integration and field trial report for AAL project nitics slovenia. In: Proceedings of the 18th International Multiconference. IJS: Ljubljana (2015)
19. Sheller, M.J., Reina, G.A., Edwards, B., Martin, J., Bakas, S.: Multi-institutional deep learning modeling without sharing patient data: a feasibility study on brain tumor segmentation. In: International MICCAI Brainlesion Workshop, pp. 92–104. Springer (2018)
20. Stafford, R., Broadbent, E., Jayawardena, C., Unger, U., Kuo, I.H., Igic, A., Wong, R., Kerse, N., Watson, C., MacDonald, B.A.: Improved robot attitudes and emotions at a retirement home after meeting a robot. In: 19th International Symposium in Robot and Human Interactive Communication, pp. 82–87. IEEE (2010)
21. Tapus, A., Maja, M., Scassellatti, B.: The grand challenges in socially assistive robotics. IEEE Robot. Autom. Mag. **14**(1), 35–42 (2007)
22. Wilkowski, A., Kornuta, T., Stefańczyk, M., Kasprzak, W.: Efficient generation of 3D surfel maps using RGB–D sensors. Int. J. Appl. Math. Comput. Sci. **26**(1), 99–122 (2016)

23. Winiarski, T., Dudek, W., Stefańczyk, M., Zieliński, Ł., Giełdowski, D., Seredyński, D.: An intent-based approach for creating assistive robots' control systems. arXiv preprint arXiv:2005.12106 (2020). http://arxiv.org/abs/2005.12106
24. Wu, Y.H., Fassert, C., Rigaud, A.S.: Designing robots for the elderly: appearance issue and beyond. Arch. Gerontol. Geriatr. **54**(1), 121–126 (2012)

Interactive Data Visualization for eHealth Retrieval System

Nesrine Ksentini, Mohamed Tmar, and Faïez Gargouri

1 Introduction

Data visualization represents the effective presentation of information and involves a multidisciplinary communication approach. Its goal is to communicate a specific message to a user. Indeed, a visual representation of data has a main goal to communicate quantitative and qualitative information clearly and effectively through graphical means which can be static, animated or interactive [1, 2].

Selecting a color schema in data visualization process is also very important. It allows the designer to set the tone of these visualizations and try to keep a consistent representation [1].

Data visualization has been used to tackle several challenges in many disciplines such as economics, medicine, and education. As eHealth is an actual topic for today and extremely important to all practitioners, we highlight in this paper the importance of data visualization in this area. In fact, many opportunities have received attention to date for supporting people to make health document sense and for supporting them in better understanding their own illnesses and their health conditions to manage them more effectively [3, 4].

Indeed, clinical-researchers are confronted today with a huge and complex patient records based on which they must study them to make sure quality control, and discover new diseases [5].

The same applies to people as they are becoming more aware of for their own health. They need to understand their own diagnostics to improve and manage their health and to better communicate with their doctors.

N. Ksentini · M. Tmar (✉) · F. Gargouri
MIRACL Laboratory, City ons Sfax, University of Sfax, Sfax, Tunisia
e-mail: mohamed.tmar@isimsf.rnu.tn; mohamed.tmar@isims.usf.tn; faiez.gargouri@isims.usf.tn

L. Chaari (ed.), *Digital Health in Focus of Predictive, Preventive and Personalised Medicine*, Advances in Predictive, Preventive and Personalised Medicine 12,
https://doi.org/10.1007/978-3-030-49815-3_13

The body of this paper will be as follows, we start with Sect. 2 to highlight earlier works related to data visualization. The Sect. 3 sheds light on our proposed data visualization system based on LSM (Least Squares Method) which is a statistical method arisen in machine learning to find semantic relationships between a set of terms and not only between a pair of terms. The Sect. 4 gives the obtained results followed by conclusions and future works.

2 Medical Visualization Systems

In this section, we review the state of the art of data visualization systems to support users (patients and clinical researchers for example) to understand personal health information. In eHealth topic, data or information visualization is part of an overall visualization field that incorporates both information and scientific visualization, which are defined in the literature separately and considered as different [3].

Scientific visualizations represent scientific concepts such as molecules, parts of the human body, or natural phenomena, mainly in 3D [6]. The goal of these visualizations is essentially the confirmation or rejection of a particular hypothesis. Information visualization is a visualization tool to represent abstract concepts or terms. Author in [7] classifies this kind of visualization as exploratory analysis visualizations, due to their goal, help user's to find a hypothesis. The power of this tool derives from its ability to represent a large information at once, including internal relations.

In our case, we focus on information visualization and through the literature review, we can find several main researches in medical field, which investigate this kind of visualization [3].

In [8] authors proposed $AsbruView$ tool, a visualization tool developed to assist in handling treatment plans in Asbru. $AsbruView$ relies on a graphical metaphor where plans are represented as a running track which the physician 'runs' along while treating the patient [3].

$LifeLines$ proposed by [9] was one of the first tools to be used for the electronic health records representation. It was originally developed as a general-purpose visualization tool to represent personal histories that was then applied for the visualization of patient records. Our aim in this paper, is to develop a visualization tool, integrated in content based retrieval system, that presents semantic relationships between medical terms appeared in patient records and not to present only patient records data. The goal is to help users to make sense of returned documents when they use content based retrieval systems and search their needs.

3 Proposed System

In this section, we present our proposed content based retrieval system that incorporates two main steps. The first step is based on a local automatic documents-analysis to define semantic relationships between query terms and terms of the top *m* returned documents deemed relevant. The second step illustrates how to visualize these relations in a graph to help users making sense of the returned documents. The process of our search system is illustrated in (Fig. 1)

3.1 *Semantic Relationships*

Measuring similarity and semantic relationships between terms in a set of documents has become a primary task and plays an important role in the natural language processing (NLP) field in order to improve and to interpret search results [10]. It is the backbone of several applications, such as query expansion, disambiguation, automatic creation of thesaurus [11].

Previous approaches that study this latter idea, can be classified into three main categories [12–14]: those based on semantic knowledge (such as ontologies, data dictionaries), those based on content-based methods documents using general statistical methods [15, 16], and hybrid approaches that combine the earlier two categories.

In our case, we will adopt statistical methods to define semantic relationships between documents terms. The choice to adopt this type of method is justified first, by the independence of this process to the used language and secondly, by its ability

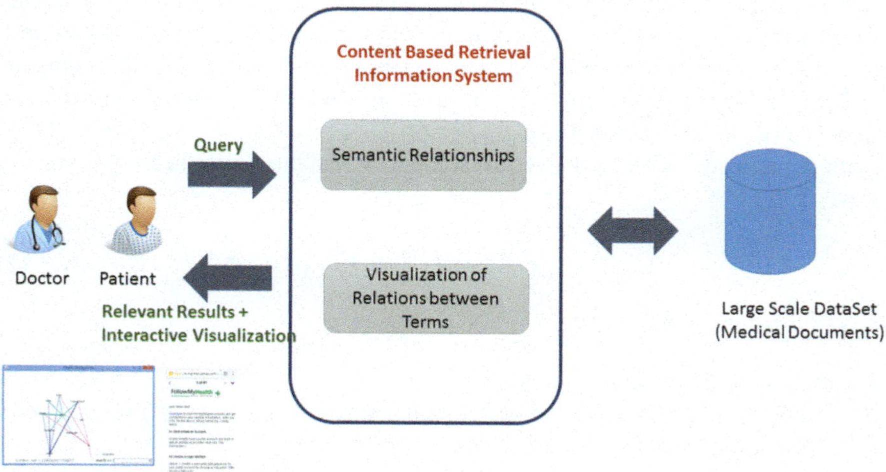

Fig. 1 Proposed content based retrieval system

to define these relations between a set of terms and not only between a pair of terms. We will apply Least Squares Method (LSM) for text analysis [17, 18] which is a method often used to define approximately relationships that may exist between many variables [17, 19–22]. Indeed, this method, known as linear regression, is the most widely used predictive model in the field of machine learning which present a particular approach to artificial intelligence [23].

Indeed, machine learning is a data analysis method which automates analytical model building process. The main idea of this method is to create algorithms that can receive input data and use statistical analysis to predict an output value.

It is an approach of artificial intelligence based on the idea that systems can learn from data and make decisions with little user intervention.

LSM tries to find the connection that may exist between an explained variable (y) and explanatory variables (x). In our case, we take a $term_j$ as an explained variable and the remaining terms in a set of documents as explanatory variables ($term_{1 \ldots n}$). The goal is to find the relation between these variables as follows:

$$term_j \approx \sum_{i=1}^{j-1}(\alpha_i term_i) + \sum_{i=j+1}^{n}(\alpha_i term_i) + \epsilon \tag{1}$$

where α represent the real coefficients of the regression model and the weights of relationships between terms. ϵ represents is the associated error.

Explanatory variables are defined from the top m returned documents that meet user's needs. As a result, for each variable which is a term in our case, we will have m measures that represent the $tf-idf$ weights. To minimize calculation complexity, we study as explained variables $term_j$ only the distinctive terms of the user's query (The process of this step is illustrated by Fig. 2).

For example, when a user sends a query with three terms (t_i,t_k,t_l), our content based retrieval system retrieves the top m returned documents which will be treated with a matrix representation. Indeed, we obtain ($terms \times documents$) matrix with ($n * m$) size where n presents the number of terms in the set of returned documents.

For each query term, if it exists in the terms set of returned documents, we calculate then its relationship weight vector $A_{term_j} = (\alpha_1, \cdots, \alpha_n)$ with other n terms. Least Squares Method gives the solution to find this vector in an approximate way:

$$A_{term_j} = (X^{jT} \times X^j)^{-1} \times X^T[., j] \times T_j \tag{2}$$

Where:

T represent TF-IDF weight vector of $term_j$.
X present the TF-IDF matrix whose columns represent the keyword set and rows represent the m returned documents.
X^j is obtained by removing the column of the term t_j in matrix X.
$X^T[j, .]$ represents the transpose of the weight vector of the term t_j in all documents.

Fig. 2 Process of defining semantic relationships

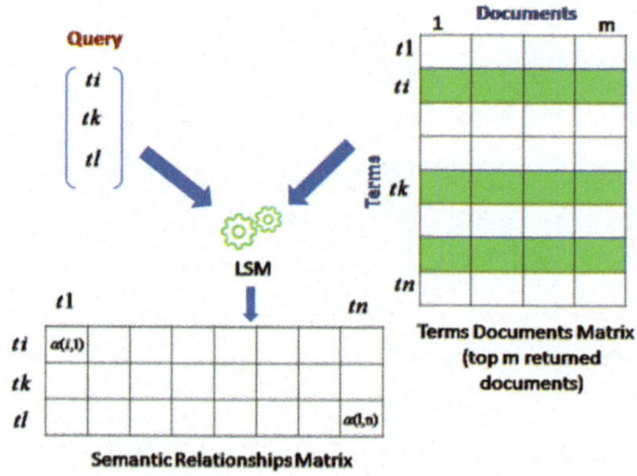

At the end of this process, we obtain terms by terms matrix (see Fig. 2) (Query-terms × terms of top m returned documents matrix) which contains the relation values founded for each query term with the remainder terms.

Once the relations are defined, we study them in order to design the graph of semantic relations with the most related terms (for example terms that have positive relations with query terms).

3.2 *Data Visualization*

Semantic relationships defined in the previous section does not make it possible to interpret the similarity between the terms in an easy way. It is thus preferable to have a comprehensive view of these semantic relationships in order to better assimilate them.

As visualization plays a very important part in the results interpretation, we propose to visualize the defined relations in a graph which will be generated after the search process for each user's query.

The generated visual graph comprises a set of nodes and a set of edges representing respectively terms and semantic relationships between these terms. We have decided to color semantic relationships defined for each query term by a different color because visual sweeping of colors takes less time and effort.

To enhance the importance of defined relations, we have modified the color intensity and the thickness of arcs which will be proportional to the similarity value. Indeed, if the defined relationship between two terms is strong, the arc becomes thicker. In order to help users interpret results, we have used the research option of the tool Prefuse[1] which makes it possible for users to easily find a term searched in the whole graph (for example term *coronari* in Fig. 3).

[1] http://prefuse.org

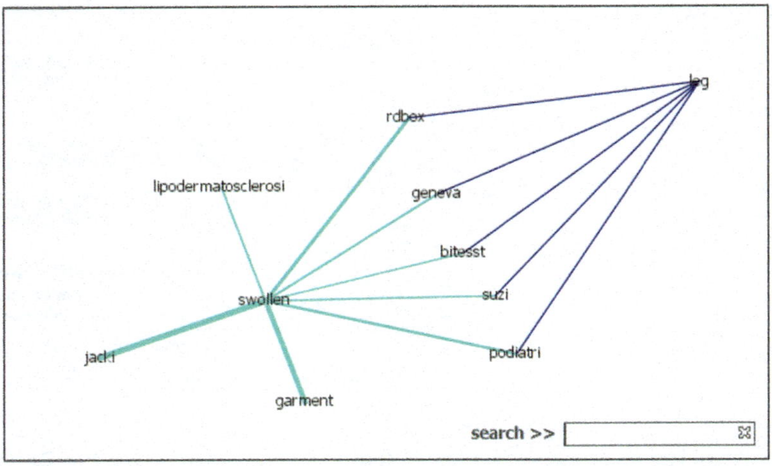

Fig. 3 Graph of Semantic Relationships: query 53 in 2015

4 Results

In order to check the performance of our proposed method, an experimental procedure was set up. This evaluation is performed on a large collection of documents provided from the CLEF company for the two successive years 2014 and 2015 [24–27].

4.1 Document Collection

The document collection is composed of a set of medical documents covering a wide set of medical topics. This collection is around of one million documents provided by the Khresmoi project [24–27] which come from different online sources such as known databases and medical sites (e.g. ClinicalTrial.gov, Genetics Home Reference, the health certified websites).

The test set in 2014 comprises 50 professional and medical queries provided by experts (clinical-researchers for example). These queries present different cases of patient diseases. In 2015, test set has 67 circumlocutory queries provided by patients when they are faced with symptoms and signs of a medical condition.

Table 1 Semantic relationships examples

Base	Query number	Some terms in relation with the query
clef2015	34	**Caviti problem** tooth cari dentistri fluoridepr dentahealth gum
clef2015	53	**Swollen leg** swell clot podiatri garment suzi lipodermatosclerosi
clef2014	1	**Coronari arteri disease** mean myocardi bypass angiograph aortic charlson cholesterol heart-attack translesion revascularis anastomos
clef2014	35	**Peptic ulcer disease** antacid food diagnos recommend gastric oesophag

4.2 LSM Results

Table 1 shows the results of defined semantic relationships for some queries. Terms that are written in bold font represent the original query terms, the other terms represent the most related terms to the original query in their root form. We notice that selected terms usually express the same context of the original query which proves the effectiveness of our proposed method.

For example we take query number 53 in 2015 and we explain some related terms like:

- podiatri: a podiatrist is a health professional who diagnoses and treats disorders of the feet.
- garment: is a pneumatic antishock garment an inflatable garment used to combat shock, stabilize fractures, promote hemostasis and increase peripheral vascular resistance.
- suzi: Extra Roomy Shoes that are cleverly designed to look slim-line but have lots of room for swollen feet.
- lipodermatosclerosi: is a skin and connective tissue disease.

Another example query 35 in 2014, related terms are in strong relation with the original query which talk about peptic ulcer. It is a disease that has long been considered chronic, defined anatomically by a loss of parietal substance not exceeding the submucosa.

4.3 Interactive Data Visualization

Interactive data visualization plays an important role in making sense process. This importance grows when we talk about the eHealth field that is a current topic that draws attention of any person which is today more aware of and take greater responsibility for his health.

The above figures show the illustrations of semantic relationships defined by the statistical method LSM. Each illustration is, as already mentioned, presented as a graph whose nodes represent the terms and the arcs represent relations between these terms.

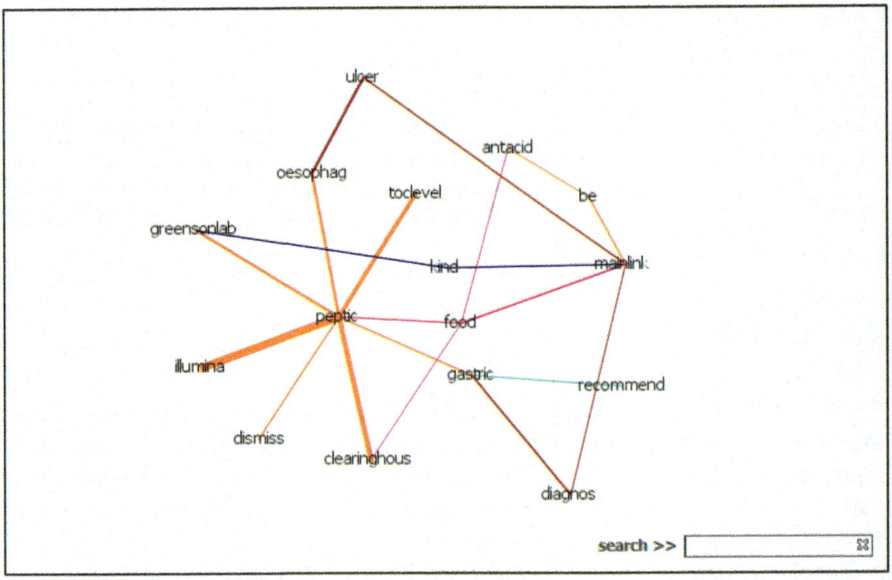

Fig. 4 Graph of Semantic Relationships: query 35 in 2014

These graphs are generated automatically and after each user's query. In fact, these types of graphs help users to understand the general context of the returned documents and to expand the knowledge on the subject later by studying the presented relationships. This study is easy to any user due to the used colors and the difference thickness edges. Indeed, if the edge between two terms is thick, the user can interpret the relation between these two terms is pertinent.

For example, in Fig. 3, edge between terms $(swollen, garment)$ is very thick, so we conclude the strong relationships between them.

In Fig. 4, we notice the presence of several relations with the term $peptic$ that can expand user's knowledge.

In the case where we end up with a rich graph with many semantic links between the terms, the research option provided by the $Prefuse$ tool makes user's easily find a specific term. Take the example shown in Fig. 5, the user looks for the word $coronari$, our visualization tool try to seek this term, if finded this term will be colored by a pink oval.

5 Conclusion and Future Works

The goal of this work is to help users making-sense when searching medical documents. Our proposed idea is to return with the search results, a graphical representation that illustrates the semantic relationships that may exist between

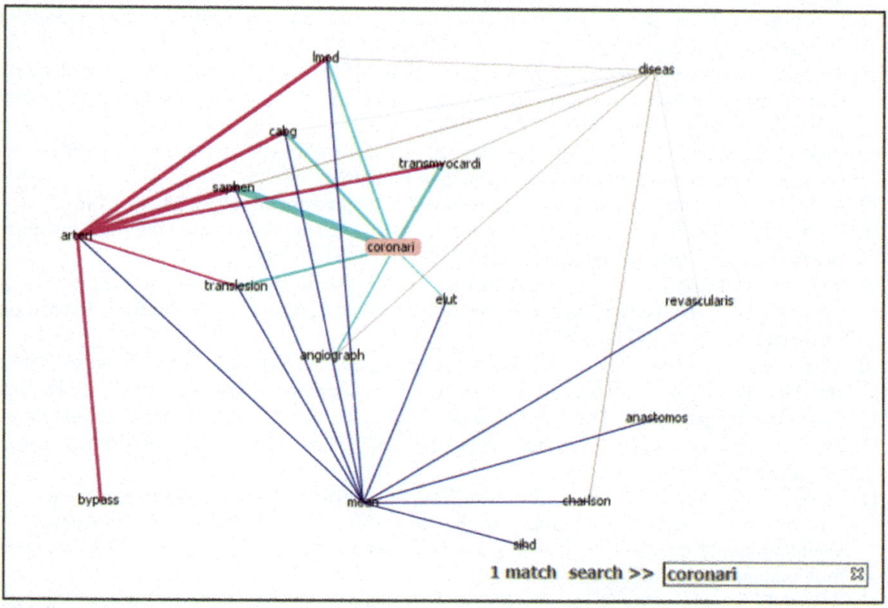

Fig. 5 Graph of Semantic Relationships: query 1 in 2014

terms in the user's query and terms of the returned documents assumed as pertinent, instead of returning only the relevant assumed documents.

Illustrated relationships in the graphs are defined by the statistical method LSM which is the most widely used predictive model in the field of machine learning that present a particular approach to artificial intelligence.

Obtained semantic relationships as well as the obtained graphs show the efficiency of the LSM method which gives significant results that help users to explore more the medical field and to ameliorate their queries with adding appropriate terms.

For future work, we try in the first time, to ask users to explain their needs (queries) based on their interpretation of provided data visualization graph. In the second time, we study the impact of query reformulation process on our content based retrieval system.

References

1. Visocky O'Grady, J., Visocky O'Grady, K.: The information design handbook. How Books, Cincinnati (2008)
2. Ksentini, N., Zarka, M., Ammar, A.B., Alimi, A.M.: Toward an assisted context based collaborative annotation. In: 2012 10th International Workshop on Content-Based Multimedia Indexing (CBMI), pp. 1–6. IEEE (2012).
3. Faisal, S., Blandford, A., Potts, H.W.: Making sense of personal health information: challenges for information visualization. Health Inform. J. **19**(3), 198–217 (2013)

4. Ksentini, N., Tmar, M., Gargouri, F.: Towards automatic improvement of patient queries in health retrieval systems. Appl. Med. Inform. **38**(2), 73–80 (2016)
5. Rind, A., Wang, T.D., Aigner, W., Miksch, S., Wongsuphasawat, K., Plaisant, C., Shneiderman, B.: Interactive information visualization to explore and query electronic health records. Found. Trends®Human-Comput. Interact. **5**(3), 207–298 (2013)
6. Card, S.K., Mackinlay, J.D., Shneiderman, B. (eds.). Readings in Information Visualization: Using Vision to Think. Morgan Kaufmann, San Francisco (1999)
7. Keim, D.A.: Visual exploration of large data sets. Commun. ACM **44**(8), 38–44 (2001)
8. Kosara, R., Miksch, S.: Metaphors of movement: a visualization and user interface for time-oriented, skeletal plans. Artif. Intell. Med. **22**(2), 111–131 (2001)
9. Plaisant, C., Mushlin, R., Snyder, A., Li, J., Heller, D., Shneiderman, B.: LifeLines: using visualization to enhance navigation and analysis of patient records. In: The Craft of Information Visualization, pp. 308–312 (2003)
10. Agirre, E., Alfonseca, E., Hall, K., Kravalova, J., Pasca, M., Soroa, A.: A study on similarity and relatedness using distributional and wordnet-based approaches. In: Proceedings of Human Language Technologies: The 2009 Annual Conference of the North American Chapter of the Association for Computational Linguistics, pp. 19–27. Association for Computational Linguistics (2009)
11. Terra, E., Clarke, C.L.: Frequency estimates for statistical word similarity measures. In: Proceedings of the 2003 Conference of the North American Chapter of the Association for Computational Linguistics on Human Language Technology, vol. 1, pp. 165–172. Association for Computational Linguistics (2003)
12. Agirre, E., Cuadros, M., Rigau, G., Soroa, A.: Exploring knowledge bases for similarity. In: LREC (2010)
13. Hassan, S., Mihalcea, R.: Semantic relatedness using salient semantic analysis. In: AAAI (2011)
14. Santus, E., Chiu, T.S., Lu, Q., Lenci, A., Huang, C.R.: Unsupervised measure of word similarity: how to outperform co-occurrence and vector cosine in VSMs. arXiv preprint:1603.09054 (2016)
15. Sahami, M., Heilman, T.D.: A web-based kernel function for measuring the similarity of short text snippets. In: Proceedings of the 15th International Conference on World Wide Web, pp. 377–386. ACM (2006)
16. Ruiz-Casado, M., Alfonseca, E., Castells, P.: Automatic assignment of wikipedia encyclopedic entries to wordnet synsets. In: International Atlantic Web Intelligence Conference, pp.380–386. Springer, Berlin/Heidelberg (2005)
17. Ksentini, N., Tmar, M., Gargouri, F.: Detection of semantic relationships between terms with a new statistical method. In: WEBIST (2), pp. 340–343 (2014)
18. Ksentini, N., Tmar, M., Gargouri, F.: Towards a contextual and semantic information retrieval system based on non-negative matrix factorization technique. In: International Conference on Intelligent Systems Design and Applications, pp. 892–902. Springer, Cham (2017)
19. Abdi, H.: The method of least squares. In: Salkind, N.J., Rasmussen, K. (eds.) Encyclopedia of Measurement and Statistics. SAGE Publications, Thousand Oaks (2007)
20. Miller, S.J.: The method of least squares. Mathematics Department Brown University, pp. 1–7 (2006)
21. Ksentini, N., Tmar, M., Gargouri, F.: Controlled automatic query expansion based on a new method arisen in machine learning for detection of semantic relationships between terms. In: 2015 15th International Conference on Intelligent Systems Design and Applications (ISDA), pp. 134–139. IEEE (2015)
22. Ksentini, N., Tmar, M., Gargouri, F.: The impact of term statistical relationships on Rocchio's model parameters for pseudo relevance feedback. Int. J. Comput. Inf. Syst. Ind. Manag. Appl. **8**, 135–44 (2016)
23. Huang, G.B., Wang, D.H., Lan, Y.: Extreme learning machines: a survey. Int. J. Mach. Learn. Cybern. **2**(2), 107–122 (2011)

24. Goeuriot, L., Kelly, L., Li, W., Palotti, J., Pecina, P., Zuccon, G., Mueller, H.: Share/clef ehealth evaluation lab 2014, task 3: user-centred health information retrieval. In: Proceedings of CLEF (2014)
25. Ksentini, N., Tmar, M., Gargouri, F.: Miracl at CLEF 2014: eHealth information retrieval task. In: Proceedings of the ShARe/CLEF eHealth Evaluation Lab (2014)
26. Palotti, J.R., Zuccon, G., Goeuriot, L., Kelly, L., Hanbury, A., Jones, G.J., Pecina, P.: CLEF eHealth Evaluation Lab 2015, Task 2: Retrieving information about medical symptoms. In: CLEF (Working Notes) (2015)
27. Ksentini, N., Tmar, M., Boughanem, M., Gargouri, F.: Miracl at Clef 2015: usercentred health information retrieval task. In: CLEF (Working Notes) (2015)

Accuracy Assessment of a Deep-Learning Based Segmentation Tool Over Right Ventricle Short-Axis Slices

Asma Ammari, Ramzi Mahmoudi, Badii Hmida, Rachida Saouli, and Mohamed Hédi Bedoui

1 Introduction

In the cardiac system, both ventricles have the role of pumping blood in the whole body. For the sake of enabling this organized role, the ventricular structure allows its function. Still, each ventricle has its own personalized morphology. Unlike the left ventricle (LV), the right ventricle (RV) has harsher trabeculae with a fibrous

A. Ammari (✉)
The National Engineering School L'ENIS, Sfax, Tunisia

Faculty of Medicine of Monastir, Medical Imaging Technology Lab - LTIM-LR12ES06, University of Monastir, Monastir, Tunisia

Department of computer science, Laboratory of Intelligent Computing (LINFI), Mohamed Khaider University, RP, Biskra, Algeria
e-mail: asma.ammari@enis.tn

R. Mahmoudi
Faculty of Medicine of Monastir, Medical Imaging Technology Lab - LTIM-LR12ES06, University of Monastir, Monastir, Tunisia

Gaspard-Monge Computer-Science Laboratory, Paris-Est University, Paris, France

B. Hmida
Radiology Service, UR12SP40 CHU Fattouma Bourguiba, Monastir, tunisia

R. Saouli
Department of computer science, Laboratory of Intelligent Computing (LINFI), Mohamed Khaider University, RP, Biskra, Algeria

Gaspard-Monge Computer-Science Laboratory, Paris-Est University, Paris, France

M. H. Bedoui
Faculty of Medicine of Monastir, Medical Imaging Technology Lab - LTIM-LR12ES06, University of Monastir, Monastir, Tunisia

L. Chaari (ed.), *Digital Health in Focus of Predictive, Preventive and Personalised Medicine*, Advances in Predictive, Preventive and Personalised Medicine 12,
https://doi.org/10.1007/978-3-030-49815-3_14

discontinuity between valves. The RV provides a thin wall and a crescent shape which makes it difficult to be modelled geometrically [1]. The assessment of the LV is widely handled using many segmentation techniques, even at the clinical practices, they segment and quantify its function automatically [2–4]. However, the RV is routinely assessed manually by expert radiologists to delineate its boundaries through the short axis several slices which are a fastidious, laborious, and time-consuming task. Therefore, automated assessment is crucial especially with the RV importance increasing for numerous pathological diagnosis. Irrefutably, its complex structure makes the segmentation task very challenging. Although many approaches have been proposed to handle those issues [5], still the problem of images variability and shape deformation from base to apex influence the accuracy of the proposed methods. In this paper, our goal is to study the impact of the RV MRI short-axis different slices on the segmentation accuracy using a commercially available cardiac MRI analysis software (CVi42, version 5.5.1, Circle Cardiovascular Imaging Inc., Calgary, Canada) [6]. Thus, we use two MRI exams of sick and healthy patients to experiment segmentation using the tool mentioned above. Based on the ground truth drawn by the expert, we compute the accuracy, the dice score metric, and other functional parameters related to the RV itself. The rest of this paper is organized as follow: We start by the state of the art in Sect. 2 followed by a description of the used image data and the experimented platform in Sect. 3. The experimental results are introduced in Sect. 4. Finally, in Sect. 5, discussion and conclusion are given.

2 State of the Art

The existing attempts to overcome the challenges related to the RV segmentation make use of many medical imaging segmentation techniques [5]. Based on prior information, in [7, 8], multi-atlas based approaches are exploited. Since atlas-based methods depend at the first stage on the database used, its results may fail to provide high accuracy when the segmented cardiac images present different structures from those used in the first place. Deformable models are also used for RV segmentation such in [9] and [10]. These methods are based on the shape information of the right ventricular. On the other hand, other works make use of graph cuts-based methods hybridized with several imaging techniques aiming thus to segment the right ventricular boundaries [11], [12]. Recently with the appearance and the augmented use of deep learning techniques to solve several imaging problems. In [12–14], deep learning methods are used for right ventricular segmentation. These methods depend on used architecture to train the model as well on the amount and the variation of used training sets. In this paper, we attempt to highlight the main issues that might hold back the adaptation of the promising deep-learning solutions for the RV challenging case considering at the first place the RV contour variation from base to apex. For that interest, we investigate the Cvi42 segmentation results, as it is based on a deep-learning approach using a fully conventional neural network trained on thousands of CMRI subjects acquired from the UK Biobank.

3 Image Data and Experiment Platform

To allow the Cvi42 cardiac segmentation tool assessment, the image data used encompasses a short-axis cine cardiac MR DICOM images which belong to two patients gathered from Fattouma Bourguiba Monastir Hospital in Tunisia. One patient presents a normal case while the other suffers from dysplasia in which the RV surface appears dilated. The manual RV delineation for both patients' sequences performed by the expert, based on the 4-chambers and the long-axis slices, is shown in Fig. 1 which is to be used as a referential segmentation. The experiment is done using a 5.10 version of Cvi42 upon an i7 ASUS platform (2.4 GHz CPU, 8GB RAM, Nvidia GeForce 920_M graphical card). The evaluation metrics are computed using MATLAB R2016a.

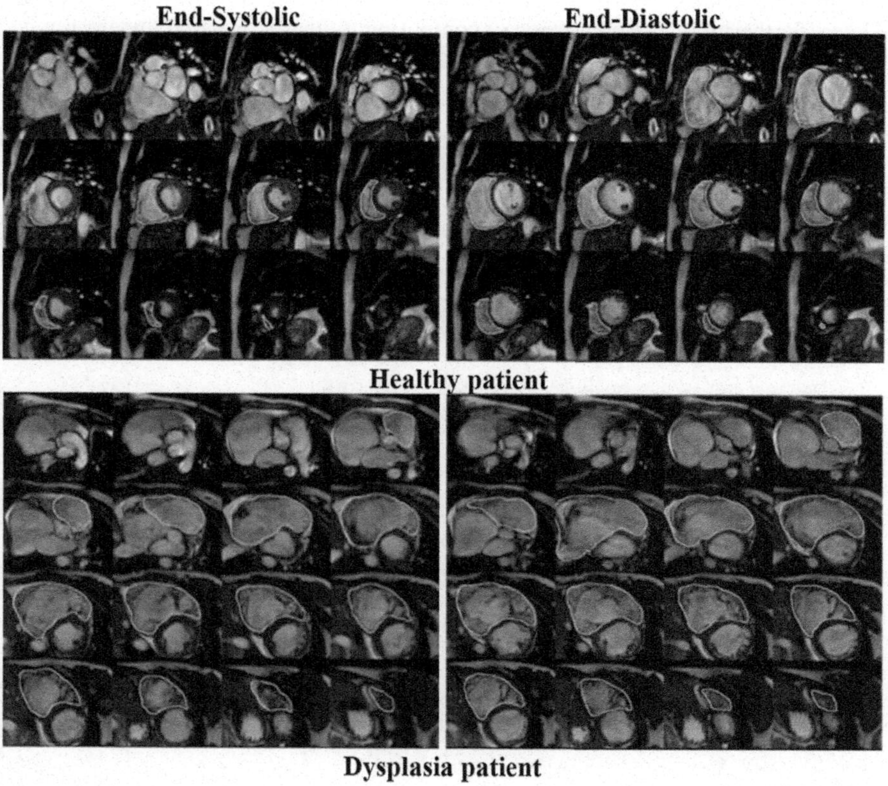

Fig. 1 Expert's manual RV endocardium delineation in end-systole and end-diastole for both healthy and diseased patient. (For interpretation of segmentation yellow color in this figure, the reader is referred to the web version of this article)

4 Experimental Results

In this section, the obtained RV boundaries automatic delineation, as well as the precession evaluation, are presented.

4.1 Segmentation Results

Figure 2 shows the segmentation results of the automated segmentation tool, in which the yellow line is the result of endocardium delineation. Compared to manual segmentation, we notice that the software has failed to detect the first basal and the last apical slices in the case of the healthy patient. However, in the case of dysplasia patient, most of the apical slices were missed out as well as some basal slices. Furthermore, the precession of contouring is clearly over and underestimated

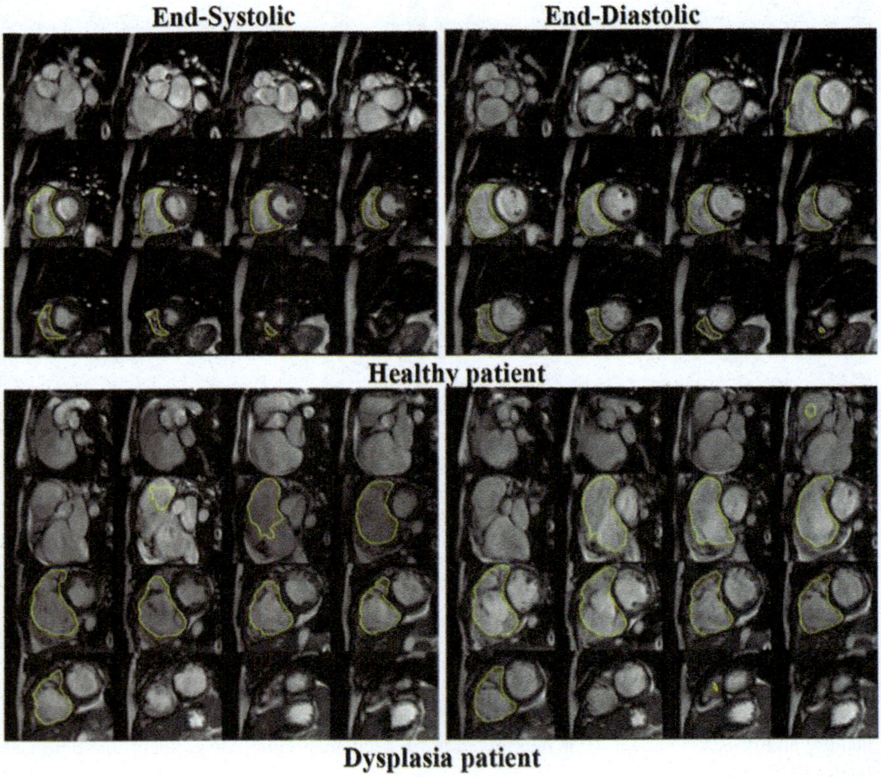

Fig. 2 Automatic Cvi42 RV endocardium delineation in end-systole and end-diastole for both healthy and diseased patient. (For interpretation of segmentation yellow color in this figure, the reader is referred to the web version of this article)

especially for the diseased case. The exact metrical evaluation of these delineation results is assessed in the following sub-section.

4.2 Empirical Evaluation

In this paper, we compute the Dice metric (DM) and the accuracy for the sake of evaluating the performance of the RV automatic segmentation offered by the tool (Cvi42). The DM is the overlap between the automatic segmentation result and the manual segmentation result computed following the Eq. (1) [5], and the accuracy computed based on true positives, true negatives, false positives and false negatives as it is described in the Eq. (2). Graphics in Figs. 3 and 4 show respectively the obtained results for the Accuracy and the DM.

$$\mathrm{DM}\,(U, V) = 2\frac{UV}{U + V} \tag{1}$$

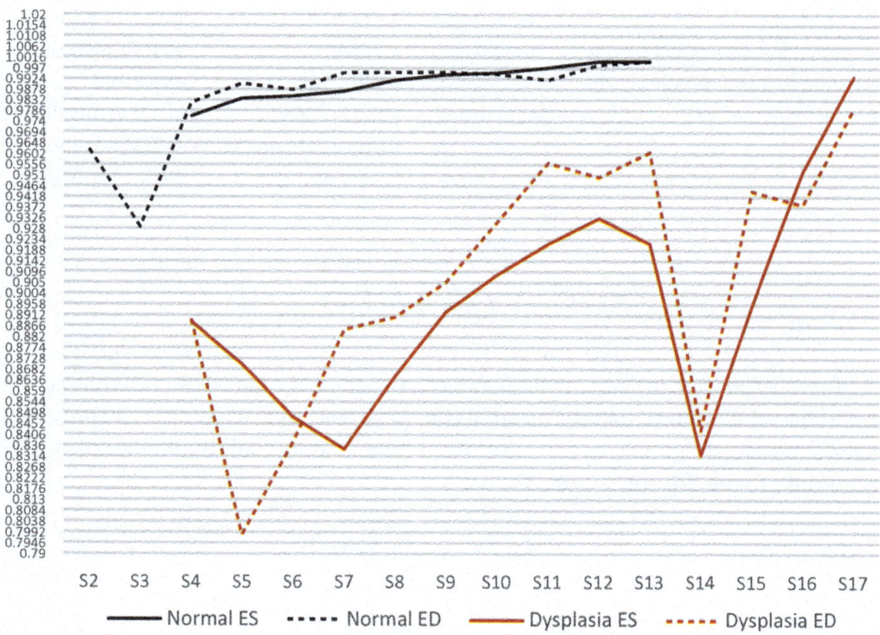

Fig. 3 Accuracy evaluation of Short-Axis Slices from (S2→S17) for both End-Systolic and End-Diastolic phases considering both normal and diseased patients

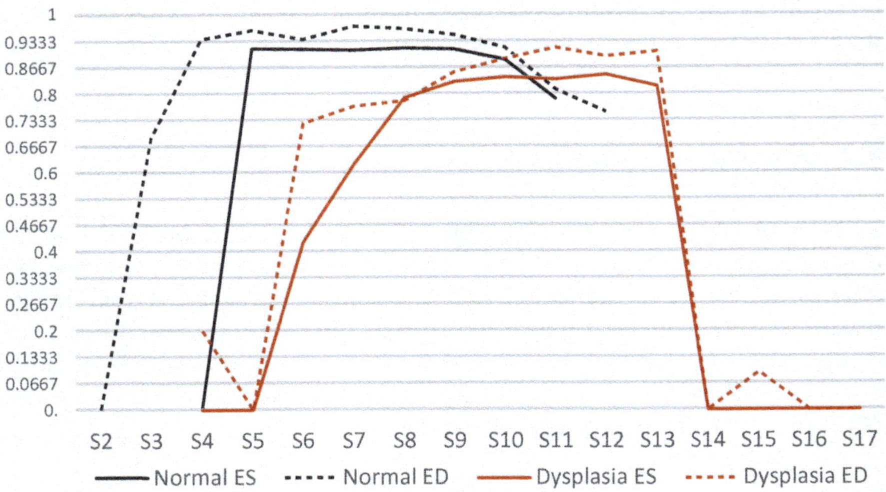

Fig. 4 Dice score metric evaluation of Short-Axis Slices from (S2➔S17) for both End-Systolic and End-Diastolic phases considering both normal and diseased patients

Table 1 Right ventricular functional parameters. (RVESV): RV End Systolic Volume, (RVEDV): RV End Diastolic Volume, RVEF): RV Ejection Fraction

	Healthy patient	Diseased patient
Ground truth	RVEDV: 75.4 ml/m^2	RVEDV: 491 ml
	RVESV: 32.2 ml/m^2	RVESV: 410 ml
	RVEF: 57%	RVEF: 6%
Automatic	RVEDV: 209.52 ml	RVEDV: 401.04 ml
	RVESV: 114.45 ml	RVESV: 276.12 ml
	RVEF: 45.37%	RVEF: 31.15%

$$\text{Accuracy} = \frac{TP + TN}{TP + TN + FP + FN} \tag{2}$$

Table 1 shows some functional parameters such as RV End-systolic Volume, RV End-Diastolic Volume, and the ejection fraction of the assessed cases. The presented values obtained by the expert and the segmentation tool might be computed according to the Eqs. (3, 4 and 5).

$$RVESV = \min_t [V(t)] \tag{3}$$

$$RVEDV = \max_t \left[V(t) \right] \tag{4}$$

$$RVEF\,(\%) = \frac{RVEDV - RVESV}{RVEDV} \times 100 \tag{5}$$

Considering both the RV-end-systolic-volume and the RV-end-diastolic-volume, the values obtained by the segmentation tool seem to be higher compared to the values obtained by the expert for the case of the healthy patient. However, in the case of the diseased patient, we find that the automatically obtained volumes show lower values than those obtained by the expert. Consequently, the resulting ejection fraction obtained by the automatic segmentation is lower for the case of the healthy patient and higher for the diseased one compared to the expert' referential results. Indeed, as the main goal of the RV boundaries segmentation is to allow accurate functional parameters computing. Thus, any under or over-estimated contours even at the basal or apical slices might influence the obtained parametrical results especially for the case of pathological patients where neither the size nor the end-systolic and the end-diastolic phases are normal.

5 Conclusion and Discussion

In this paper, a deep-learning-based cardiac segmentation tool is considered for evaluating the impact of CMRI slice from base to the apex on the effectiveness of the segmentation. The metrical presented results in Fig. 3 and Fig. 4 show respectively the computed Accuracy and Dice metric values for each short-axis slice from base to apex (S2, S3 . . . S17). The very first basal slice is excluded as it doesn't belong to the RV space. For the healthy patient, the included slices are S2, S3 . . . S12. However, the pathological patient covers the whole 16 slices as the RV is dilated. For both patients, the very first basal and the very last epical slices associate low accuracy and DM. Besides, the accuracy and the DM results are low for the entire pathological patient' slices compared to the healthy slices. Thus, the segmentation results show that from central to basal and apical slices the effectiveness of the delineation decreases. Also, the case of dysplasia illustrates how widely the effectiveness decreases and how do the diseased cases influence the accuracy of segmentation. As a perspective, we attempt to tackle the basal and apical segmentation issues as well as the pathological problem toward a better effective segmentation process based on deep-learning approaches.

References

1. Sheehan, F., Redington, A.: The right ventricle: anatomy, physiology and clinical imaging. Heart. **94**, 1510–1515 (2008). https://doi.org/10.1136/hrt.2007.132779
2. Irshad, M., Sharif, M., Khan, M.Y.: A survey on left ventricle segmentation techniques in Cardiac Short Axis MRI, https://doi.org/10.2174/1573405613666170117124934, Last accessed 2019/06/12

3. Sami, S.M., Elfawal, S.K., Abdelgawad, M.S., Zidan, M.A., Zaki, A.M., Mowaki, A.F.: MDCT in the study of left ventricular function compared with MRI in patients with myocardial ischemia. Egypt. J. Radiol. Nucl. Med. **49**, 29–41 (2018). https://doi.org/10.1016/j.ejrnm.2017.11.004
4. Epstein, F.H.: MRI of left ventricular function. J. Nucl. Cardiol. Off. Publ. Am. Soc. Nucl. Cardiol. **14**, 729–744 (2007). https://doi.org/10.1016/j.nuclcard.2007.07.006
5. Petitjean, C., Zuluaga, M.A., Bai, W., Dacher, J.-N., Grosgeorge, D., Caudron, J., Ruan, S., Ayed, I.B., Cardoso, M.J., Chen, H.-C., Jimenez-Carretero, D., Ledesma-Carbayo, M.J., Davatzikos, C., Doshi, J., Erus, G., Maier, O.M.O., Nambakhsh, C.M.S., Ou, Y., Ourselin, S., Peng, C.-W., Peters, N.S., Peters, T.M., Rajchl, M., Rueckert, D., Santos, A., Shi, W., Wang, C.-W., Wang, H., Yuan, J.: Right ventricle segmentation from cardiac MRI: a collation study. Med. Image Anal. **19**, 187–202 (2015). https://doi.org/10.1016/j.media.2014.10.004
6. Cardiac MRI and CT Software – Circle Cardiovascular Imaging – Cardiac MRI, https://www.circlecvi.com/cvi42/cardiac-mri/. Last accessed 17 Oct 2019
7. Ou, Y., Doshi, J., Erus, G., Davatzikos, C.: Multi-Atlas segmentation of the Cardiac MR right ventricle. Presented at the (2012)
8. Bai, W., Shi, W., Wang, H., Peters, N.S., Rueckert, D.: Multi-atlas based segmentation with local label fusion for right ventricle MR images. Presented at the (2012)
9. Sun, H., Frangi, A.F., Wang, H., Sukno, F.M., Tobon-Gomez, C., Yushkevich, P.A.: Automatic cardiac MRI segmentation using a biventricular deformable medial model. In: Jiang, T., Navab, N., Pluim, J.P.W., Viergever, M.A. (eds.) Medical Image Computing and Computer-Assisted Intervention – MICCAI 2010, pp. 468–475. Springer, Berlin/Heidelberg (2010)
10. Yang, X., Yeo, S.Y., Su, Y., Lim, C., Wan, M., Zhong, L., Tan, R.S.: Right ventricle segmentation by temporal information constrained gradient vector flow. In: 2013 IEEE International Conference on Systems, Man, and Cybernetics, pp. 2551–2555 (2013). https://doi.org/10.1109/SMC.2013.435
11. Maier, O.M.O., Jiménez, D., Santos, A., Ledesma-Carbayo, M.J.: Segmentation of RV in 4D cardiac MR volumes using region-merging graph cuts. In: 2012 Computing in Cardiology, pp. 697–700 (2012)
12. Quispe, A.M., Petitjean, C.: Shape prior based image segmentation using manifold learning. In: 2015 International Conference on Image Processing Theory, Tools and Applications (IPTA). pp. 137–142. (2015). https://doi.org/10.1109/IPTA.2015.7367113
13. Zotti, C., Luo, Z., Lalande, A., Jodoin, P.-M.: Convolutional neural network with shape prior applied to cardiac MRI segmentation. IEEE J. Biomed. Health Inform. (2018). https://doi.org/10.1109/JBHI.2018.2865450
14. Jang, Y., Hong, Y., Ha, S., Kim, S., Chang, H.-J.: Automatic segmentation of LV and RV in cardiac MRI. In: Pop, M., Sermesant, M., Jodoin, P.-M., Lalande, A., Zhuang, X., Yang, G., Young, A., Bernard, O. (eds.) Statistical Atlases and Computational Models of the Heart. ACDC and MMWHS Challenges, pp. 161–169. Springer (2018)

Big Data Analytics in Healthcare

Wayne Matengo, Ezekiel Otsieno, and Kelvin Wanjiru

1 Introduction

Personalised, Preventive, Predictive and Participatory (P4) medicine is on the rise due to the following factors: (1) increasing capacities and capabilities of systems biology and systems medicine, (2) digital revolution and (3) changing consumer demands in healthcare. The increasing capabilities of systems biology has seen clinical medicine shift from a reductionist approach to a more holistic approach where the human body is seen as an interconnection of different systems all together. On the other hand, the increasing levels of technological advancements has amplified the possibilities for collecting, integrating, storing, analysing and communicating data and information, including conventional medical histories, clinical tests and the results of the tools of systems medicine [4, 5]. Lastly, consumers are increasingly becoming more and more cognizant of their healthcare status and interested in managing their own health.

Since the advent of P4 medicine, various research has shown that the healthcare environment will undergo a paradigm shift under which the industry will be driven by technological buzzwords such as 'big data', 'genomics', 'digital health' and 'personalised medicine' [3, 14]. For this paper, we pay attention to the digital revolution in the healthcare industry and the limitless scope for promoting P4 medicine using Wearable technology. The first section looks at the current craze of big data, followed the trends in the healthcare industry. We further look at the various research publications around big data and wearable technology at large which helps us develop our methodology and analysis procedures and lastly, we present a call to action for the implementation of P4 medicine.

W. Matengo · E. Otsieno (✉) · K. Wanjiru
Strathmore University, Nairobi, Kenya

L. Chaari (ed.), *Digital Health in Focus of Predictive, Preventive and Personalised Medicine*, Advances in Predictive, Preventive and Personalised Medicine 12,
https://doi.org/10.1007/978-3-030-49815-3_15

2 Big Data

Big data refers to data, which is large in volume, high in velocity and in different varieties that can be computationally analysed for insights that lead to better decisions, predictions and strategic business moves. It is used by industry analysts, business users and executives who ask the right questions, recognise patterns, make informed assumptions and predict behaviour. The idea of big data was first embraced by online start-up firms such as Google, eBay, LinkedIn and Facebook. It has grown rapidly, permeating almost every sector. Notably, big data is applied widely in psychographics. This is a qualitative methodology used to describe individuals based on psychological attributes, which is then useful in targeted engagement such as politics, marketing, advertising and now to be used in medicine. It is also applied in weather observatory by repurposing sensors in mobile devices such as android mobile phones to map special readings. Finally, it has applications in sports. For example, in football, sports data analytics Sci-Sports has developed a camera called Ball James to capture big data from all players in the field who don't have the ball. This generates player data such as precision, direction and speed of the passing, sprinting strength and jumping strength. This could be used by football managers to make substitution decisions. These are just but a few of the numerous applications.

With the increasing interest in big data analytics around the world, the big data market is equally booming. According to Forbes, the big data market which was estimated at $ 42 billion in 2018 is expected to grow to $103 billion by 2027. Statista on the other hand estimates that the market will grow to $ 70 billion by 2022. These projections on growth prospects underscore how the use of big data is expected to take a centre stage in decision making across many spheres. If fully adopted in the healthcare industry, the growth in its market size may outrun the current projections.

Big data in healthcare refers to these various large and complex data that includes physician notes, lab reports, X-ray reports and case history, used to capture essential information about a patient for complete insights useful in health management and patient engagement [1]. This data is often difficult to analyse and manage with traditional software or hardware. Big data analytics covers integration of heterogeneous data, data quality control, analysis, modelling, interpretation and validation. Application of big data analytics provides comprehensive knowledge discovering from the available huge amount of data. Particularly, big data analytics in medicine and healthcare enables individual analysis of the large datasets from thousands of patients, identifying clusters and correlation between datasets, as well as developing predictive models using data mining techniques. This integrates the analysis of several scientific areas such as bioinformatics, medical imaging, sensor informatics, medical informatics and health informatics. A survey of big data cases in healthcare institutions is given in [1]. The authors acknowledge the reliance of healthcare institutions on big data technology to improve care coordination and develop outcome-based reimbursement models. The new knowledge discovered by big data analytics techniques should provide comprehensive benefits to the patients, clinicians and health policy makers.

In healthcare, big data's strength is in finding the associations and not showing whether these associations have meanings. Therefore, the intervention of medical practitioners is required to attach meaning to such associations derived from data analytics. While doing so, care must be taken to avoid spurious results. Otherwise, "Big Error" may lead to inaccurate and hence inappropriate decisions [9].

3 Healthcare Trends

In the recent times, the increasing prevalence of non-communicable diseases together with aging population in different parts of the world has led to increased mortality as well as rising costs of healthcare provision. Non-communicable diseases such as cardiovascular diseases (CVDs), cancer, diabetes mellitus and respiratory diseases are now identified as among the world's leading cause of death, disability, diminished quality of life and a key contributor to the rising costs of healthcare. In response to this, traditional reactive approaches to medicine are now being shunned and instead replaced with a proactive approach which encompasses predictive, preventive, personalised and participatory (P4) medicine [13] Aided with advancement in technologies and digitization of medicine, electronic health records (EHRs) are gaining momentum. This is geared towards helping physicians and healthcare providers at large to be able to detect potential diseases early enough and intervene in good time, as well as monitoring the health of a patient.

Since the majority of these diseases are preventable or can be delayed to a significantly later stage in life, notable focus has to be placed on monitoring the lifestyle of individuals by obtaining actionable data about some important health metrics of the individuals. To collect such data continuously and in real-time, adoption of wearable technology in medicine provides a good opportunity to improve disease monitoring, provided that big data analytics are performed on the enormous amount of data stored to derive actionable insights for prediction and timely intervention to prevent the diseases [10].

4 Related Literature

With the rise in popularity of Internet of Things (IoT), big data analytics has found its demand in healthcare as providers seek to analyse unstructured data and recognise trends and patterns that can inform decision making [11]. It stands to improve health by providing insights into the causes and outcomes of disease, better drug targets for precision in medicine, and enhanced disease prediction and prevention [7] Moreover, citizen-scientists will increasingly use this information to promote their own health and wellness. This supports P4 medicine, whose premise is to transform the approach of medicine from being largely reactive and population based practice to an individual-based approach focused on wellness. If wellness can be quantified, diseases can be demystified.

In healthcare, the use of smart wearable devices has gained traction to the extent that an estimated 245 million units of wearable devices will be sold by the end of 2019 (CCS Insight's Forecast on wearable devices). These devices are used to continuously record useful individual health metrics in real-time which facilitates continuous out-of-clinic health monitoring as well as in-home disease management through lifestyle monitoring. The enormous amounts of data recorded is storable on google cloud and can be analysed using certain algorithms to give predictions of diseases. Medical researchers note that diseases are usually a result of perturbed networks in the body cells and that there are usually early signals that can be tracked even before any symptoms are manifested. Thus, it is the early prediction of such diseases through careful analysis of health metrics data from individuals that will lead to appropriate preventive measures being undertaken. For instance, Sagner et al. [12] reports that monitoring and maintaining of normal values for key health metrics such as blood pressure and blood glucose play a primary role in reducing chronic disease risk.

Whereas the use of smart wearables to record data on health vitals of individuals is novel, there are a few challenges faced. Notably, data privacy and security issues remain the biggest question that could slacken their adoption. These devices are feared as being likely to lead to identity fraud, especially when the manufacturers of the devices (who are deemed to be owning the data) sell it to third parties who are likely to abuse it. Similarly, some researchers argue that sophisticated algorithms have the ability to reveal user identity from anonymous data. We believe that data protection rules will be made in different territories and regions to prevent abuse of personal data [8].

5 Methodology

The study was conducted to examine the wearable devices, their systems architecture, and the data they collect and to investigate any emerging patterns and predictive insights. The main source of the data used for this project is Kaggle website.

Our goal was to observe the risk of Cardiovascular Disease (CVD). Research from the Framingham Heart Study indicate that healthcare officials can use the Framingham Risk Score algorithm to estimate the 10-year Cardiovascular Disease risk of an individual. The key risk factors under CVD include: Gender, Age, Total Cholesterol, Systolic Blood Pressure, Smoking, Family History and Diabetes [6].

Such tools address the need for preventive, predictive, personalised and participatory (P4) medicine. The underlying foundation of P4 Medicine lies in the presence of big data. Wearable biometric monitoring devices (BMDs) allow for remote, high frequency and high-resolution monitoring for patients' health outside the hospital. Coupled with progressive advancements in artificial intelligence (AI), the data collected from wearables will help in informing diagnosis, predicting patient outcomes and helping care professionals elect the best treatment for their patients. As one of the constituent pillars of P4 medicine, wearable devices heavily contribute to personalized medicine. Individual health status can be uniquely monitored using the continuous key health metrics that these devices are able to record, which can be tracked over the long term to identify any patterns. This is important to aid detection of any deviation from the norm and thus take a remedial action. The devices should not be shared among individuals at any time so that data which is only attributable to one individual can be measured, recorded and accumulated over time. This is crucial in addressing the different health needs of various individuals. Finally, wearables can promote primary prevention measures that aim for reducing the probability or risk of CVD. Secondary prevention measures are also applicable to help reduce the impact of the presence of CVD in an individual.

6 Data Analysis and Results

The examination of wearable data on the first phase only represented a single subject. The data collected had the following parameters:

1. Date time
2. Steps
3. Distance covered
4. Calories
5. Minutes per Activity
6. Weight
7. BMI
8. Fat level

The results were based on various parameters of observations and visualized using ggplot2 library in R-Studio (Fig. 1).

The figure below shows that the user did not take any steps within the years 2013–2014. This could be attributed to various reasons such as: the user might have lost their Fitbit watch, the user might have not worn their watch for that period for various reasons, the user could have actually not been moving around (this is too abnormal though).

To take a new look at the steps of the user, we further analysed the steps taken per day, every year. The figure is shown below (Fig. 2).

This gives us a look into the days in which the patient is taking more steps than average, against the days that the user is taking less steps than average. A further visualisation was made in order to get more sense from the daily steps made and what interventions can be put in place to ensure that the user takes the minimum required steps each day (Fig. 3).

To dig deeper into the steps taken by the user, the fat levels and BMI levels were evaluated with regards to the steps.

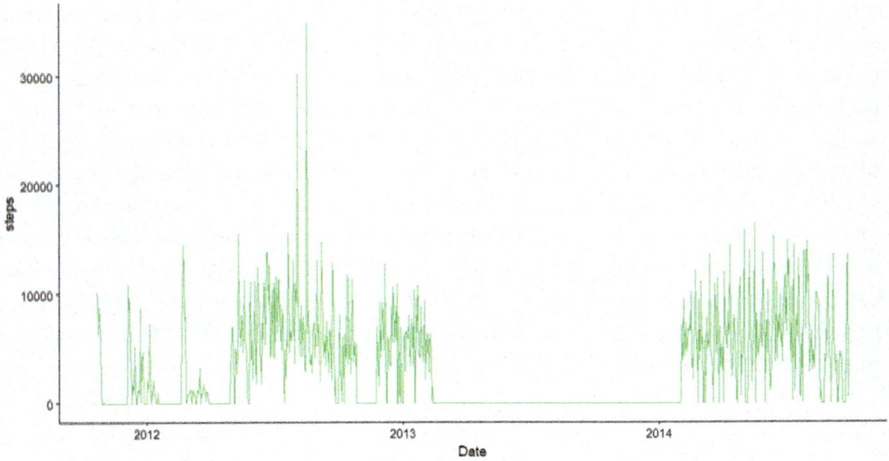

Fig. 1 Variation of Steps taken by the user over a timeline

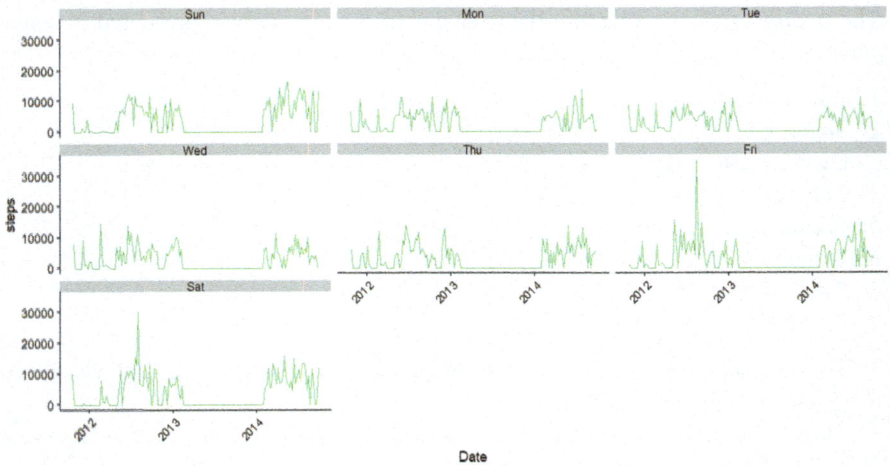

Fig. 2 Variation of steps taken by the user on each day of the week over the time period

It is observed that the fat level and BMI level show almost equal levels of variations over the time period. It is however worth noting that during the period 2013–2014 where there was no record on the number of steps taken, there was an increase in the levels of BMI and Fat, as shown in the figure below (Fig. 4).

These insights, when coupled up with the various electronic health records (EHRs); such as the Blood Pressure of the specific user, would really mean a lot to the health and care professionals. They would be able to predict diseases before they actually come and therefore provide preventive interventions to the user.

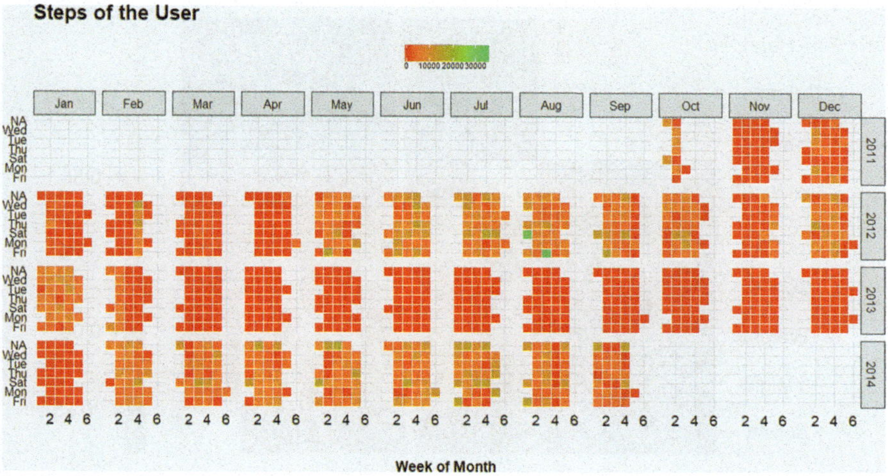

Fig. 3 Analysis of the daily steps taken by the user over the time period

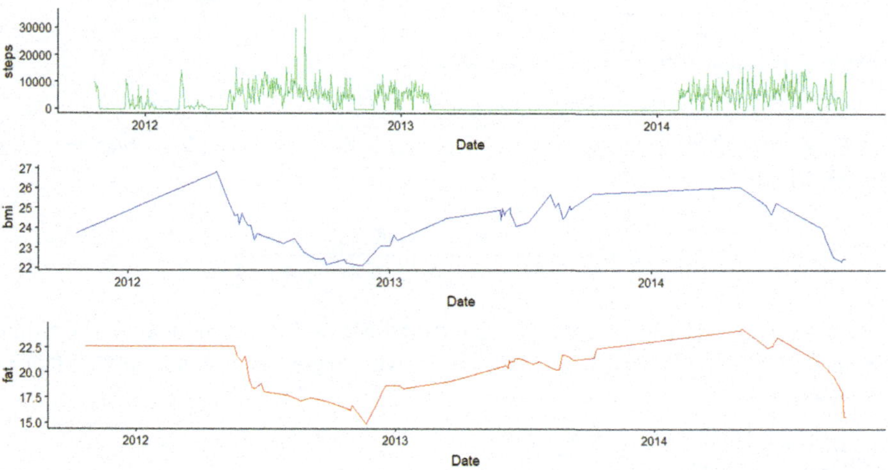

Fig. 4 Fat and BMI Levels against the number of steps of the user

Onto the second phase of our analysis, the examination of the Fitbit data was based on various number of subjects. It was a collective dataset representing the records for various individuals.

We first visualised the correlation between the different variables in the dataset, and came up with the correlation matrix below (Fig. 5).

This informs us that the variables – Heart, Calories and Steps are strongly positively correlated to each other. Also, the presence of Age, Gender, Weight, and Height also indicate a strong correlation.

Having this in mind, we developed a Logistic Regression model to predict the probability of an individual within the dataset contracting heart disease (also known

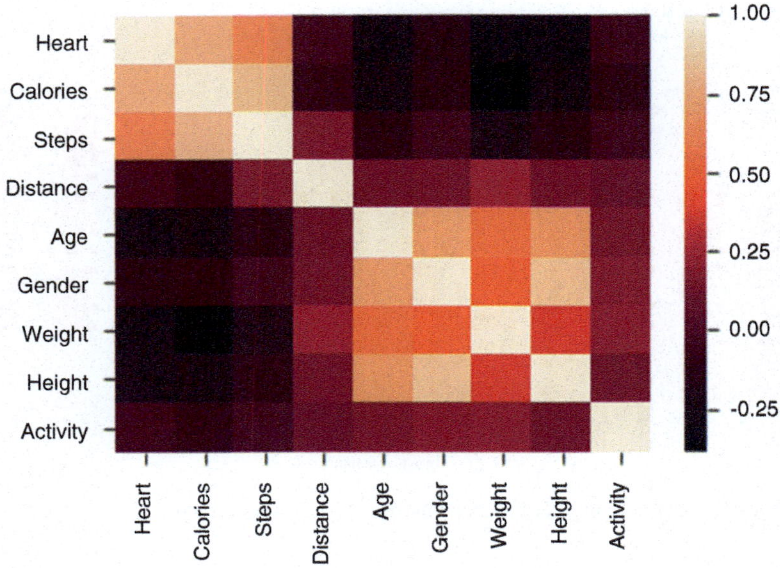

Fig. 5 Correlation Matrix of the Collective Data

as Cardiovascular Disease). First, we came up with a new variable and defined it as BMI; where:

$$BMI = \frac{Weight\ in\ Kilograms}{Height\ in\ Meters\ squared}$$

Various research has indicated the use of BMI as a better indicator of Cardiac Risk Factors [2]. Once BMI was calculated, we categorised it in a binary format as follows:

- BMI between 18.5 to 29.9 = 0
- BMI above 29.9 = 1

Our classification was such that a person is either obese or not, hence the classification format as stated above. However, the conventional way of classifying BMI is as follows:

- BMI <18.5 = Underweight
- BMI 18.5–24.9 = Normal Weight
- BMI 25.0–29.9 = Overweight
- BMI 30–34.9 = Class I Obesity
- BMI 35–39.9 = Class II Obesity
- BMI > 40 = Class III Obesity

```
                           Logit Regression Results
==============================================================================
Dep. Variable:               bmi_pred   No. Observations:                21489
Model:                          Logit   Df Residuals:                    21478
Method:                           MLE   Df Model:                           10
Date:                Sun, 09 Jun 2019   Pseudo R-squ.:                   1.000
Time:                        20:53:46   Log-Likelihood:            -0.00016464
converged:                      False   LL-Null:                        -14325.
                                        LLR p-value:                     0.000
==============================================================================
                 coef    std err          z      P>|z|      [0.025      0.975]
------------------------------------------------------------------------------
const        812.9701        nan        nan        nan         nan         nan
Heart         -0.0528      6.074     -0.009      0.993     -11.958      11.853
Calories       0.0702     64.068      0.001      0.999    -125.501     125.642
Steps         -0.0011      3.969     -0.000      1.000      -7.780       7.778
Distance       0.0165     10.093      0.002      0.999     -19.766      19.799
Age          -13.0688        nan        nan        nan         nan         nan
Gender       -19.0417        nan        nan        nan         nan         nan
Weight        11.3264        nan        nan        nan         nan         nan
Height      -619.0515        nan        nan        nan         nan         nan
Activity      -0.2843    142.304     -0.002      0.998    -279.195     278.627
BMI          -10.4263        nan        nan        nan         nan         nan
==============================================================================
```

Fig. 6 Logistic Regression Results

Our predictor variable was therefore a binary type with the 0's and 1's. We run the model using Sci-Py library in Python 3.6 environment. The results are as shown above (Fig. 6):

The results indicate that the variables: Heart, Calories, Steps, Distance and Activity are significant in determining the changes in BMI, which would ultimately impact the probability of one getting CVD. We went ahead to split the dataset into testing dataset and training dataset and the model achieved an accuracy score of 69%.

7 Conclusion

Apart from the rapidly advancing genomics, metabolomics, single-cell analysis, phenotyping, micro-fluids and imaging technologies used for early detection of chronic illnesses, wearable technology is a change agent in the entire healthcare industry. The data gotten from wearables present tremendous opportunities for healthcare practitioners to promote a proactive approach to preventing and treating such diseases. The capabilities behind big data tracking and system analytics will ultimately result in personalised actionable health insights. However, it is worth noting that these devices should undergo proper tests and validation to ensure that the data used for the clinical operations is of good quality. Various measures should be put into place to ascertain the levels of data privacy too [8].

P4 medicine presents a myriad of opportunities for research and development. This has been accelerated due to the technological advancements that has led to the explosion of massive amounts of data. The shift from traditional reactive medicine to P4 medicine will only be possible when various stakeholders from the healthcare and other industries form strategic partnerships to work together towards the common goal of attaining sustainable healthcare.

References

1. Archenaa, J., Mary Anita, E. A.: A Survey of Big Data Analytics in Healthcare and Government. International Symposium on Big Data and Cloud Computing (ISBCC'15). (2015)
2. Debnath, S.: BMI is a better indicator of cardiac risk factors, as against elevated blood pressure in apparently healthy females and young adult students: Results from a cross-sectional study in Tripura. Indian J. Community Med. **41**, 292 (2016)
3. ESF: Personalised Medicine for the European Citizen—Towards more Precise Medicine for the Diagnosis, Treatment and Prevention of Disease. European Science Foundation, Strasbourg (2012)
4. Flores, M., Glusman, G., Brogaard, K., Price, N.D., Hood, L.: P4 medicine: how systems medicine will transform the healthcare sector and society. Pers. Med. 565–576 (2013)
5. Hood, L.: Systems biology and P4 medicine: past, present, and future. Rambam Maimonides Med. J. (2013)
6. Jia, X., Baig, M. M., Mirza, F., Gholam Hosseini, H.: A cox-based risk prediction model for early detection of cardiovascular disease: identification of key risk factors for the development of a 10-Year CVD risk prediction. Advances in Preventive Medicine. (2019)
7. Khoury, M.J., loannidis, J.P.: Big data meets public health. PubMed Central. 1054–1055 (2014)
8. Lymberis A.: Smart wearables for remote health monitoring, from prevention to rehabilitation: current R&D, future challenges. Proceedings of the 4th Annual IEEE Conference on Information Technology Applications in Biomedicine, UK (2003)
9. Raghupathi, W., Raghupathi, V.: Big data analytics in healthcare: promise and potential. Health Info. Sci. Syst. **2**, 3 (2014)
10. Ristevski, B., Chen, M.: Big data analytics in medicine and healthcare. J. Integr. Bioinform.. De Gruyter (2018)
11. Rodriguez C., Barrow A., Dangore S., Pathak U., Talledo J.: Applying Data Analytics to Big Data Obtained from Wearable Devices. In Proceedings of Student-Faculty Research Day, CSIS, Pace University, Pleavantville, New York (2018)
12. Sagner et al.: The P4 Spectrum – a predictive, preventive and personalised and participatory continuum for promoting Healthspan. Progress in Preventive Medicine. (2017)
13. Tian, Q., Hood, L.: Systems Cancer Medicine: Towards Realization of Predictive, Preventive, Personalized and Participatory (P4) Medicine. Journal of Internal Medicine, Seattle (2011)
14. Topol, E.J.: The Creative Destruction of Medicine: how the Digital Revolution Will Create Better Health Care. Basic Books, New York (2012)
15. Vogt, H., Hofmann, B., Getz, L.: The new holism: P4 systems medicine and the medicalization of health and life itself. Med. Healthcare Philos. 307–323 (2016)

Towards an Oversampling Method to Improve Hepatocellular Carcinoma Early Prediction

Mahbouba Hattab, Ahmed Maalel, and Henda Hajjami Ben Ghezala

1 Introduction

Knowledge discovery in medical databases has become an attractive and crucial complement for clinical research. Survival and disease prediction are of a highly important task addressed by the medical research communities due to its direct effect on doctor's decisions [1]. Using KDD (Knowledge Discovery in Databases), efficient and important knowledge can be extracted from these data sets. The principal steps in the KDD process are as follows: (1) Data selection, (2) Data management and pretreatment, (3) Transformation, (4) Data mining, and (5) Assessment and interpretation. Ideally, from a computer science perspective, data mining is one of the ultimate steps in the KDD process. Indeed, Data Mining is a discipline resulting from combining statistics and computer science such as Machine Learning algorithms. Data mining aims to extract new and useful knowledge from a large amount of data (i.e.: applied to have an effective and preferment predictive model [2]). However, each of the aforementioned domains has its specifics, therefore it is

M. Hattab (✉)
Higher Institute of Applied Sciences and Technology of Sousse, University of Sousse, Sousse, Tunisia

A. Maalel
Higher Institute of Applied Sciences and Technology of Sousse, University of Sousse, Sousse, Tunisia

National School of Computer Sciences, RIADI Laboratory, University of Manouba, Manouba, Tunisia
e-mail: ahmed.maalel@ensi.rnu.tn

H. H. B. Ghezala
National School of Computer Sciences, RIADI Laboratory, University of Manouba, Manouba, Tunisia

L. Chaari (ed.), *Digital Health in Focus of Predictive, Preventive and Personalised Medicine*, Advances in Predictive, Preventive and Personalised Medicine 12,
https://doi.org/10.1007/978-3-030-49815-3_16

important to wisely choose the best data optimization and pre-treatment algorithm to achieve state-of-the-art classification accuracy.

Due to the abundance of data in the biomedical domain, this latter has a high potential in improving the well being of humankind. Nevertheless, it is very complex to process and analyze such data by traditional methods [1]. As a result, the interest of data mining and machine learning is increasing considerably with a wide range of medical applications. They become useful instruments in bioinformatics thanks to their capability to convert this vast resource into information and knowledge that helps achieve better decision making in several disease areas including cardiovascular disorders, Parkinson's, Alzheimer's, etc. [3].

Cancer is a generic term for a large variety of diseases that can affect any person and any part of the body and it represents one of the leading causes of morbidity and mortality worldwide after heart diseases [4, 15]. Globally, according to the World Health Organisation (WHO) [4], one in six deaths are due to cancer. Relatable to cancer, Hepatocellular carcinoma (HCC) also referred to as malignant hepatoma [3] is a malignant tumor, and represent the sixth most common type of cancer and the third leading cause of cancer-related deaths globally according to [5].

2 Related Works and Motivation

Over the past years, several research works have been conducted on HCC and liver-related diseases. For instance, **Santos et al. (2015)** [5] studied HCC data set using a new cluster-based oversampling algorithm. The proposed methodology is based on the data pre-treatment process considering appropriate distance metrics for both heterogeneous and missing data by applying the Heterogeneous Euclidean-Overlap Metric (HEOM) distance. Then Kmeans clustering algorithm is applied for the first sampling step within the HCC database and SMOTE oversampling algorithm to build a representative balanced data set and use it for Leave-One-Out cross Validation (LOO-CV) assessment with different machine learning algorithms such as logistic regression (LR) and neural networks (NN) classifiers. The results indicated that the proposed approach can achieve efficient results.

In another work, **Sawhney et al.** (2018) [6] explored the performance of the firefly algorithm by adding a penalty function to the existing fitness function. Afterward, they modify the existing wrapper feature to reduce the feature set to an optimal subset. Furthermore, the influence of the method is proved on the classification accuracy as well as feature reduction using a Random Forest classifier for the Hepatocellular Carcinoma dataset in comparison to other contemporary methods such as Deep Learning methods and Information Gain. However, the above-mentioned works, are of a highly computationally expensive and require a large amount of data in order to generate a satisfying model. Moreover, real-world data tends to be incomplete, noisy, and inconsistent and the important task is to fill in missing values, smooth out noise and correct inconsistencies. To address these issues, previous works have relied on applying feature selection [7] to eliminate the redundant and inconsistent data and thus improve the capacity of the classifier. Other studies used multiple scaling methods such as normalization and standardization to improve the classification model [5, 6]. Despite the good *theoretical* approach of these methods, the delivered results can be tremendously inconsistent as each of the feature selection or the normalization/standardization methods can deliver a different result and thus selecting the best approach is a time consuming and exhausting process. Another important issue that could be found which is:

- outliers: "*Observation which deviates so much from other observations as to arouse suspicion it was generated by a different mechanism*" Hawkins(1980)

In Data Science, an Outlier is an observation point that is distant from other observations on data that diverges from an overall pattern on a sample. They may indicate variability in measurement, experimental errors or a novelty. The quality and the prediction speed of classifier depend on the input data set for the training thus, the more outliers existing in the training set is, the less accurate the prediction is [7, 8]. In fact the most common causes of outliers on a data set are: (1) Incorrect data entry, (2) Data processing errors: application of inappropriate missing values methods in a dataset, (3) Outliers case did not come from the intended sample and (4) Not an outlier, just a novelty in data.

Instance selection is a recommended technique that was developed to overcome the limitations related to noise and outliers. The aim behind using instance selection is to improve the prediction accuracy of the classifier. To achieve that goal these algorithms are designed to remove outliers and noisy instances. The ensemble learning has become one of the most promising machine learning approaches during the last decade. It takes advantage of combining several models, which when grouped together, can outperform each method with only a linear increase in computational complexity [8]. Several states of the art were included in these groups of algorithms. We include, in the first one, an ensemble of C different models trained on the same training set of data T vote for the output of the instance being classified t. In another state of the art, an extension of the voting approach is presented; where c independent models of different types are trained on the same data set T, then all models outputs are combined for an extra model for the final prediction. Also, a third approach consists of c models of the same type, where each of them is trained on the data set T* that is obtained from T by sampling. The final prediction is obtained by voting. Finally, a similar approach to the previous, but the probability of selecting an instance from T depends on a classification error of the previous models so that an instance that was incorrectly classified by the current models is more likely to be selected.this method called Boosting [8].

For small data sets, noise filtering can be used as a step in the pre-processing of training data; on the other hand, the sampling process which selects a subset of the training set may include or followed by noise and outliers filtering.

In machine learning, Data clustering is frequently used in many fields, such as sampling of data (Stratified sampling) [9]. The mechanism of dividing a set of data to a particular set of groups is termed as clustering, and one such prominent methodology is the k-means clustering. Due to the nature of our available data, its efficiency and its usefulness in several fields of pattern recognition particularly for clustering cancer data, K-means is a well-known unsupervised learning algorithm for data partition with a low computational cost. K-means iteratively reduces the Sum of Squared Error (SSE) from every object to their cluster centroids for every cluster Ck. (SSE) indicates the compactness of the cluster, the lower is, the better is.

Generally, to achieve success ensemble modeling, it recommended ensuring the diversity of the obtained results of each model, which are then combined into a final predictive one. The diversity of the results can be attained in several ways:

- Guarantee diversity of the models: Several different algorithms are used or the same algorithms but with different hyper-parameters or setup.
- Guarantee diversity of the data: we keep the same model, and each subset of the data used for training generates diversity.

In this paper, we address the issue of existing of outliers and noise in small datasets, so that data sampling, the instance selection and data oversampling are combined to ensemble methods and the diversity is obtained by manipulating different algorithms such as K-mean clustering and SMOTE. Our goal is that the ensemble of instance selection algorithm and the Oversampling technique allow us to manipulate the trade-off between the problem of small data sets and prediction accuracy. Moreover, improve both which grouped can outperform each method without an increase of computational complexity. This paper is organized as follows: the next section describes the basic algorithms used in the experiments. The following section describes the testing environment and presents numerical experiments. The last section summarizes the results and presents their interpretation.

3 Model Description

In the presented section, the different stages that compose the followed methodology to construct our approach, as well as the approach itself, are described.

First of all Fig. 1 represent the methodology applied in this work: Data imputation, Data partitioning, Clustering and finally classification. The main aspects of each stage are briefly described.

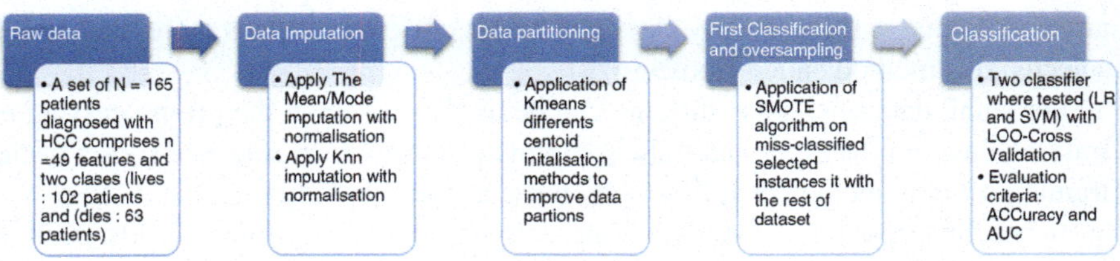

Fig. 1 Followed methodology

We used a HCC dataset composed of N = 165 patients diagnosed comprises n = 49 features provided by UCI machine learning repository.[1] The dataset's class distribution presents 63 cases labeled as 0 (dead) and the remaining 102 cases as 1 (alive) [5]. In the Data Imputation phase, two well-known imputation techniques (Mean/mode and K nearest neighbor) are used to handle missing values with Normalization. According to [10] Cross-validation is a common way of avoiding over-training. Nonetheless, the fundamental problem with this method is the proper partition of data. Simple random sampling is used for most applications. However, a variety of sophisticated methods of statistical sampling suitable for different types of datasets are available. The stratified sampling is one of these methods. The fundamental idea is to investigate the internal structure and distribution of the T dataset and to split T into relatively homogeneous sample groups. The samples were selected from each cluster separately [9]. Various clustering algorithms can be used to divide dataset T into clusters including K-means. For instance, The data sampling phase, in this work, aims to partition the initial data set into a set of tow different partitions by applying classification via clustering method with K-means algorithm for different seed values and three different centroid initialization methods (Random; Kmeans++; Canopy and Farthest first) to ensure diversity of the data. After the data partitioning phase, different resulting partitions are presented and the selection process was based mainly on the SSE that indicates how compact a cluster is: The lower the value, the better. then a manual review is applied to the chosen partitions: correctly labeled instances are kept to learn the classifier, then miss-labeled are used as a supplied test set for the next phase. Once final samples are produced, Our proposed method for selecting the outliers, which is based on the classification error of the previously built model, is performed and the resulting set is oversampled With the SMOTE algorithm. Thus, the oversampled partition is added to the initial dataset and duplicates instances are removed. The final phase consists of fit the classifier with the new augmented dataset. tow classifiers were engaged in this step, which are Logistic regression [11] and Support Vector Machine [12].

Our proposed approach is presented in Fig. 2. It starts by loading the data, then the data imputation is applied on missing values followed by Normalization for features scaling. After the pre-treatment phase, the stratified sampling with k-means is processed with different centroid initialization methods to find better subsets. For the following, and for rigorous scalability, reproducibility, and generalizability, the rest of the process was wrapped by the leave one out cross-validation for underlying subsets selection and the prediction process. It's important to note that the cross-validation strategy guarantees the best performance of the model [13] Step (C) is repeated several times in order to refine the resulting subset. Since the data set is relatively small, each instance is important for the prediction task.

[1]UCI Machine learning Repository, URL: https://archive.ics.uci.edu.

4 Experimental Results and Discussion

Considering the description presented above we have decided to conduct the experiments, which empirically verify the influence of the ensemble learning method on the quality of the instance selection. In the experiments we examine the influence of different parameters on the compression of the training data and the accuracy of the final prediction model.

In our study, we used the Waikato Environment for Knowledge Analysis (WEKA) software V3.8.2 [14] to construct and evaluate the different models. The Weka machine learning workbench offers a general-purpose framework for automated classification, regression, clustering, and selection of features that represents common bioinformatics research data mining issues. This provides a comprehensive collection of machine learning algorithms and data pre-processing methods accompanied by graphical user interfaces for software exploration and practical comparison of various machine learning techniques on the same problem.

For the ensemble of the different used algorithms, basic hyper-parameters were fixed based on several previous tests, such as Number of Nearest neighbor for KNN Imputation n = 1, Number of clusters for the classification via clustering with K-means k = 2 and with different seed numbers (1 to 10); number of iterations of Step (c) in the approach was fixed to t = 5, so each time a new model is created with LOO-CV, then tested with the selected supplied test subset. As shown in Fig. 2; for each iteration of (C): correctly classified subjects are extracted from the test subset and added to the training subset then the process is repeated. For the SMOTE algorithm that based on the similarity between the available minority samples and represents the most popular and applied oversampling procedure, generates synthetic minority

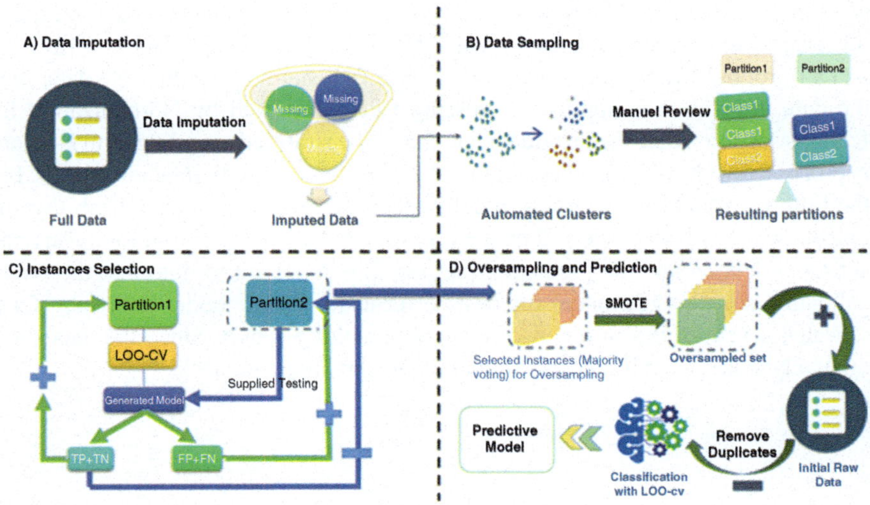

Fig. 2 Schematic representation of the proposed approach

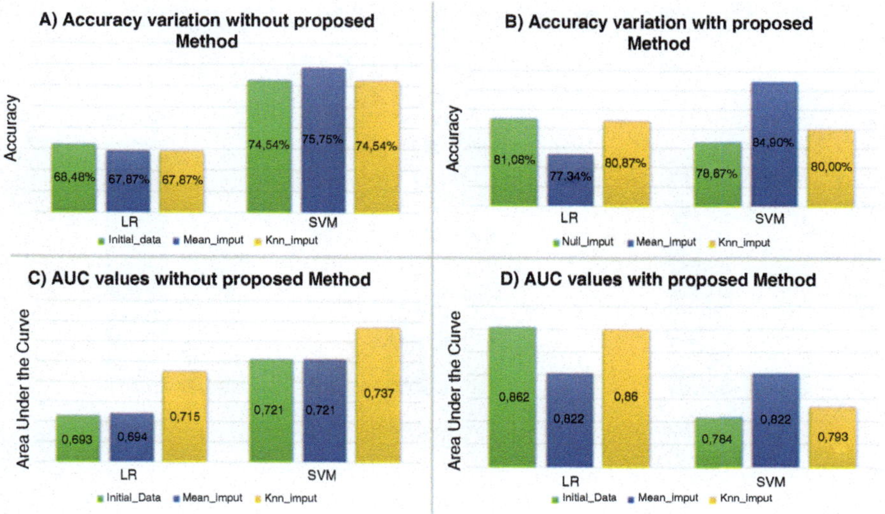

Fig. 3 Comparison the accuracy and AUC of the proposed approach achieved by the instances manipulation for different data imputation and K-means centoid Initialization

samples considering K-nearest neighbors. Thus, different nearest-neighbor values were tested nn = [1,2,3]. Logistic Regression model with ridge estimator = 1.0E-4. Support vector machine model with polynomial kernel and C = 1.0.

All of the experiments were performed on a HCC dataset composed of N = 16 patients diagnosed comprises n = 49 features [4]. Both of the tested algorithms; LR and SVM were tested independently and the results are presented using the Accuracy-Classifier plot and AUC-classifier plot to simplify the interpretation.The obtained results are presented in Figs. 3, 4, and 5. An excellent model with an AUC near to 1, means that it has a good measure of separability. Contrariwise, a poor model with an AUC near to 0 means incapability of separability between classes. When AUC equals to 0.5, it means that the model has no class separation capacity whatsoever.

Hence, in this study, several data mining and machine learning technique were applied; therefore, results were evaluated according to these applied technique. The obtained results show that our approach achieves good results coupled with imputed datasets. In several essays, data imputation didn't ameliorate the model accuracy Fig. 3a with the LR model, instead of the AUC that shows a good response to the imputation with Knn method Fig. 3c. Moreover, the SVM algorithm was sensitive for the applied imputations in terms of ACC and AUC Fig. 3a. The algorithm behaves differently when applying the proposed approach Fig. 3b, d; the accuracy increases remarkably.

Different situations were observed for the LR and SVM algorithms due to the data imputation, the centroid initialization for K-means clustering and SMOTE

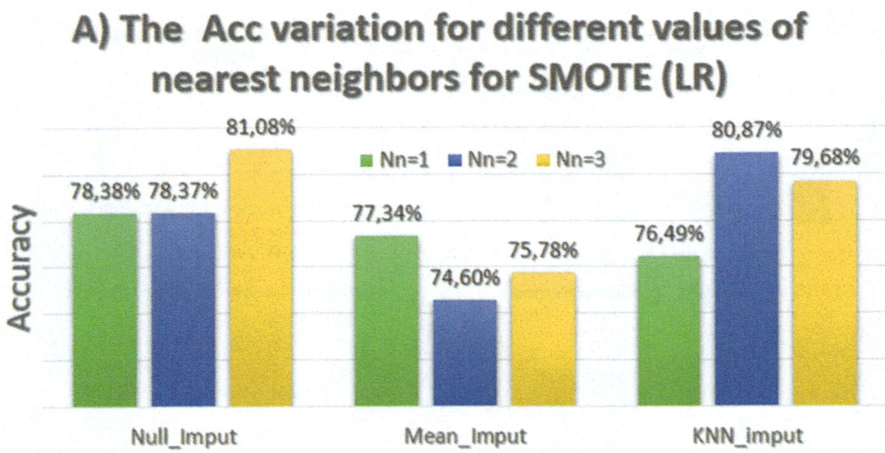

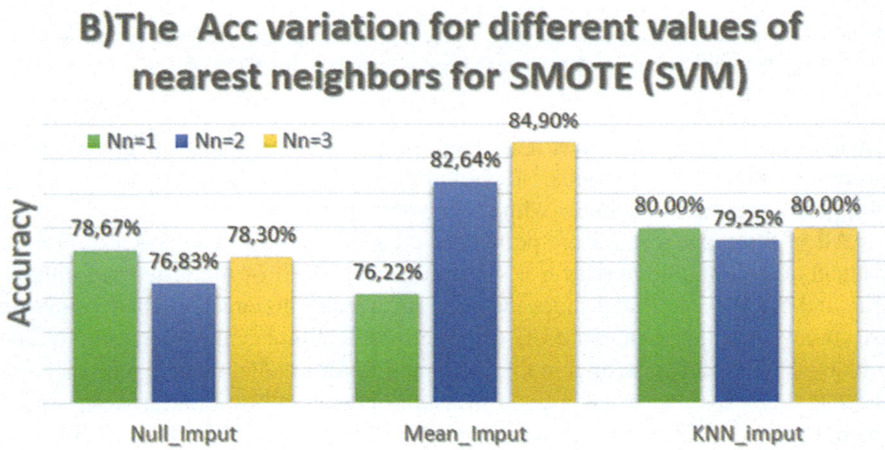

Fig. 4 Comparison the accuracy and AUC of the proposed approach achieved by the instances manipulation for different SMOTE nearest neighbor values

nearest neighbor number Fig. 4; that led to an important diversity of selected instances, hence, conducting to improve the final accuracy.

It can be seen from Fig. 4 that, our method obtained much better performance in the Accuracy and the AUC than the other methods used in [4, 5]. For different parameters of the models, we can improve the accuracy up to 84,90% without any loss of instance or features numbers. It is not possible to define a universal and optimal set of parameters. They must be chosen in each case independently, and based on several experimentation to avoid the wrong choice that cause a significant deterioration in the performance of the model. The advantages of the proposed method are as follows:

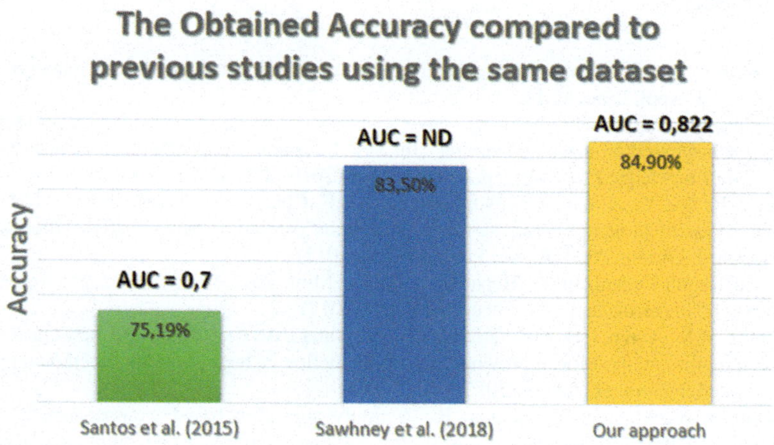

Fig. 5 The Accuracy and AUC achieved by the proposed approach other studies working on the same data set

- Obtained the highest performance (accuracy and AUC).
- Proposed method is robust and accurate as we have employed LOO-CV cross-validation twice (for the Instance selection and the prediction)
- Easy to implement and with a low computational cost.
- Instances selection was used for outliers detection and data oversampling instead of data compression.

5 Conclusion

Nowadays new possibilities open for the use of instance selection methods, in particular in limited and small data sets. These types of applications have two objectives: to improve or maintain the accuracy of the prediction model created on the selected data and to achieve the compression as high as possible. This study aimed to analyze the possibility of using ensemble learning methods to improve the efficiency of instance selection without reducing the size of data. Different data pre-processing techniques associated with learning models were used for this objective. The empirical experiments were performed with the proposed approach, which was based on instances management. The results indicate that it is possible to improve the Accuracy and the AUC while maintaining the initial data size. The approach was able to achieve preforming results compared to other approaches using the same data set.

References

1. El Houby, E.M.F.: A survey on applying machine learning techniques for management of diseases. J. Appl. Biomed. **16**, 165–74 (2018)
2. Maalel, A., Hattab, M.: 'Literature review: overview of cancer treatment and prediction approaches based on machine learning'. In: Smart Systems for E-Health, Advanced Information and Knowledge Processing, p. 324. Springer (2019). ISBN: 978-3-030-14938-3
3. Wu, C.F., Wu, Y.J., Liang, P.C., Wu, C.H., Peng, S.F., Chiu, H.W.: Disease free survival assessment by artificial neural networks for hepatocellular carcinoma patients after radiofrequency ablation. J. Formos. Med. Assoc. **116**, 765–773 (2017)
4. World Health Organization.: Hepatitis C. [online] [cit. 2017-10-15]. Available from: http://www.who.int/mediacentre/factsheets/fs164/en/ (2017)
5. Santos, M.S., Abreu, P.H., García-Laencina, P.J., Simão, A., Carvalho, A.: A new cluster-based oversampling method for improving survival prediction of hepatocellular carcinoma patients. J. Biomed. Inform. **58**, 49–59 (2015)
6. Sawhney, R., Mathur, P., Shankar, R.: A firefly algorithm based wrapper-penalty feature selection method for cancer diagnosis. In: International Conference on Computational Science and Its Applications, pp. 438–449. Springer, Cham (2018)
7. Gamberger D., Lavrač, N.: Filtering noisy instances and outliers. In: Liu, H., Motoda, H. (eds.) Instance Selection and Construction for Data Mining. The Springer International Series in Engineering and Computer Science, vol. 608. Springer, Boston (2001)
8. Blachnik, M.: Ensembles of instance selection methods based on feature subset. Proc. Comput. Sci. **35**, 388–396 (2014)
9. Reitermanova, Z.: Data splitting. In: WDS, pp. 31–36 (2010)
10. Korjus, K., Hebart, M.N., Vicente, R.: An efficient data partitioning to improve classification performance while keeping parameters interpretable. PloS one **11**(8), e0161788 (2016)
11. Kourou, K., Exarchos, T.P., Exarchos, K.P., Karamouzis, M.V., Fotiadis, D.I.: Machine learning applications in cancer prognosis and prediction. Comput. Struct. Biotechnol. J. **13**, 8–17 (2015). https://doi.org/10.1016/j.csbj.2014.11.005
12. Chang, C-C., Lin, C-J.: LIBSVM: a library for support vector machines. ACM Trans. Intell. Syst. Technol. **2**(3), 27 (2011). Article 27. https://doi.org/10.1145/1961189.1961199
13. Nebli, A., Rekik, I.: Gender differences in cortical morphological networks. Brain Imaging Behav. (2019). https://doi.org/10.1007/s11682-019-00123-6
14. Han, J., Kamber, M., Pei, J.: Data Mining: Concepts and Techniques, 3rd edn. Morgan Kaufmann Publishers Inc., San Francisco (2011)
15. Schutte, A.E.: Global, regional, and national age-sex specific mortality for 264 causes of death, 1980–2016: a systematic analysis for the Global Burden of Disease Study (2017)

Towards a Chatbot Based Smart Pervasive Healthcare Medical Emergency Cases

Nourchène Ouerhani, Ahmed Maalel, and Henda Ben Ghézela

1 Introduction

The rise of chatbots inspired many researches to adopt chatbots into healthcare to avail of their multiple advantages. One of the oldest examples includes Eliza [10]. However, to the best of our knowledge, very few works [1–3] use them to manage medical emergencies. In fact, when facing a medical emergency case and human lives are on the line, there is a need of performing an immediate treatment to the victim. Unfortunately,the current prehospital emergency process [6] shows that the emergency medical staff would take a lot of time to locate the emergency incident spot [6]. Even worse, people who are present in the emergency spot may not interfere because most of them have no skills in first aid. Even more severe, there are persons who take advantage of such situations to share it on social media. Given the previously outlined circumstances, a chatbot based smart pervasive healthcare is proposed in this paper in order to save time during medical emergencies and to provide care starting immediately to the victim or his companions. The remainder

N. Ouerhani (✉)
Higher Institute of Applied Sciences and Technology, University of Sousse, Sousse, Tunisia

A. Maalel
Higher Institute of Applied Sciences and Technology, University of Sousse, Sousse, Tunisia

National School of Computer Sciences, RIADI Laboratory, University of Manouba, Manouba, Tunisia
e-mail: ahmed.maalel@ensi.rnu.tn

H. B. Ghézela
National School of Computer Sciences, RIADI Laboratory, University of Manouba, Manouba, Tunisia
e-mail: henda.benghezala@ensi.rnu.tn

L. Chaari (ed.), *Digital Health in Focus of Predictive, Preventive and Personalised Medicine*, Advances in Predictive, Preventive and Personalised Medicine 12,
https://doi.org/10.1007/978-3-030-49815-3_17

of the paper is organized as follows: First, we explain our approach in Sect. 2. Then, we evaluate our work by a test case in Sect. 3. And finally in Sect. 4, we conclude the work and give some future works for interesting research directions.

2 Proposed Approach

The proposed chatbot is designed to be able to help victims or companion perform first aid work properly.

Our proposed chatbot's architecture is depicted in Fig. 1. It is divided into several modules as follows: Input Pre-processor module (IPM), Natural Language Pipeline, Storage module (SM) and Response Engine (RE).

When the chatbot receives a message (text/voice) that will be pre-processed by the IPM to bring out a text whatever is its initial form. In case of a voice input, IPM should convert the speech to text through the speech recognition [4].

Then, the Natural Language Pipeline's main task is to convert the natural language text received form the IPM into a structured format consisting of intents and entities. Thus, to properly realize the natural language processing (NLP), it is required to transform the text to the vector domain which is referred as word embedding [5, 7]. Our solution is to simply train the pre-trained model GloVe [5] on our domain specific medical data. Since the embeddings are already trained and entities are extracted [9], our intent classifier [8] requires only little training to make confident intent predictions that are relative to the ongoing emergency case.

In order to be more efficient our chatbot is able to store all information the user provided once he/she starts communicating with the platform such as location, as well as information gathered during the ongoing discussion in order to influence

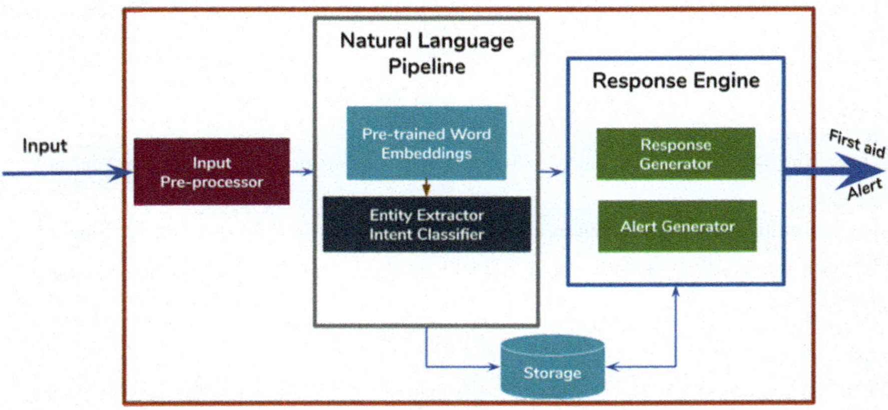

Fig. 1 Architecture of the chatbot based smart pervasive healthcare

how the dialogue progresses. All these data will be consulted later on by the RE in order to respond to the user, or request more information if required.

The RE's task is formulated as a classification problem, over a predefined list of actions for each emergency case. The generated answers are based on the information stored in the SM. An immediately response is generated once there are sufficient information describing the emergency situation, otherwise, if there are some missing information which are crucial for the bot better understand the situation, it will keep requesting information from the user according to the St John DRSABCD action plan[1] that we learnt before having a first aid certification from the civil protection in our Tunisian government. This process will be repeated until the bot has enough knowledge of the emergency victim's state to generate helpful first aid tips. More over, the chatbot is able to send a real time alert to the emergency medical service when the situation presents high risk to the victim and individuals on the scene.

3 Experimental Set Up: Application Development and Deployment

We have developed two separate but inter-dependent applications: The mobile application that will be used by the user and the chatbot back-end. However, the implementation of health information management via mobile devices poses many problems, such as storage and data management so we used the cloud, where each of the proposed modules is written as web services which are exposed as REST API micro services on the cloud, as shown in Fig. 2.

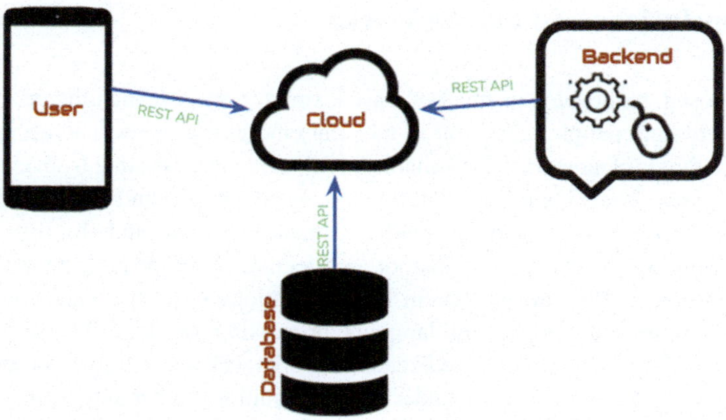

Fig. 2 Implementation of chatbot based smart pervasive healthcare

[1] https://www.stjohnnsw.com.au/drsabcd-action-plan/

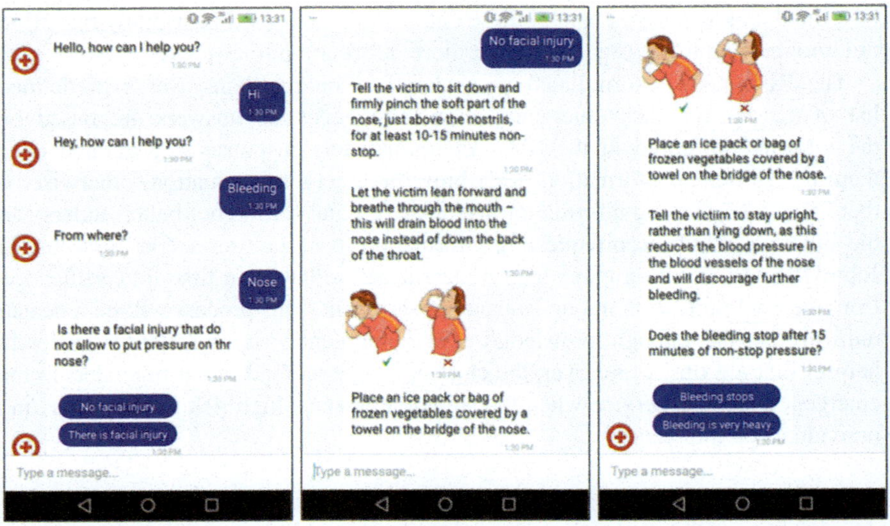

Fig. 3 Responses of Chatbot based Smart Pervasive healthcare amongst a victim suffers from epistaxis (nosebleed)

The chatbot asks specific questions to understand the victim's condition. The user is free whether to write his own answer or to choose one of the answers suggested by the chatbot, this method allows a faster response time from the user. Once the chatbot understands the victim's situation, first aid is performed before aid arrives. The implemented process is shown in Fig. 3.

4 Conclusions and Future Works

We proposed to develop a chatbot based smart pervasive healthcare, which is designed to help people react well in medical emergency cases. The pervasiveness of our chatbot is clear since it is available anytime and is accessible from everywhere and for every body including experts or normal people and it's context-aware since its response differs on the medical emergency case and the user supplies information. We introduced the chatbot architecture by proposing the notion of its several modules. The current system has foundations in each domain including a response engine and other natural language processing tool-kits. We used GloVe to solve the NLP problem in our case because it works well according to our evaluation experiments. The work is still under implementation and much further work is needed to improve our chatbot's capability to manage more emergency cases.

References

1. Tsai, M-H., Chen, J.Y., Kang, S-C.: Ask Diana: a keyword-based chatbot system for water-related disaster management. Water **11** (2019). https://doi.org/10.3390/w11020234, http://www.mdpi.com/2073-4441/11/2/234
2. Chung, K., Park, R.: Chatbot-based heathcare service with a knowledge base for cloud computing. Clust. Comput. (2018). https://doi.org/10.1007/s10586-018-2334-5
3. Srivastava, M., Suvarna, S., Srivastava, A., Bharathiraja, S.: Automated emergency paramedical response system. Health Inf. Sci. Syst. **6**, 22 (2018). https://doi.org/10.1007/s13755-018-0061-1
4. Mohammed, M., Badruddin Khan, M., Bashier, E.: Machine learning: algorithms and applications. Mach. Learn. Algorithms Appl. (2016). https://doi.org/10.1201/9781315371658
5. Pennington, J., Socher, R., Manning, C.: Glove: global vectors for word representation. In: Proceedings of the 2014 Conference on Empirical Methods in Natural Language Processing (EMNLP), pp. 1532–1543, Association for Computational Linguistics, Doha (2014). https://doi.org/10.3115/v1/D14-1162, http://aclweb.org/anthology/D14-1162
6. Söderström, E., van Laere, J., Backlund, P., Maurin Söderholm, H.: Combining Work Process Models to Identify Training Needs in the Prehospital Care Process. In: Johansson, B., Andersson, B., Holmberg, N. (eds.) Perspectives in Business Informatics Research, pp. 375–389. Springer International Publishing, Cham (2014)
7. Mikolov, T., Chen, K., Corrado, G., Dean, J.: Efficient estimation of word representations in vector space, CoRR, abs/1301.3781 (2013). http://arxiv.org/abs/1301.3781
8. Chang, C-C., Lin, C-J.: LIBSVM: a library for support vector machines. ACM TIST **2**, 27:1–27:27 (2011)
9. Lafferty, J.D., McCallum, A., Pereira, F.C.N.: Conditional random fields: probabilistic models for segmenting and labeling sequence data. In: Proceedings of the Eighteenth International Conference on Machine Learning, pp. 282–289. Morgan Kaufmann Publishers Inc., San Francisco (2001). http://dl.acm.org/citation.cfm?id=645530.655813
10. Weizenbaum, J.: ELIZA & Mdash; a computer program for the study of natural language communication between man and machine. Commun. ACM **9**, 36–45 (1966). ACM, New York. http://doi.acm.org/10.1145/365153.365168

A Tool for Multi-scale Modeling of Software Architectures: Application to the Smart Home for Telemonitoring Elderly People at Home

Ilhem Khlif, Mohamed Hadj Kacem, Khalil Drira, and Ahmed Hadj Kacem

1 Introduction

The design of a software architecture is a complex task. On the one hand, we have to describe the system with enough details for understanding without ambiguity and implementing in conformance with architects requirements and users expectations. On the other hand, we have to master the complexity induced by the increasing model details both at the human and automated processing levels. So, there is a need for a new approach that automates the construction of the design architecture and guarantees its correctness. An iterative modeling process that helps architects to elaborate complex but yet tractable and appropriate architectural models and specifications can be implemented by successive refinements. Providing Rules for formalizing and conducting such a process is our objective, which we implemented in visual modeling notations. For this purpose, we propose to consider different architecture descriptions with different levels of modeling details called **"the scales"**. We define a step-wise iterative process starting from a coarse-grained description and leading to a fine-grained description. We propose a modeling solution to describe software architectures using a visual notation based on the UML graphic language [1]. UML is a standard modeling language defined by the OMG. These diagrams are submitted to vertical and horizontal transformations. The intermediate models provide a description with a given abstraction that

I. Khlif · M. H. Kacem (✉) · A. H. Kacem
University of Sfax, ReDCAD Research Laboratory, Sfax, Tunisia
e-mail: ilhem.khlif@redcad.org; mohamed.hadjkacem@isimsf.usf.tn; ahmed.hadjkacem@fsegs.rnu.tn

K. Drira
LAAS-CNRS, Université de Toulouse, Toulouse, France
e-mail: khalil.drira@laas.fr

L. Chaari (ed.), *Digital Health in Focus of Predictive, Preventive and Personalised Medicine*, Advances in Predictive, Preventive and Personalised Medicine 12,
https://doi.org/10.1007/978-3-030-49815-3_18

allow the validation to be conducted significantly while remaining tractable w.r.t. complexity. The validation scope can involve intrinsic properties ensuring the model correctness w.r.t. the UML description. To ensure model consistency, our approach supports model transformation and validation of UML models with OCL constraints. In order to experiment our approach, we tested it with a predictive and preventive system dedicated to the smart home application for maintaining personalized medicine at home. This system is helpful for people with loss of autonomy, exposed to risks of accidents or needing a precise daily medical follow-up. The remainder of the paper is organized as follows. In Sect. 2, we describe the multi-scale approach in Sect. 2. Section 3 presents the e-health application dedicated to the smart home for the homecare of elderly people. We conclude and outline some perspectives in Sect. 4.

2 Approach in a Nutshell

We propose a multi-scale modeling approach for software architectures [2, 5]. The proposed design approach is founded on UML notations and uses component diagrams. The diagrams are submitted to vertical and horizontal transformations for refinement; this is done to reach a fine-grain description that contains necessary details. The model transformation ensures the correctness of UML description, and the correctness of the modeled system. UML provides a formal language, the Object Constraint Language (OCL), to define constraints on model elements. Our approach supports model transformation and validation of UML models with OCL constraints [4].

The approach supports the modeling of multi-scale architectures using the semi-formal language UML. We propose a modeling solution to describe software architectures using a visual notation based on the UML graphic language. UML is a standard modeling language defined by the OMG [6]. The UML diagrams make it possible to present the structural properties as well as the behavioral properties of the multi-scale architecture. These diagrams are submitted to vertical and horizontal transformations. The intermediate models provide a description with a given abstraction that allow the validation to be conducted significantly while remaining tractable w.r.t. complexity. The validation scope can involve intrinsic properties ensuring the model correctness w.r.t. the UML description. To achieve this, we propose a set of model transformation rules. The rules manage the refinement and abstraction process (vertical and horizontal) as a model transformation from a coarse-grain description to a fine-grain description. To ensure model consistency, our approach supports model transformation and validation of UML models with OCL constraints. The choice of using OCL is motivated by its wide adoption in the MDE approach and the fact that it is a standard formal language supported by OMG. The second phase ensures validation of the model with the OCL language. Consequently, we have defined constraints on the elements of the model using OCL language. Tools are used to check and validate OCL constraints such as the

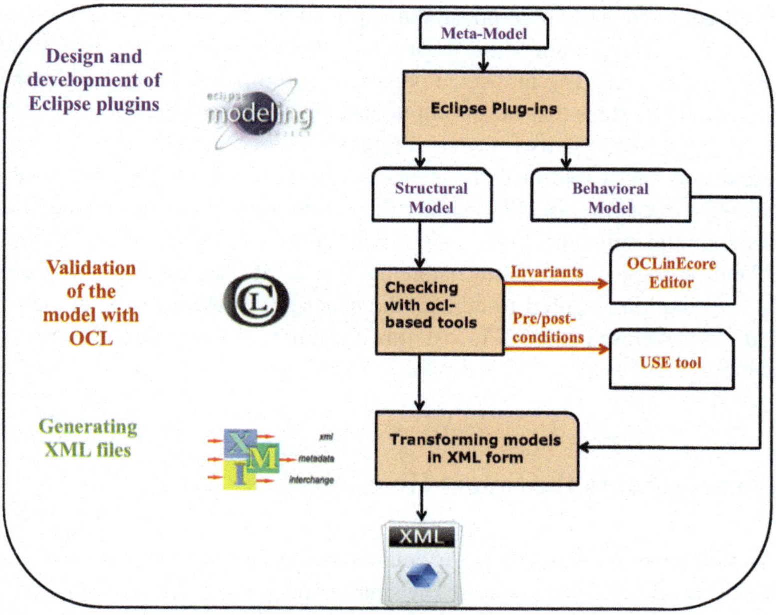

Fig. 1 Description of used tools for multi-scale modeling

OCLinEcore Editor to validate the invariants and the USE tool to validate the pre/post conditions. The third phase allows XML files to be generated using XMI, which transforms the models into XML. So we can get the XML file of the templates that we created. Figure 1 shows the different used tools during the design process.

2.1 Multi-scale Modeling

We present the multi-scale approach by a two-dimensional array describing vertical and horizontal scales [3]. The top-down scale transformation process, much like regular refinement, begins with a high level description of a system which we describe as a whole. Then, scale changes are applied to obtain a more detailed description, by describing components and connections. An iterative modeling allows to refine software systems descriptions. The vertical scales add the architecture decomposition details to obtain a more detail on the internal architecture of previously defined components. The horizontal scales describe or give details on the interconnections between components and their interfaces. We iterate on the architecture until reaching the details necessary to verify the associated architectural properties. The first scale Sv_0 begins with specifying the application requirements. It defines the whole application by its name. Two horizontal refinements called horizontal scales are associated with the first scale Sv_1. The first horizontal scale shows all components that compose the application. The second one describes the links between those components. Four horizontal refinements are associated with the second scale Sv_2. The first scale presents subcomponents for components, and enumerates all the roles that each component can take. The second one identifies the list of communication ports for each component, and refines those roles. The third one shows the list of interfaces for communication ports. The last one is obtained by successive refinements while adding the list of connections established between components and subcomponents. This scale allows us to define the architectural style. With a graphical modeling language like UML, we are not able to express all the information required to convey the exact information of the domain in the diagram. We propose to use OCL to define constraints on models to define the well-formedness rules of our iterative design process.

3 Application to the Smart Home System

This section focuses on modeling the smart home system for the homecare monitoring of elderly and disabled persons. The smart home constituent elements are largely distributed in the house area. The main issue is to ensure efficient management of the optimized comfort, and the safety of the elderly and disabled person at home. We specify the essential information architecture and we illustrate, in (Fig. 2), the constituent elements of the smart home System. The monitoring center is

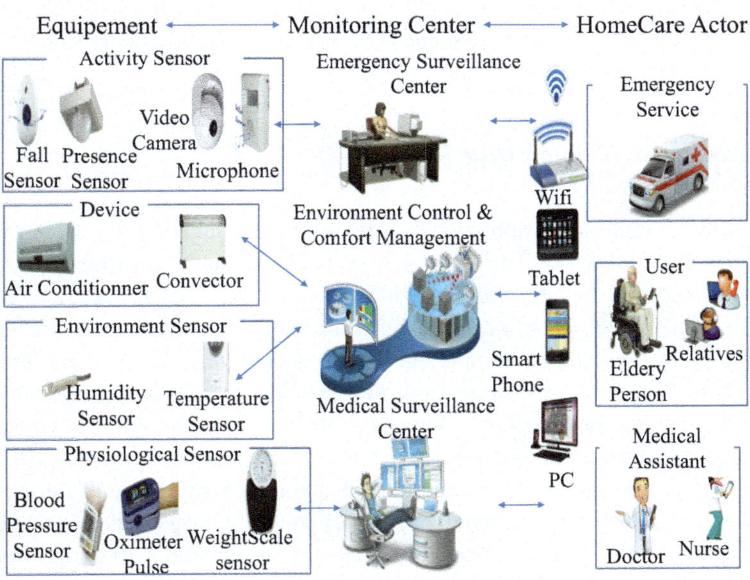

Fig. 2 Smart home system

composed of three systems:the Environment Control and Comfort Management, the Emergency Surveillance Center, and the Medical Surveillance Center. Thus, the actors selected who interact with other entities of the system are: The Home Care Actor, who interacts with the monitoring center, by setting medical or emergency conditions. The Equipment, that includes sensors and house devices. The emergency surveillance center controls critical situations using the activity sensors. In order to track the presence, activity sensors can be installed in each room. Activity sensors include fall sensors, presence sensors, video camera and microphone. The sensors send urgent signals to the center which treats immediately the received information. Once the signal is correct and the situation is critical, the center call the Emergency Medical Service to react and help the person. The medical surveillance center monitors physiological sensors. To track the medical information, physiological sensors can be installed in the bed, the chair, and on the body to detect the O2 level, the blood pressure, and the weight. The functions are achieved by the Oximeter, the Pressure Sensor, and the Weight Scale Sensor, classified as physiological sensors. While there are problems, the center requires the medical assistant intervention (the doctor, the nurse). The comfort management and the environment control system guarantees a comfort life for the users which are the elderly person and his relatives. This center enables communications between users, control the environment sensors (Humidity and Temperature Sensors), and commands the house devices (Convectors, Air conditioners). We are interested in studying the smart home system established for the home monitoring of elderly and disabled persons at home.

3.1 Structural Features

We experiment our approach by applying successive iterations to the smart home SoS. We illustrate the implemented iterative process applied to the smart home system. We obtained then the following results: In $S_{0.0}$, we define the application named "*SmartHome*". The constituent systems of the smart home are described (in $S_{1.1}$): *HomeCare-Actor*, *Equipment*, and *MonitoringCenter*. Those systems communicate with each other via the monitoring center. Those participants communicate with each other via the monitoring center. Those relationships are represented (in $S_{1.2}$) as links. UML associations. We also illustrate instances obtained in the next scale. We apply successive model transformation operations to add the following composites: *MedicalAssistant, EmergencyService, User, Physiological-Sensor, Activity-Sensor, Environment-Sensor, House-Device, MedicalSurveillance-Center, EmergencySurveillanceSystem, and EnvironementControlAndComfortManagement*. The *MonitoringCenter* plays the role of an "*EventDispatcher*". The *HomeCare-Actor* and *Equipement* play roles of "*Producer-Consumer*" in the application. $S_{2.1}$ allows to add the list of the ports for each component. We briefly describe the list of required/provided services of the *HomeCare-Actor* component. The *MedicalAssistant* receives information about the patient's situa-

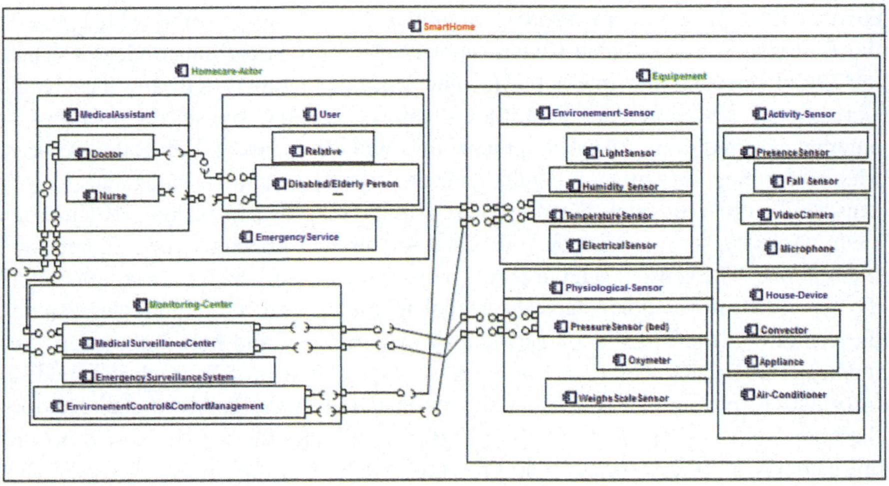

Fig. 3 Structural modeling applied to the smart home (Scale Sv_3/Sh_3)

tion from the *MedicalSurveillanceCenter*, he manages the patient's medical care (provides) and return a report after the care. The *EmergencyService* receives information about a critical situation *EmergencySurveillanceCenter*, reacts to save the patient (provides), and return a report after the intervention. The *User* receives not only emergency and medical services but also comfort services like online communication or house device command provided by the *EnvironementControl And ComfortManagement* component. $S_{2.2}$ assigns to each port an interface of the type provided or required according to the type of service. Finally, we indicate at the scale $S_{2.3}$ connections established according to the used topology and we define the "*Publish-Subscribe*" style. We implemented Eclipse plugins that allow multi-scale modeling of a software architecture based on the component diagram and the sequence diagram. We have checked and validated the OCL constraints under Eclipse (the structural part) and with the USE tool (the dynamic part). Finally, we have presented the level of instances of our case study using the Eclipse plugins (Fig. 3).

4 Conclusion

In this paper, we applied the multi-scale modeling approach on a case study for a predictive and preventive system dedicated to the smart home application for maintaining personalised medicine at home. This system is helpful for people with loss of autonomy, exposed to risks of accidents or needing a precise daily medical follow-up. We have experimented and evaluated the functional and the performance aspect of our approach as well as the functional aspect of our developed tool supporting the multi-scale modeling approach for software architectures. In our future work, we expect to apply the multiscale modeling approach to other complex use cases for e-health applications for public health.

References

1. Khlif, I., Hadj Kacem, M., Hadj Kacem, A.: Iterative multi-scale modeling of software-intensive systems of systems architectures. In: Proceedings of the Symposium on Applied Computing, SAC 2017, Marrakech, 3–7 Apr 2017, pp. 1781–1786 (2017)
2. Khlif, I., Hadj Kacem, M., Hadj Kacem, A., Drira, K.: A multi-scale modelling perspective for SoS architectures. In: Proceedings of the 2014 European Conference on Software Architecture Workshops, ECSAW 14. Association for Computing Machinery, New York (2014)
3. Khlif, I., Hadj Kacem, M., Hadj Kacem, A., Drira, K.: A UML-based approach for multi-scale software architectures. In: 17th International Conference on Enterprise Information Systems (ICEIS), pp. 374–381 (2015)
4. Khlif, I., Hadj Kacem, M., Stolf, P., Hadj Kacem, A.: Software architectures: multi-scale refinement. In: 14th IEEE International Conference on Software Engineering Research, Management and Applications, SERA 2016, Towson, 8–10 June 2016, pp. 265–272 (2016)
5. Khlif, I., Tounsi, I., Hadj Kacem, M., Eichler, C., Hadj Kacem, A.: A refinement-based approach for specifying multi-scale software architectures: application to sos. In: Proceedings of the 33rd Annual ACM Symposium on Applied Computing, SAC '18, pp. 1660–1667. ACM, New York (2018)
6. UML, O.M.G.: Unified modelling language: Infrastructure (2011)

Index

L. Chaari (ed.), *Digital Health in Focus of Predictive, Preventive and Personalised Medicine*, Advances in Predictive, Preventive and Personalised Medicine 12,
https://doi.org/10.1007/978-3-030-49815-3

The manufacturer's authorised representative in the EU is Springer Nature Customer Service Centre GmbH, Europaplatz 3, 69115 Heidelberg, Germany. If you have any concerns regarding our products, please contact ProductSafety@springernature.com

Printed and bound by CPI Group (UK) Ltd, Croydon, CR0 4YY
28/09/2026
02224092-0012

Bioregional Planning and Design: Volume I

David Fanfani • Alberto Matarán Ruiz
Editors

Bioregional Planning and Design: Volume I

Perspectives on a Transitional Century

Springer

Editors
David Fanfani
Architecture Department-Dida
Florence University
Florence, Italy

Alberto Matarán Ruiz
Urban and Spatial Planning Department
University of Granada
Granada, Spain

ISBN 978-3-030-45869-0 ISBN 978-3-030-45870-6 (eBook)
https://doi.org/10.1007/978-3-030-45870-6

This Springer imprint is published by the registered company Springer Nature Switzerland AG.
The registered company address is: Gewerbestrasse 11, 6330 Cham, Switzerland

Contents

Contributors

Dimas Wisnu Adrianto School of Environment, Education and Development, The University of Manchester, Oxford, UK

Christides Anastasios Bureau of Environment and Civil Protection (GPDE), GR, Elefsis, Greece

Mavrakis Anastasios Institute of Urban Environment and Human Resources, Department of Economic and Regional Development, Panteion University, GR, Athens, Greece

Tasopoulos Anastasios Institute of Urban Environment and Human Resources, Department of Economic and Regional Development, Panteion University, GR, Athens, Greece

Stefano Bocchi Department of Environmental Science and Policy, State University of Milan, Milan, Italy

Gianluca Brunori Department of Agrarian, Food and Agro-environmental Sciences, University of Pisa, Pisa, Italy

Agata Cabanek Curtin University Sustainability Policy (CUSP) Institute, School of Design and the Built Environment, Curtin University, Perth, Australia

Michela Chiti Architecture Department, Florence University, Florence, Italy

Papavasileiou Christina Secondary Education Directorate of West Attica, Greek Ministry of Education, GR, Mandra, Greece

Andrea Colantoni Department of Agricultural and Forestry Sciences (DAFNE), Tuscia University, Viterbo, Italy

Anna Maria Colavitti DICAAR – Department of Civil and Environmental Engineering and Architecture, University of Cagliari, Cagliari, Italy

Pavel Cudlin Global Change Research Centre, Academy of Sciences of the Czech Republic, České Budějovice, Czech Republic

Sergio De La Pierre School of Architecture, Florence University, Milan, Italy

Manuel Delgado Cabeza AREA Research Group, Department of Applied Economics II, University of Seville, Seville, Spain

Roselyne de Lestrange Faculté d'architecture, d'ingénierie architecturale, d'urbanisme (LOCI) & Metrolab.brussels, Université catholique de Louvain, Ottignies-Louvain-la-Neuve, Belgium

Pierre Donadieu École Nationale Supérieure du Paysage de Versailles, Marseille, France

Verouti Eleni Bureau of Environment and Civil Protection (GPDA), GR, Aspropyrgos, Greece

David Fanfani Architecture Department-Dida, Florence University, Florence, Italy

Dominique Gauzin-Müller Architect, école nationale supérieure d'architecture de Strasbourg, Strasbourg, France

Maria Rita Gisotti Architecture Department-Dida, Florence University, Florence, Italy

Joseli Macedo School of Design and the Built Environment, Curtin University, Bentley, Australia

Alberto Magnaghi Architecture Department, Florence University, Florence, Italy

Liakou Margarita Bureau of Environment and Civil Protection (GPDA), GR, Aspropyrgos, Greece

Alberto Matarán Ruiz Urban and Spatial Planning Department, University of Granada, Granada, Spain

Peter Newman Distinguished Professor of Sustainability, Curtin University Sustainability Policy (CUSP) Institute, School of Design and the Built Environment, Curtin University, Perth, Australia

Antonio Ortega Santos Department of Contemporary History, Faculty of Bachelor and Arts, Granada University, Granada, Spain

Coline Perrin UMR INNOVATION, Univ Montpellier, CIRAD, INRAE, Institut Agro, Montpellier, France

Daniela Poli Architecture Department-Dida, Florence University, Florence, Italy

Paolo Prosperi Department of Agrarian, Food and Agro-environmental Sciences, University of Pisa, Pisa, Italy

Joe Ravetz Manchester Urban Institute, The University of Manchester, Oxford, UK

Juan Requejo Liberal At Clave, Seville, Spain

Luca Salvati Department of Economics and Law, University of Macerata, Macerata, Italy

Claudio Saragosa Architecture Department, Florence University, Florence, Italy

Cividino Sirio Department of Agriculture, University of Udine, Udine, Italy

Marta Soler Montiel AREA Research Group, Department of Applied Economics II, University of Seville, Seville, Spain

Kyvelou Stella Institute of Urban Environment and Human Resources, Department of Economic and Regional Development, Panteion University, GR, Athens, Greece

Robert L. Thayer Department of Human Ecology, University of California, Davis, CA, USA

Mingjie Wang Zhejiang International Studies University, Hangzhou, China

Carolina Yacamán Ochoa Department of Geography, University Complutense of Madrid (Es), Madrid, Spain

Ilaria Zambon Department of Agricultural and Forestry Sciences (DAFNE), Tuscia University, Viterbo, Italy

Maria Elena Zingoni de Baro School of Design and the Built Environment, Curtin University, Bentley, Australia

About the Editors

David Fanfani PhD, is Associate Professor of Urban and Regional Planning in the Department of Architecture at Florence University and lecturer in the Master of Science Course in Regional Planning and Design and the Master of Science Course in Architecture of Florence School of Architecture. His research activity focuses especially on analysis and design at the regional scale, addressing matters mainly related to peri-urban areas and reconnection between city and countryside, which, according to an integrated and cross-disciplinary bio-regional approach, aims to the recovery of a co-evolutionary relation between urban and rural domain. On these subjects, Prof. Fanfani authored several publications and articles at national and international level.

Alberto Matarán Ruiz is PhD in Environmental Science and Associate Professor at the University of Granada. Prof. Ruiz has been researching and teaching at the University of Granada since 2003. He is a professor in several postgraduate programs including Urbanism, Regional Planning and Environment, Agroecology, and International Cooperation. In the professional field, Prof. Ruiz is environmental specialist in the local administration and previously worked for the Environmental Agency of the Province of Cordoba, Argentina. He is researching visitor at the University of Manchester, UK; University of Central Lancashire, UK; Florence, Italy; Buenos Aires, Argentina; Universidad de la República, Uruguay; and Universidad Santo Tomás, Colombia. Prof. Ruiz has authored more than 100 publications within his research interests, initially centred on water and spatial planning, and more recently on landscape and planning, food planning and short food supply chains, and local sustainability in peri-urban contexts all around social participation.

Introduction to Bioregional Planning. Relocalizing Cities and Communities for a Post-oil Civilization

David Fanfani and Alberto Matarán Ruiz

1 The Crisis of Civilization: From Development to Post-development

The last global economic crisis, which affected much of the planet since it broke out in 2008, is just one of the many representations of a civilization crisis which threatens to extinguish the very existence of the human species. It is increasingly clear that the problem is not due to a lack of development but to the capitalist and predatory nature of development itself, a concept that has always been linked to the idea of progress. This idea, in turn, is connected to the value system created within the history of the Western civilization (López and Matarán 2011).

The current notion of development implies, among other issues, the colonization of the world by the Global North, the economic war (Testot 2014, pp. 441–446) and the plunder of nature, as shown by Latouche (2007). By drawing a parallel between medical science and the notion of development, Naredo (2009) suggests that the unhealthy striving for economic growth and the available technologies within globalization intensify and 'turn the human species into a terrestrial pathology, similar to cancer in its effects on territory'.

It is thus important, in the current situation, to return to the idea that the crisis goes far beyond a concept or discourse of development to be modified. As stated by Edgar Morin:

The chapter is the result of a shared reflection and conception; nevertheless, paragraphs 1, 2, 4, 7 have to be attributed to Alberto Matáran Ruiz, whereas David Fanfani wrote paragraphs 3, 5, 6, 8.

D. Fanfani (✉)
Architecture Department-Dida, Florence University, Florence, Italy
e-mail: david.fanfani@unifi.it

A. Matarán Ruiz
Urban and Spatial Planning Department, University of Granada, Granada, Spain

D. Fanfani, A. Matarán Ruiz (eds.), *Bioregional Planning and Design: Volume I*,
https://doi.org/10.1007/978-3-030-45870-6_1

> … it is indeed an auto-partial crisis, a cultural crisis of civilization, an industrial-economic crisis, Western crisis, Eastern crisis, Southern crisis and planetary crisis. The ecological crisis concerns just one aspect, one symptom of a much more radical crisis. This affects the principles of intelligibility of the settled beliefs and driving force myths of our civilization. In this very sense we are allowed to name it as a crisis of civilization. (Morin 1995)

2 The Global Ecological Crisis as a Matter Related to the Human Settlement Rift with Nature

According to Toro Sànchez (2011), the ecological crisis could be defined as «an exponential change in human ecological involvement in the Biosphere as a whole». It entails two fundamental defining facts:

> Human beings are capable of producing changes and alterations on environmental variables with a planetary scale effect, because of their development and activity on environment.

On the one hand, "Human beings are capable of producing changes and alterations on environmental variables with a planetary scale effect, because of their development and activity on environment. [On the other hand], we define it as a crisis because it is an emerging situation with no appearance of being sustainable. It can be described as a shortage between the material demand of planetary human metabolism and the supplies nature can provide in quantitative terms. But this shortage must be assessed in more complex terms, in view of the fact that the risk does not only derive from the depletion or deterioration of resources but from a loss in physical and environmental functions and mechanisms which are necessary for human development" (Toro 2011).

It is then a systemic crisis, stemming from an economic growth model whose unsustainability—in material, energetic and ecological terms—had already been envisioned with precision some years earlier, though not properly taken into account (Meadows et al. 2004; Georgescu-Roegen 1976). Its main feature is a high entropy level, meaning an irreversible deterioration of the relation between energy and matter and a deep alteration of complex ecosystems (Odum 1988). A model which is now showing the limits of the immoderate trust paid by modernity in technology.

Unfortunately, based on the tangible effects, can we appraise in retrospect the accuracy of those anticipatory considerations?

It is clear that we are currently suffering from the effects of environmental system inertia and previous impact accumulation. This is the reality in spite of the modest governmental attempts to reduce the causes of the environmental crisis in the future (Riechmann 2018).

Built environment and human settlements are therefore affected by such factors and processes that heavily damage the ecosystem. The amplification of the crisis itself is fostered by processes of growing concentration and exponential growth of urban domain (UN 2015; EEA 2006). These features, in turn, are strongly led by productive specialization at the global level (Polanyi 1944) and by the unbalanced prevailing 'extractive' model of capitalistic accumulation (Sassen 2012, 2014). Unsustainable and unmanageable manifold forms of urban and metropolitan agglomeration are then developed at regional level (Soja 2000; Wheeler 2011). That even under the phenomenology of a 'global gentrification' process that affects human settlements as a whole—also blurring, in spatial and functional terms, urban rural divide (Brenner and Schmidt 2015)—as one of the main (spatial) tools to cope with the financial crisis and perpetuate the capital accumulation mechanism (Lees et al. 2016).

3 Issues for Sustainable Settlements Patterns and Design

Built environment produced by anthropogenic actions is being called into question by the global geo-climatic drift, not only as a field affected by the global warming effects but also as a tool which has proven ineffective in reversing the described processes.

In this framework, then, climate change, desertification, inundations, droughts, extreme weather conditions, sea-level rise, massive extinction of species and loss of fertile soil merge and mutually reinforce with the above-mentioned urbanization patterns. That raises up many issues that represent a huge set of challenges and set up a remarkable endeavour in recovery and designing a balanced, sustainable and fair human settlement. A commitment that should aim for a twofold objective:

On the one hand, it should contribute to developing strategies aiming to reverse the long-term trends which led to the ongoing environmental crisis. On the other hand, it should strive to connect the former issue to an endeavour to mitigate the global change effects, primarily the climate change ones, through pro-active, adaptive and defensive strategies of the human settlements. That also envisioning sustainable settlement patterns, models and design solutions at the various scales.

Consequently, planning must address this twofold problem—joint issues of development and spatial forms—and revise its methodologies and approaches. Both the traditional and current 'modern' knowledge which define the care of the historic environment must be taken into account; moreover, these sources of information ought to be connected and revitalized through a proper and contextual use of either 'appropriate' or innovative technologies.

Territory and human settlement matters, and the related environmental, social and economic dimensions, should then be considered a crucial factor in re-building and recovery of a life-supporting environment and no longer a destructive one. A renewed co-evolutionary relationship between nature and culture, and among technology, natural environment and shared social values, must be established (Norgaard 1994), resulting in newly-recovered capabilities to reproduce territory as a 'high complexity living being' structured and composed by 'neo-ecosystems' (Magnaghi 2011, p. 97) as results of a balanced mankind/nature interaction.

Thus, human settlements and the redefinition of territory interpretation and design models have a central and strategic role related to the possibility of reversing previously described trends and the general framework—as well as including a strong bottom-up mobilization in the territories themselves.

On the basis of these assumptions and before introducing the urban bioregion model in the context of the bioregional approach, a recall of some specific points may be helpful in showing the ways modernity and the recent global financial drift of the capitalist model of accumulation have involved human settlements, influencing their features. Features that are also conceived and managed as a tool for reproducing the aforementioned development model.

4 The Crisis of the City and the Territory: Deterritorialization

As we just pointed out, modern mentality has had a deep impact on the urban area and the territory, reductionism being one of its key components. The humanist Greek conception, which is still valid today (De Manuel 2007), included and integrated the concepts of *urbs, polis* and *civitas*, aiming for a balance between the settled entity and the settlement. But the Modern Age specialization upset that balance.

In Ancient Roman culture, a balance among *firmitas* (firmness—strength), *utilitas* (commodity—utility), and *venustas* (delight—beauty) was subsumed in the *ars aedificandi* (art of edifying). Then, in Leon Battista Alberti's view, that balance had to be revised during the Renaissance, according to the needs of human activities, resulting in *necessitas*, *commoditas* and *concinnitas* (necessity, utility, harmony). Nevertheless, the increasing influence of economy and technical, scientific and financial powers has reduced the current mentality to only *utilitas* and *necessitas*.

The main reason for this is a limited understanding of the nature of the urban and territorial phenomenon, which is confined to the mere management of shapes and volumes in space, and to the organization of objects and artefacts, such as buildings, streets, canals, networks and other infrastructures, with the belief that—above all thanks to technologies, matter and energy disposal—it may be the solution to all human problems.

Although widely criticized, this reductionism can be found nowadays. The origin of some current principles in planning can be traced back, at least in part, to Le Corbusier conceptions. In the words of the prominent Rationalism promoter within the Modern Movement, territory 'as a tormented entity must be flattened and regulated in order to build the essential functions of a rational city in every country of the world'. (Corbouisier 1963).

In this way, contemporary cities are tending to an unprecedented condition, influenced by technological development and the use of non-renewable energy sources (mainly fossil sources). It is the megalopolis form, a pattern which is endlessly repeated and told to be the climax of the urban and human evolution by institutionalized media, but which is, in fact, proving unsustainable in current use (Magnaghi 2011 cit., Davis 2006).

The growing tendency to lose autochthonous territorial values in cultural processes—such as planning and the territory project which lies behind—is at the basis of the *deterritorialization of metropolis* (Magnaghi 2011, cit, pp. 23–44). Its origins can be traced back to the hegemonic replication of an unsustainable development model, resulting in a loss of cultural and ecologic diversity. In other words, while technology—it seems—'liberates' human society from territory and culture, severe environmental impact and social inequalities are produced in the process, due to the unequal access to technology, inter alia.

The loss of the 'circular' and co-evolutionary relationship between urban and surrounding environmental domain is well represented by modern productivist agriculture model and farmland exploitation. In fact, agriculture is 'de-territorialised, that is, carried on without any reference to protection and reproduction of regional land, soil quality and ecosystem viability, with no commitment to supplying local market with fresh and healthy food, and finally with a complete lack of local knowledge, competence and skill enhancement' (Altieri 1989; Gliessman 1997). Land, soil, environment and farmers' capabilities had to adapt to the myths—and connected equipment and inputs—of the so-called 'green revolution' and of its supposed increasing crops. Such processes, which have appeared from the outset of the industrial market economy, originated with the disintegration of the ecological and productive 'proximity' connections between urban domain and surrounding region area. The consequence is a critical 'ecologic rift' between city and countryside, which was first envisioned and well described in Marx's seminal writings (Bellamy Foster 1999).

This model is widely represented by the disciplinary approaches of planning, historically based on a developmental view (Fariña Tojo 2011) that is completely unaware of agro-environmental and ecological matters. The strongly sectorial methodology of this approach has proved neither able to mitigate nor reduce the severe impact on the landscape and the environment, which is a consequence of the territorial transformations due to the economic dynamics and planning.

5 Energetic and Socio-ecologic Transitions as the Main Issue in the 'Century of the Great Challenge': Recovering the Centrality of 'Place'

The above-mentioned multidimensional crisis determines a high degree of unsustainability in the current world system, where the possibility of a civilization's breakdown does not seem to be remote (Diamond 2005).

An integrated and multidisciplinary approach is thus necessary in order to set out a reinterpretation of planning and multiscalar tools in territorial project. Connections among different areas of activity should be considered, in order to face the aforementioned problems and by adopting a place-based focus.

In this framework, the energy matter must be considered as a fundamental one. As a matter of fact, the above mentioned progressive detachment between cities and surrounding regions was triggered and fostered by the 'fossil energy regime' as the driving force behind modernity, and its apparently everlasting and cheap supply of power (Jancovici 2013). That detachment was one of the main bases on which local and global development set off. Consequently, the energy, matter and information proximity flows that had previously characterized—although not exclusively—such a relationship were substantially weakened.

As a result, city and settlement forms started to base on private car hyper-mobility, ecosystem destruction and the concentration of directional activities in a few world 'core cities', both—albeit with different features—in the global North and in the global South (Sassen 2012, cit.). Two seemingly opposing joint processes were then entailed: a strong polarization of the human settlements in some 'city regions' or 'megalopolis' on a planetary scale (Neumann and Hull 2011), alongside with a remarkable spreading of residential, tertiary and commercial activities, featuring 'low density' and quality urban habitat.

In this context, the degradation of peri-urban rural spaces is noteworthy. These areas, which used to be an essential part of cities and towns' living system, being a key element for the survival and prosperity—now for sustainability—of settlement systems, have been and are being destroyed, irrevocably at times. Causes can be found in residential, commercial and industrial urban growth, as well as in the constant construction of infrastructures, in a twofold way: directly, with the physical occupation of the space, and indirectly with the degradation processes engendered by this growth-based territorial model on the surrounding areas. Some examples of these processes include areas which are abandoned in view of a possible 'urbanization', territory fragmentation, destruction of the heritage and agricultural infrastructures, dispersion of pollutants and waste, and the pressure of the population on open spaces among others. Furthermore, 'fossil energetic turn' also triggered another important driver in this direction that relates to the hyper-productivity and globalization aims of food system productions. In this framework, peri-urban farming has undergone a strong loss of profitability owing to its weakness in the context of the globalized and specialized agri-food system that also transformed food production in the framework of commodities market.

In the energy domain, a large-scale transition is then a crucial demand: it would mean a solution for the problem of carbon sink depletion and the climate crisis it produces, as well as for the depletion of energy sources related to different peaks of availability in fossil fuels. Furthermore, an analogous transition is highly necessary in order to deal with the problems of an ever-growing part of the population, whose access to natural resources is being reduced by the overexploitation caused by the voracity of the global consumer class (Sachs 2011).

Based on the aforementioned considerations about the energy regime of modernity, the change of this regime itself could entail a radical shifting towards more sustainable economies and settlement patterns (Rickwood 2009; Hopkins 2008;

Newman 2009; Thayer 2013, Jancovici, *cit* 2012, pp. 203–215). In these, the territorial framework is conceived and featured as a system where the information, energy and matter flows are continuously exchanged between built and natural environment, at a regional and local scale primarily.

Conceptualizing the socio-ecological transitions in spatial terms, that is, focusing on the place they are planned to occur, is one of the fundamental tasks in this 'Century of the Great Challenge' (Riechmann 2013) we are facing. It is, in fact, a key approach, since all social processes have an effect on space and the transition alternatives must find their way to connect with the place they set in.

6 The Bio-regional Model and the Urban Bioregion as a Basis for the Re-localization of Local Development and Human Settlements

As we have seen, the contemporary metropolitan model, which has been shaping the territory for more than a century, is characterized by a voracity which is «topophagous» (place-destroying), hypertrophic (producing an exacerbated growth) (Magnaghi 2011, *cit.*) and carcinogenic (Naredo 2009).

As we have seen, recovering the environmental quality and sustainability of the built environment implies the necessity of regenerating and rebuilding some underpinning relationships of proximity and co-evolution between urban settlement and the relative 'eco-regions'. That, especially, requires inhabitants and communities to recover not only the sovereignty principle but, as well, the willingness and wisdom to use and administer territory resources in a regenerative way. Thus, according to this goal, the different articles in the present volume intend to explore the hypothesis of a regionalist approach recovery and, mainly the bioregionalist one. This can be defined as a cross-disciplinary paradigm suitable to conceive, analyze and design a territorial context fitting with the recovery and enhancement of the complementary relationships between geo-ecosystems and anthropogenic factors, city and countryside, nature and culture.

In pursuing that aim, the volume mainly refers to the contribution inherited in the planning domain by the seminal works proposed in the twentieth century by Patrick Geddes' activity and writings, the American regionalism of Regional Planning Association of America of Mumford and McKay and W. Odum's Southern Regionalism (Friedman and Weaver 1979, pp. 29–41), up to the most recent works and ideas proposed—in a meaningful, although not complete, continuity with the former—by the North American bioregional movement, especially by authors, planners and social activists, such as K. Sale, P. Berg, R. Dasmann and others (Sale 1991; Berg and Dasmann 1977; McGinnis 1999; Thayer 2003).

This extensive and multifaceted legacy left by the aforementioned 'bioregional' authors serves here as a theoretical, methodological and practical framework that the book primarily aims to recover and adopt. That with the aim to point out some principles and methodological issues that may prove strategic in facing the problematic framework which has been described. They can be summarized as follows:

- *co-evolutionary approach between natural environment and anthropogenic action.*

This point refers to the need to recover an operational, complementary and balanced relationship between natural environment and anthropogenic action. During civilization's history, the 'proximity' interactions' between nature and culture, technology and cultural progress, communitarian values and political principles of government and development were featured as a whole in a specific regional domain. It had been the most common relationship before the advent of the fossil energy era, which introduced the 'de-territorializing' factors in former 'discursive communities' (Norgaard 1994 cit.pp. 165–167). The co-evolutionary view overcomes the risk to adopt a deterministic environmental approach—that could be pointed out in some recent bioregional contributions—privileging a 'possibilistic' model of human development. In our view, the interaction between technical capabilities, environment and culture originates territorial structures and forms as complex 'neo-ecosystems' (Magnaghi 2011 cit., p. 91) or a 'second-nature' (Clement 2012): innovative elements ruled by a joint action of natural laws and of the human 'eso-somatic' tools and knowledge capabilities (Beatley 2011).

From this perspective, sustainability of human environment refers to the construction of systems of virtuous relationships between the territory components (natural environment, built environment and anthropic environment). In this way, as Magnaghi points out (2011, *cit*), 'territory' stands as a reference for sustainability, while 'natural environment' is considered a part of it. Hence the requirements for sustainability are modified by including the enhancement of the relationships among culture, nature and history, which lies at the heart of the bio-cultural memory as defined by Víctor Toledo and Narciso Barrera-Bassols (2008).

- *self-reliance and self-provisioning* vs self-sufficiency: towards a circular bioregional economy

The prospect of the regional re-embedding of human settlement doesn't entail the research of new forms of fanciful bounding and autarchic parochial closure. In the bioregional view, the ideal territorial level should host forms of settlement whose life is guaranteed, to the greatest extent possible, by the circular relationships and flows of matter, energy and information, which is achievable within their surrounding 'proximity' territory. This evidently implies an economic principle of both *self-reliance* and cooperation, in conceiving bioregionally settled urban domain and regions (Scott Cato 2013; Thayer 2013), based also on a principle of import-replace economic development innovative model (Jacobs 1984). Obviously the self-reliance principle, although excluding the self-sufficiency idea, entails a strong commitment on behalf of local communities to the recovery of sovereignty on their reproductive principles and to the fair and balanced use of regional resources and endowments (Pezzoli and Leiter 2016) without excluding a mutual and cooperative exchange with other regions lacking and not producing *loco* goods and artefacts.

- *governance bottom-up and federal cooperation, local willingness and universal values*;

The recovery of sovereignty in the use and management of regional resources of the settlement areas entails the support and enhancement of the administrative political control over the territory itself, at the local level. Nevertheless, the current expulsive and 'extractive' processes and mechanisms that global economy triggered worldwide (Sassen 2014, cit) lead the deliberative and decision-making power at the regional/local level to be increasingly taken over by the central—national or transnational— one. Such forces are usually characterized by an 'extra-territorial' nature, so that the set up international and national public bodies and rules of control are not able to deal with them.

These public bodies and rules do not seem to be capable anymore of competing against the financial drift of globalization. On several occasions, they actually resemble the simulacrum of the legitimacy and legal principles that they were created to ensure. Obviously, the much needed change of political prospect and policy practice would not automatically create ideal local communities: the bioregional principles of sovereignty, subsidiarity and shared responsibility will only be followed thanks to a governance and deliberative approach commitment. The self-government and federalist idea that underpins the bioregional political model, as well as the transition processes in general (Foxon 2011), have an 'incremental', piecemeal growth and 'constructive' nature. That is to say, they imply starting from the existing practices of self-government, even if they may be restricted in scope and may raise only limited issues. Those practices, especially the ones related to the use of commons, may work as an initial enzyme posed at an appropriate scale (Sale 1991, cit. pp. 52–66) for starting a process of empowerment, awareness-building and sense of belonging to places on behalf of the inhabitants and local communities as a whole. The principal aim would be, according with the bioregionalism basic principles, re-learning rules and inhabiting place rules in a shared, responsible and participated way. Consequently, the bioregion is not to be generally conceived as a matter of fact, especially on the post-metropolis horizon. Rather, it should be considered a project or a 'concrete utopia' and a process of democratic, participative and deliberative empowerment in the territory government and use forms.

Finally, it is worth noting, as argued by Mumford, such a principle of participative democracy and regional collaboration or subsidiarity is not the antithesis, but a complement of the more general shared legacy of universalistic and ruling principles of mankind on earth (Mumford 1938). This is a guarantee against risks of selfish parochial closure and, moreover, it aims to foster and protect plurality, differences and solidarity between different communities and cultures.

- *From the bioregion to the urban bioregion*

The bioregional model emphasizes the historical role of mankind and the organizational forms of settlement in modelling basic endowments of geo-ecosystemic nature. Related to this, the growing pervasive role of the urban development, at the planetary scale, leads to conceive such a paradigm or territorial model not only as an 'underpinning image' in supporting new plans, projects and practices to inhabit places. Besides that, it also serves as a tool to regenerate and recover the built environment as an already configured whole, characterized by heavy de-structuring phenomena in social, functional and environmental aspects of everyday landscape. In this sense, in these volumes, a shift is stressed, passing from the possible drift of the bioregionalism as a philosophy mainly committed with ecologically-minded visions where the issue of settlements stands in the background, to the more integrated concept of *urban bioregion* (Atkinsons 1992; Magnaghi 2014), according to which the bioregional paradigm is conceived as a set of ruling references, even for the urban domain, strongly connected to the agro-ecosystemic and long-lasting geo-structures of the surrounding areas (Calthorpe 1993, Church 2014).

The starting premise is that urban matters and domain still remain a non-negligible condition of the social, cultural and economic organization of the human communities, even if they require to gain a deep revision and criticism in their recent development patterns. An urban condition that, besides, in the late modernity, has assumed plurality of forms in spatial and social qualitative terms. And, as well, a dimensional prevalence in terms of land-taking and demographic thickness. That either considering its quantitative expansion—frequently under the unsustainable patterns of urban sprawl—and, moreover, referring to its capacity to exert a form of "remote control" and exploitation on area spatially far from urbanized systems.

7 Volume Aims, Topics and 'Spirit'

The analyses and proposals collected in this book that we have edited in two volumes under the name *Bioregional planning and design*, are written by a group of internationally recognized authors who are working, although not exclusively, on bioregional planning, especially in the European context. Our aim is not one to present an exhaustive theoretical and methodological body about bioregional planning. It turns out to be impossible at this stage of practices and reflections. More modestly, we try to collect some key points of view and practices that seem to converge—more or less explicitly and at least for some elements—towards a bioregional way of approach in planning and regional/urban design. That of trying to trigger and foster—mainly in the European context—a possible vision and debate about a place-based, bottom-up approach to planning, viable to jointly focus on endogenous local development and sustainably built environment design. As we explain below, volume I of the book reflects some general and preliminary approaches to bioregionalism. They are complemented by different ways of combining planning with bioregionalism, making reference to some basic concepts like commons, justice, biophilia, and the urban-rural relation. Whereas in volume II, sectoral approaches are presented, addressing some key points as energy, soil protection, urban ecosystem, heritage, agroecology and food sovereignty. To end this volume, we include some practical examples, where some 'bioregional-like' approaches are being adopted either in a social or political framework, mainly in the European context.

In this volume I *Bioregional Planning and Design. Perspective on a transitional century*, Part I, 'Rethinking places for community life', aims to render a framework of development visions that imply and require a new co-evolutionary relationship between human settlements, place resources and environment. In those visions, the bioregional approach is the main reference, although it is articulated in different, yet complementary, points of view (see Thayer and Magnaghi articles). The pivotal issue is the special attention to be paid to the recovery of a regional economy based on a self-sustainable, reproductive use of resources on behalf of localized human societies (Soler and Delgado Cabeza chapter) according with metabolic and ecological principles that underpin a low entropy model of settlement development, as shown in the Saragosa and Chiti chapter.

Finally, a critical review of the dimension of spatial fairness and justice as the pivotal component of a bioregional approach to be explored is then carried on by Colin Perrin in her Chapter. In this contribution is assessed the way how bioregional paradigm relates to justice conceptions and theories, concerning especially environmental resources, spaces and land access. The contribution highlights how—although with possible threat of some parochial closures—a bioregional approach is basically endowed and suitable to foster an inclusive planning model for a redistributive and fair process of resources distribution to cope with socio-spatial inequalities. A model that contrasts with the current, top-down and 'extractive' development and planning models.

In a nutshell, this part intends to set the general reference points of a bioregional idea of development that will be afterwards better evaluated, through some general issues, about spatial planning domain, in Part II.

Then, Part II—'Reframing planning in bioregional sense'—aims to deal with some general spatial matters that strongly connect with the practice of the spatial planning domain. These matters lead to a general integrative, place-based and re-territorialized approach to planning and design. They explore the following questions:

- The biophilic approach, conceived as a methodological and practical vision where nature and wildlife newly integrate with built environment. As a result, quality improvement of settlements is supported, and the challenges of climate change impacts at different scales are took on as well (Newman, Cabanek chapter).
- The wide and multidimensional perspective stemming from a new transitional and relational conception of the urban/rural interface as a domain to be explored for the recovery of an innovative urban/rural mutual support according a multi-scale vision (Fanfani chapter).
- The role of 'commons' as shared and heritage goods on which underpin a regenerative, shared, and bioregional practice of landscape planning and design and territory social reconstruction (Donadieu chapter).
- Analysis methods, design and planning for regional food delivering schemes or systems which contribute both to a lasting and circular post-oil re-localization of energy and matter flows, and to a wider reconstruction of a fair and healthy

bioregional economy. The main point being how to best interact with spatial features, city/countryside relationships and with the general planning system in the context of a cross-disciplinary dialogue (Brunori chapter).

Finally, a conclusive Short Glossary chapter by Gisotti is aimed to provide an integrative contribution to allow readers better comprehension of several key conceptual/disciplinary categories and technical/special terms adopted in the Italian territorialist planning approach and which have been used/introduced especially in the Magnaghi chapter. Categories that are of background reference for many other chapters in this book. The main goals are firstly to deepen and best contour the meanings that such categories convey, mainly relating to the cultural milieu where they originate, and second, to let readers appraise similarities and differences of their use in such a context with the ones possible in Anglophone cultural/disciplinary domain, conceived in a wider sense. We hope that terms and categories included in the glossary section would help readers better understand their meaning and contribute to bridging communication gaps that might be caused by misunderstanding in translation from Italian to English words, hopefully enhancing and underpinning a fruitful international dialogue.

As mentioned, this volume—as part of a whole unique book—has a continuation in a second one published under the title: *Bioregional Planning and design, Issues and Practices for a Bioregional Regeneration*. This complementary volume aims to describe and select some matters that represent compelling elements to be treated in planning domain—also several European and international experiences of innovation for that field—and well-fitting with a bioregional approach.

8 Final Remarks. Recovering a New Relationship Between Regional Development and Spatial Planning: A Prospect for Bioregional Governance

As shown by the previous points, the bioregional approach represents a paradigm in the field of physical planning, as well as a reference framework aiming to support self-reliant communities and local bottom-up development schemes. Therefore, the bioregional project refers not only to the domain of spatial planning and regional and urban design but also to a new approach towards the goals and methods in public policy creation, in the field of local and socioeconomic development. Without this kind of awareness and scope, the bioregional model would represent, at best, a good repository or toolkit for the mitigation of some of the problems that affect regions and cities as a whole.

Accordingly, the strong connection between territory and landscape amenities is acknowledged, together with the call for a sustainable management of regional endowments and the fostering of local development processes. Furthermore, we highlight the unavoidable socioeconomic decline threat for regions and communities that were not able to cope with a suitable control over global dynamics of transnational financial power and to 'engage' global capital at the local level (Power 1996). In this sense, reversing the point of view makes it possible to point out that the construction of resilient regions under the economic-productive prospect necessarily means to foster 'proto-bioregional' settlement frameworks based on endogenous development processes. Especially, according to Cato and Cato and James, innovative and fair production-consumption connection schemes have to be enhanced at the regional scale (Scott Cato 2013; Scott Cato and James 2014).

Within this perspective, it is worth indicating that the bioregional approach to planning deeply affects—and interacts with—the policy sciences, political economy and local development governance domains. This approach means to set out and aspire to a shared governance model of deliberative and participative democracy for the enhancement of the increasingly weakened forms and institutions of the representative democracy. The aim is to give back to local communities the non-negligible commitment to practice willingness and sovereignty, with the purpose of the protection and stewardship of their own life-places.

In this direction, the educative and didactic commitment, aimed to promote self-help and self-development, acknowledged to planning in the regionalist and bioregional approach (Mumford 1938 *cit.*, Friedmann and Weaver 1979: cit. pp. 37–40, Sale 1991, *cit.*, Thayer 2003: pp. 52–70), becomes a pivotal factor and value, and underpins the volumes' aims. Nevertheless, on occasion, this implies the opportunity and the necessity to adopt critical and 'radical' planning approaches (Friedmann 1987; Forrester 1989). These are suitable to pursue and achieve the necessary empowerment in reframing decision-setting on the part of local communities, in the direction of a model of community-led local development (CLLD) practices, which have been positively recognized even by the EU commission (EU 2014).

In conclusion, the aim is to pursue, through regional planning and design practices, an alternative local and urban development approach, which may best fit and foster sustainability targets, fixed by many global government bodies. As a consequence, the current problems, originated by climate change effects and economy unfairness, may be tackled. Whereas, on the side of the territorial settlement structure, the growing polarization and hierarchization of the urbanizing processes, which overwhelm the capabilities of regional and local governance and decision level, may be reversed.

References

Altieri, M. (1989). Agroecology: A new research and development paradigm for world agriculture. *Agriculture, Ecosystems and Environment, 27*(1–4), 37–46.

America Planning Association. (2007). *APA Policy guide on community and regional food planning,* https://www.planning.org/policy/guides/adopted/food.htm. Accessed 3 Mar 2019.

Atkinsons, A. (1992). The urban bioregion as sustainable development paradigm. *Third world Planning Review, 4*(14), 327–354. (Liverpool University: Liverpool).

Beatley, T. (2011). Biophilic cities. In *Integrating nature into urban design and planning.* Washington D.C: Island Press.

Bellamy Foster, J. (1999). Marx's theory of metabolic rift: Classical foundations for environmental sociology. *American Journal of Sociology, 105*(2), 366–405. University of Chicago.

Berg, P., & Dasmann, R. (1977). Reinhabiting California. *The Ecologist, 7*(10), 399–401.

Brenner, N., & Schmidt, C. (2015). Towards a new epistemology of the urban? *City, 19*(2–3), 151–182.

Calthorpe, P. (1993). *The next American Metropolis: Ecology, community, and the American dream*. Princeton: Princeton Architectural Press.

Church, S. P. (2014). Exploring urban bioregionalism: A synthesis of literature on urban nature and sustainable patterns of urban living. In *S.A.P.I.E.N.S.* 7(1) http://sapiens.revues.org/1691. Accessed 12 Jan 2020, 1–11.

Clement, T. G. (2012). *Jardin, Paysage et génie naturel*, College de France. Paris: Fayard.

Corbouisier, L. (1963). *Manière de penser l'urbanisme*. Geneve: Éd. Gonthier.

Davis, M. (2006). *Planet of slums*. London/New York: Verso.

De Manuel, E. (2007). (2007). Participar para recuperar la Polis. In J. Encina et al. (Eds.), *La ciudad a escala humana. Democracias participativas 5* (pp. 89–102). *Sevilla*: Atrapasueños, Unilco, ACS.

Diamond, J. (2005). *Collapse*. London: Penguin.

European Commission. (2014). *Community-led local development*. http://ec.europa.eu/regional_policy/sources/docgener/informat/2014/community_en.pdf. Accessed 12 Jan 2020.

European Environmental Agency. (2006). Urban sprawl the ignored challenge, EEA Report n.10/2006, Luxembourg.

Fariña Tojo, S. (2011). El plan de urbanismo ante los límites del crecimiento. Necesidad de nuevos instrumentos para organizar la ciudad del siglo XXI. In A. Matarán Ruiz & F. López Castellano (Eds.), *La Tierra no es muda: Diálogos entre el desarrollo sostenible y el postdesarrollo* (pp. 259–271). Universidad de Granada: Granada.

Forrester, J. (1989). *Planning in the face of power*. Berkeley: University of California Press.

Foxon, T. J. (2011). A coevolutionary framework for analysing a transition to a sustainable low carbon economy. *Ecological Economics, 70*(12), 2258–2267.

Friedmann, J. (1987). *Planning in the public domain*. Princeton: Princeton University Press.

Friedmann, J., & Weaver, C. (1979). *Territory and function. The evolution of regional planning*. Chicago: Edward Arnold.

Georgescu-Roegen, N. (1976). *Energy and economics miths*. New York: Pergamon Press.

Gliessman, S. R. (1997). *Agroecology: Ecological processes in sustainable agriculture*. New York: CRC, Press/Taylor & Francis.

Hopkins, R. (2008). *The transition handbook. From oil dependency to local resilience*. Dartington: Chelsea Green Publishing.

Jacobs, J. (1984). *Cities and the wealth of nations. Principles of economic life*. Vintage, New York.

Jancovici, J. M. (2013). *Transition energetique pour tous*. Paris: Odile Jacob.

Latouche, S. (2007). *Decrecimiento y posdesarrollo: El pensamiento creativo contra la economía del absurdo*. Barcelona: El Viejo Topo.

Lees, L., Shin, H. B., & López-Morales, L. (2016). *Planetary gentrifications*. Cambridge: Polity Press.

López, F., & Matarán, A. (2011). *La Tierra no es muda: Diálogos entre el desarrollo sostenible y el post desarrollo*. Granada: Universidad de Granada.

Magnaghi, A. (2011). *Il progetto locale*. Bollati Boringhieri, Torino (2th edition enhanced, English edition, 2005, *The urban village. A charter for democracy and local self sustainable development*. London: Zed Book).

Magnaghi, A. (2014). *La bioregion urbaine. Petit traité sur le territoire bien commun*. Paris: Eterotopia France-Rhizome.

McGinnis, M. V. (Ed.). (1999). *Bioregionalism*. London: Routledge.

Meadows, D., Meadows, D., & Randers, J. (2004). *Limits to growth: The 30-year update*. Vermont: Chelsea Green Publishing Company.

Morin, E. (1995). *Principios de los cambios sociales del Siglo XX, Sociología*. Madrid: Tecnos.

Mumford, L. (1938). *The culture of the cities*. New York: Harcurt Brace.
Naredo, J. M. (2009). *Luces en el Laberinto: Autobiografía intelectual*. Madrid: Los Libros de la Catarata.
Neumann, M., & Hull, A. (Eds.). (2011). *The future of the city regions*. London/New York: Routledge.
Newman, P. (2009). A vision for resilient cities. In P. Newman (Ed.), *Resilient cities. Responding to peak oil and climate change* (pp. 55–85). Washington D.C.: Island Press.
Norgaard, R. B. (1994). *Development betrayed. The end of progress and a coevolutionary revisioning of the future*. London/New York: Routledge.
Odum, H. T. (1988). Self-organization, Transformity, and information. *Science, 242*(4882), 1132–1139. https://doi.org/10.1126/science.242.4882.1132.
Pezzoli, K., & Leiter, R. A. (2016). Creating healthy and just bioregions. *Reviews on Environmental Health, 31*(1), 103–109.
Polanyi, K. (1944). *The great transformation*. New York: Farrar& Rinehart.
Power, T. (1996). *Lost landscapes and failed economies, the search for a value of places*. Washington D.C.: Island Press.
Rickwood, P. (2009). *The impact of physical planning policies on households energy use and greenhouse emissions*, PhD thesis, Faculty of Design., Architecture and Building, Faculty of Technology, Sydney, https://opus.lib.uts.edu.au/handle/10453/35060. Accessed 15 May 2019.
Riechmann, J. (2013). *El siglo della gran prueba*. Tegeste (Tenerife): Baile del Sol.
Riechmann, J., Carpintero Redondo, O. Mataràn Ruiz A. (eds) (2018). Para evitar la barbarie: Trayectorias de transición ecosocial y de colapso. Granada: Universidad de Granada.
Sachs, W. (2011). Globalización, convergencia y modelo de desarrollo euro-atlántico. En López, F. y Matarán, A. *La Tierra no es muda: Diálogos entre el desarrollo y el postdesarrollo*. Granada. Editorial Universidad de Granada. España.
Sale, K. (1991). *Dwellers in the Land. The bioregional vision*. Gabriola Island (BC): New Society Publisher/New Catalyst
Sassen, S. (2012). *Cities in a world economy*. Los Angeles: Sage Publishing.
Sassen, S. (2014). *Expulsion. Brutality and complexity in the global economy*. Cambridge: Cambridge University Press.
Scott Cato, M. (2013). *The bioregional economy, land, liberty and the pursuit of happiness*. London: Routledge.
Scott Cato, M. & James F. R. (2014). From resilient regions to bioregions: An exploration of green post-keynesism. *Post Keynesian study group, working paper* 1407, www.postkeynesian.net
Soja, E. (2000). *Postmetropolis: Critical studies of cities and regions*. Oxford: Blackwell Publishing.
Testot, L. (2014). *Cataclysmes. Une histoire environnementale de l'humanité*. Paris: Payot.
Thayer, R. L. (2003). *LifePlace. Bioregional thought and practice*. Berkley: University of California Press.
Thayer, R. L. (2013). The world shirks the world expands: Information, energy and relocalisation. In E. Cook & J. Lara (Eds.), *Remaking METROPOLIS. Global challenges of the urban landscape* (pp. 39–59). London, Routlege.
Toledo, V. M., & Barrera-Bassols, N. (2008). *La memoria biocultural: La importancia ecológica de las sabidurías tradicionales*. Barcelona: Ed. Icaria.
Toro Sànchez, F. J. (2011). Crisis ecológica y Geografía: Planteamientos y propuestas en torno al paradigma ecológico-ambiental. Tesis doctoral. Universidad de Granada. 2011.
United Nations. (2015). Department of Economic and Social Affairs, Population Division (2015). World population prospects: *The 2015 Revision, Key Findings and Advance Tables*. Working Paper No. ESA/P/WP.241, https://esa.un.org/unpd/wpp/Publications/Files/Key_Findings_WPP_2015.pdf. Accessed 5 Jan 2020.
Wheeler, S. (2011). Regions, megaregions and sustainability. In M. Neuman & A. Hull (Eds.), *The futures of the City region* (pp. 95–105). Milton Park: Routledge.

A Bioregional Bridge Across the Urban-Rural Divide

Robert L. Thayer Jr

1 Premise

One of the most important, yet often overlooked, philosophical questions of today is: What should be global, and what should be local? Another way of asking might be: At which scales, in which places, and by what means are the most important human endeavors appropriate? It is, perhaps, the most crucial question in all of human geography, yet its answer, or *answers*, will bear upon the lives of all other living things, and maybe even the future of life itself.

For the past 40 years, various individuals and groups have dedicated their careers from different perspectives, and by different means, to one singular conclusion: that the best way to ensure a sustainable and resilient future for human and non-human life is through thoughtful consideration and dedicated "reinhabitation" of one's life-place, or *bioregion*. Over time, a recognized body of theory and practice has evolved that recognizes the limitations of globalism. Instead, a relatively new social movement, with both a theoretical framework and multiple examples of grounded application, offers an alternative, geographic-centered approach to life on earth by approaching and solving environmental and social problems one natural region at a time.

In a book published in 2003 (*LifePlace: Bioregional Thought and Practice)*, I wrote:

> A *bioregion* is literally and etymologically a "life-place"[1]—a unique region definable by natural (rather than political) boundaries with a geographic, climatic, hydrological, and ecological character capable of supporting unique human and nonhuman living communities. Bioregions can be variously defined by the geography of watersheds, similar plant and animal ecosystems, and related, identifiable landforms (e.g., particular mountain ranges, prairies, or coastal zones) and by the unique human cultures that grow from natural limits

R. L. Thayer Jr (✉)
Department of Human Ecology, University of California, Davis, CA, USA
e-mail: rlthayer@ucdavis.edu

D. Fanfani, A. Matarán Ruiz (eds.), *Bioregional Planning and Design: Volume I*,
https://doi.org/10.1007/978-3-030-45870-6_2

> and potentials of the region. Most importantly, the bioregion is emerging as the most logical locus and scale for a sustainable, regenerative community to take root and to *take place*. (Thayer 2003, p. 3)

Various authors in this book will elaborate on the concepts I mentioned above. However, "Bioregional thought and practice" is just a name; a label to make description easier. Most of the actions on the ground that are truly "bioregional" do not self-refer to that name at all. However, just because a label for the activity is not often mentioned in practice does not mean the activity itself and the thought behind it are not happening. Before I wrote *LifePlace,* there were no professional schools of "bioregional planning"; now, several have renamed their regional planning programs or departments as "bioregional planning," as they acknowledge that there is something essential to such natural place-based theory.

This particular geographic focus has emerged from a wide variety of theoretical origins: "tributaries," if you will, or domains of endeavor that contribute to the main channel of bioregional practice. In the United States, contributors to this "watershed" of theory include the original bioregionalists, Ray Dasmann, Peter Berg, Kirkpatrick Sale, and the poet, Gary Snyder; regional planners, such as Ebeneezer Howard, Patrick Geddes, Lewis Mumford, and Ian McHarg; geographers (abiotic, plant and animal), like Alfred Wallace, Miklos Udvardy, C. Hart Merriam, Frederick Clements, and Robert Bailey of the US Forest Service; economists, such as E. F. Schumacher and Jane Jacobs; social theorists, like Canada's John Ralston Saul and Montana's Daniel Kemmis; and place-based writers, such as Wendell Berry, Wes Jackson, Ursula LeGuin, Terry Tempest Williams, and David Robertson.

Fundamentally, a life-place approach begins from two perspectives: the *land* and the *individual.* One must first understand that all life flows from the stuff beneath our feet and above our head: rock, soil, water, and air. In a stair-step fashion, life gradually builds upon that ultimate foundation to include weather patterns, plant and animal ecosystems, age-old human survival and living strategies, artistic and celebratory practices, trading and economic structures, land planning and building, and finally, personal and social responsibility, leading to stewardship and resilience. Inherent in a bioregional or territorialist approach is a sense of intimate *practice:* enacting the skill, knowledge, and dedication necessary to permanently dwell on, or inhabit, the landscape in its fullest context.

Nearly a half century has passed, wherein countless examples of this kind of practice have taken place throughout regions of the world. Watershed stewardships are routinely established; "friends of …." groups have formed to protect vast marshlands, mountain ranges, coastlines, forest regions, expanses of tundra, and every other conceivable unique geographic feature. Ancient crop-growing or fish-catching regions are defended by those who have learned their stewardship over generations. Non-profit foundations have been established to teach urban citizens that they are part of a larger, natural region. All of these phenomena recognize the essential role human behavior plays in the practice of permanence and reverential inhabitation.

However, in the past several decades, a growing philosophical and political gap between rural and urban populations of the United States has arisen. As a long-time

American proponent, author, and formerly cheerful booster of bioregional thought and practice, I will confess to be intensely concerned by what I have called the "Great American Divide." While similar developments may be occurring elsewhere in the world, I can only address the problem from the vantage point of my own country: The United States.

2 The Great American Divide

What is the problem? In the United States, rural populations, mostly white, are becoming more politically conservative. Urban populations, ever more diverse, are growing more liberal. Even the largest cities in Texas now vote Democratic, while the Republicans own the physical and philosophical territory just beyond nearly every metropolitan city limit sign in the country. Each constituency listens to different opinion leaders and lives within its own communication echo chambers.

This widening ideological gap makes collaboration across the urban-rural threshold in any bioregion a very difficult proposition. But since bioregions extend from urban centers to suburbs to rural farms and ranches all the way to wild lands, they call for cooperative effort between two major American populations who are otherwise drifting farther apart. On either side of this Great American Divide are some actions quite inimical to the essence of bioregional consensus.

3 My Definition of Bioregional Practice

There are a number of meanings of the word "bioregion," and several interpretations of the concepts of bioregional theory and practice. For some, a bioregion is strictly an ecological concept that should, therefore, define and direct "appropriate" human behavior. For others, a bioregion is a territory defined by certain cultural life ways practiced by humans over a long period of time. Still another interpretation is that the bioregion is a territory of appropriate scale and efficient physical, entropy-fighting relationship between the sources, uses, and distribution of essential living systems, such as food, fiber, water, energy, and material flows.

My concept of a bioregion combines all of the above, but especially includes a shared system of human values, where local stakeholders take on an active role in the social construction and physical caretaking of the region itself. In this view, no one person or group has complete dominion over the management direction of the place. Countless examples of this process still abound. Watershed stewardships and local food movements remain two of the most potent approaches to bring urban and rural constituencies together. However, the Great American Divide threatens the future of such efforts.

What follows are three examples of recent and current activities which could be construed as "bioregional," but I will argue that only one fulfills the definition and purpose I believe is worthy of the label.

3.1 The State of Jefferson

In 1941, some disgruntled residents of the borderlands of northern California and southern Oregon put up a roadblock of protest, rifles at the ready, handed out pamphlets, and declared themselves to be residents of the independent state of Jefferson. Their protest was largely fueled by what they felt was complete inattention by state governments in Salem (Oregon) and Sacramento (California) to their desires for more local economic control over mining, timber harvesting, and ranching. While Pearl Harbor, World War II, and the sense of national purpose that followed soon overshadowed their efforts, the conceptual State of Jefferson rose again during the last two decades. At first, the concept was local and inclusive. The regional National Public Radio station, broadcasting from the liberal city of Ashland, labeled itself "Jefferson Pubic Radio," and a wide group of citizens shared a common sense of place (ijpr.org).

Unfortunately, as of this writing, one finds significant and dire changes in the media face of the State of Jefferson, with ultra-right-wing white nationalism rising to the fore. The "Jefferson State Militia" (jeffersonstatemilitia.com) rants that the "Shit Storm is Approaching," declares that they are "One nation, under revolt," rails against the federal and state governments, champions the "Coming American Revolution," runs images of Confederate flags and other extreme-right-wing paranoid positions. Another website, the soj51.org, states that "We the people of the Jefferson Counties are not the playthings of the criminals who rule over California" (soj51.org).

A curious geography has evolved: what was once a movement centered around the Klamath-Siskiyou borderlands of southern Oregon and northern California has expanded steadily southward and eastward, and one now sees State of Jefferson flags and decals all over northern California east of the coastal mountains. Many of the northern California counties have had referenda or supervisorial actions addressing the question of succession. While most of these referenda have failed or been tabled, some, like Tehama County's, have passed. The State of Jefferson movement, having originated in a regional context, has become somewhat of a right-wing political philosophy that is spilling far beyond the confines of its original region (https://en.wikipedia.org/wiki/Jefferson_(proposed_Pacific_state). The original website, (stateofjefferson.com), still aims to give an inclusive and objective view, but is ignored by the angry, various, now-competing websites and hard right political spin-offs. The current State of Jefferson movement is no longer bioregional and is dominated by rural, white nationalist conservatives who fear the government and the urban regions. Consequently, the State of Jefferson represents one extreme, polar rampart of the Great American Divide.

3.2 *The Berryessa Snow Mountain National Monument*

In 1997, an organization was formed at the conjunction of Lake, Napa, Colusa, Yolo, and Solano Counties called the Blue Ridge–Berryessa Natural Area Conservation Partnership (BRBNACP). This mouthful-named organization was established as an all-inclusive volunteer group of those private and public partners who had an interest in conservation of the part of the inner Coast Range that formed the headwaters of Putah and Cache Creeks. The monthly meetings attracted ranchers, wildlife managers, environmentalists, boaters, range specialists, professors, mining interests, rafting guides, and entrepreneurs. Care was taken to not to create political boundaries, and few disputes over philosophy reared up (http://brbna.org/library/).

However, in 2005, a group of Sierra Club and wilderness advocates from Davis, California, formed a new organization ("Tuleyome," ironically named after a paragraph in my book, *LifePlace*), joined BRBNACP, stirred up political and philosophical differences, and finally left the Conservation Partnership to launch a competing movement whose aim was to create a conservation area in the Putah-Cache headwaters from land federally owned by the United States Forest Service, the Bureau of Reclamation, and the Bureau of Land Management (BLM). Opposition was strong from private landowners and those county governments with conservative boards of supervisors. Oddly, one of the driving factors motivating the Tuleyome "environmental" group was its fear that a wind farm would be established on Walker Ridge on BLM land in the region. They also objected to the inclusion of a "Working Landscapes" assessment in the GIS analysis being prepared by BRBNACP, fearing that it would give landowners and ranchers too much legitimacy. By usurping the role of the stakeholder group and replacing it with an environmental advocacy group driven by liberal environmentalists from Davis, California, roughly 10 years of social capital developed by BRBNACP was destroyed.

By cultivating relationships with the Democratic Party majorities on county boards of supervisors, by lobbying California state senators and assembly members, and by gaining the support of one of California's United States senators, Tuleyome succeeded in having a motion placed on President Obama's desk, which he signed, to designate the area as the "Berryessa-Snow Mountain National Monument."(https://en.wikipedia.org/wiki/Berryessa_Snow_Mountain_National_Monument)

Ironically, the newly-named national monument does not include "Lake" Berryessa, a reservoir under the control of the US Bureau of Reclamation (Reservoirs are not allowed in National Monuments, apparently). Furthermore, the monument boundaries only include those portions of federal land lying in counties with Democratic-majority boards of supervisors. Federal lands on the Republican-dominated Colusa County side of a major mountain range were left out of the boundaries. Hence, the monument is a political, not an ecological, construction. Half of the land originally considered for wind energy development lies in Colusa County.

The upshot: a national monument many private landowners did not want was superimposed on a bioregion in which they lived, by a government they did not trust—exactly the kind of action that lends fuel to rural right-wing movements like the State of Jefferson. I have had a lengthy interest and involvement in this (my home) bioregion, yet I consider the creation of the Berryessa-Snow Mountain National Monument to be a case of a twentieth century organization using twentieth century tactics to solve a twentieth century "problem" in a twenty-first century world crying out for a different approach.

Berryessa-Snow Mountain National Monument therefore stands on the opposite rampart of the canyon of the Great American Divide from the State of Jefferson. There are similar impositions occurring elsewhere in the country where federalized national park or monument proposals are met with keen resistance from local rural residents. In the case of Berryessa-Snow Mountain, the land in question was already in the federal public domain, so the designation as a monument does little in the way of "protecting" it further. When compounded by the confusion that Lake Berryessa is not included within the monument named after it, and that major portions of the US Forest Service Land and BLM land lying within Republican-dominated counties were not included, the bioregional integrity of the monument designation seems flawed and overtly political in nature. Lastly, the designation of a monument does little in the way of lifting the livelihoods of those rural residents who make their living from working landscapes surrounding the federal lands. Since no federal dollars will be allocated by a Republican-dominated US Senate to "improve" the management of the new national monument, nothing much will change other than a label for the place. Was the designation of Berryessa Snow Mountain as a national monument an example of bioregionalism at its best? My answer is no. When the voices of various stakeholders in a particular bioregion are silenced by the one-sided domination of an activist group, the region is not well served, and the Great American Divide is exacerbated. The Berryessa Snow Mountain National Monument and the State of Jefferson, in my view, are both extreme examples of the Great American Divide.

3.3 The Klamath River Accords

In contrast to the two examples above (one driven by rural conservatives and one by urban environmentalists), there is a stellar example of a natural region doing the genuine, hard trench-work of local bioregional management. The "Klamath Water Wars" is a story about a conflict over water and food in a bioregion and a resolution to that conflict. The Klamath River rises in the Cascade mountains north of Klamath Lake in southern-central Oregon, flows through volcanic soils into northern California, crossing the Scott Valley, skirting the Marble and Siskiyou mountains, passing through several ancestral native American territories, through redwood groves, and empties into the Pacific ocean at Requa, California. In 2001, during a drought, irrigation from federal projects normally delivered to the Klamath Basin farmers of potatoes, strawberries, and other crops had to be restricted for the health of endangered salmon. Farmers broke the locks on a federal diversion gate and took what they considered "their" water. As a result, eighty-thousand salmon died downstream in early 2002, infuriating both native tribes and commercial salmon fishermen. Both sides lawyered up and set their respective Republican (upstream) and Democratic (downstream) representatives against each other in Washington. Lawsuits were filed, and animosity ensued. More than thirty organizations were party to the early attempts to reach a watershed-wide solution. At least one salmon fisherman in downstream Orrick and one potato farmer in upstream Tulelake each put up signs in their yards, declaring themselves as "endangered species."

After years of wrangling, acrimony, and legal procedures, a breakthrough was reached when upstream farmers and downstream fishermen decided they must actually travel to each other's domains and meet where each made their living. PacificCorp, the utility owning four rather outdated dams along the river, agreed to remove those dams, as the costs of relicensing them outweighed the small energy benefit received, which the utility could easily make up elsewhere. For participants and observers alike, the accord was marked by a celebratory barbeque attended by farmers and fishermen, who roasted salmon and potatoes on the same sticks.

As of this writing, the former Republican US Congress failed to provide funding for Klamath River dam removal (which will be the biggest dam removal project in the world). However, the participants, not wishing their decade-and-one-half effort to be for naught, conceived a plan to ask the Federal Energy Regulatory Commission to decommission the dams, obviating the need for congressional action. While there is still some political friction, actual watershed stakeholders have worked too hard at reconciliation to see angry polarization spoil a decade or more of creating "social capital," and there is still considerable potential left for creative solutions. Also, a more favorable US House of Representatives has been seated that may help speed up the accord along its intended trajectory (https://en.wikipedia.org/wiki/Klamath_Basin_Restoration_Agreement).

Ironically, the 15-year effort by the 30-plus separate partner organizations resulting in the Klamath Accords took place in the very bioregion that State of Jefferson claims as its original birthplace. Furthermore, the breakthrough occurred when the federal agencies themselves realized they were getting in the way of real dialog between aggrieved private and tribal parties both upstream and down, and stepped back from the fray. The participating Klamath partners have demonstrated by hard work, diligence, and compromise the true nature of a bioregion. As Daniel Kemmis outlined in his seminal volume, *Community and the Politics of Place,* a region is the "table" around which the sense of a true natural community can gestate (Kemmis 1990). A bioregion effort, then, should be considered as an open hand, not a clenched fist.

4 The Geography of the Great American Divide

To extrapolate from the three examples of regional identity mentioned above, it is necessary to talk about the evolving geography and nature of the "Great American Divide."

Two graphics illustrate that geography perfectly: the 2016 presidential election map results from both Hillary Clinton and Donald Trump. The map of territories won by Clinton territory is a rough approximation of liberal-leaning America, while Trump's is indicative of rural America. Both parties' presidential candidates were considered to have strong negatives; one won the popular vote, the other won the Electoral College. Therefore the voting patterns for each represent a reasonable template for the geographic divisions in American culture. (For much more detailed information on this division, readers should search the Pew Research Center data and maps, www.pewresearch.org.)

With minor exceptions, liberal America is a geographic archipelago of "islands" concentrated around major metropolitan areas (even those contained in "red," or conservative-tending states). If one were to translate this into the language of landscape ecology, these liberal areas would be called *patches*. On the other hand conservative, Republican territory occupies most of the land area of the United States, or, in landscape ecological terms, the *matrix*. Anyone with even a vague notion of bioregions or any form of systematic regional geography will immediately recognize that, as these geographic divisions harden and become more ideologically separate and antagonistic, cross-regional cooperation becomes that much more difficult.

5 Causes of the Great American Divide

While entire books have been written about how American culture arrived at this point, I will venture my own take on the origins of the Great American Divide. The first place I will lay blame is on growing economic inequality. The authoritative tome on this subject is Thomas Piketty's "Capital in the twenty first Century." While both urban and rural constituencies blame different causes for this trend (rural: multiculturalism and government policy; urban: corporate hegemony and runaway capitalism), the percentages of rural poor and urban poor are roughly the same. Both rural and urban constituencies have been mostly treading water economically, while those at the top of the pyramid grab the spoils. However, as Piketty lays bare, inequality has been growing globally, and not just in the United States. We have all heard of the statistics of the percentage of world's or the US wealth that is accumulated in the top 1% of the population, but there is a plethora of other related statistics that support the reality of growing inequality. Two different political belief systems, however, have exploited the discomfort felt by the growing cadres of rural and urban "have nots" such that scapegoats like undocumented foreign workers are blamed instead (Piketty 2014).

The second culprit I would argue to be a cause for Great American Divide is the advent of social media and personalized technological communication. We have lost many, if not most, of the real-time, real-place spaces where we once rubbed shoulders with one another. Instead, we communicate only with our "friends." We read only the news media we trust not to be "fake" (each side considers the other's news sources to be illegitimate). Truth slips away, and we believe much unverified information. In such a supersaturated media reality, we each create our own echo chambers in which we dwell, dismissing information not deemed compatible with what we have constructed as our own realities.

6 Trump

It is widely assumed by many observers that current US President Donald Trump has caused the angry divisiveness now prevalent in the United States. However, like a number of others, I would argue that Trump is the *result*, not the cause, of that divisiveness. The Great American Divide fractured long before Trump emerged; he merely became the bellwether of that growing divide. The Great American Divide caused Trump, not the other way around. Trump has merely given many Americans surrogate permission to lay bare their simmering prejudice, even hatred, in ways heretofore considered impolite or impermissible. I need not mention the specific and manifold violent examples of this hatred, as they have been thoroughly examined in global news.

I believe that the United States suffers from a strong reaction by white people to losing their grip on political power, much as South African whites did during the death throes of apartheid. Many white Americans could not stand the idea of a black president, and have acted out accordingly ever since Obama was elected. Trump's subsequent election has only facilitated the overt expression of this racial prejudice. We knew that recalcitrant white people would not give up their presumed position of superiority without a fight, and they are fulfilling that expectation now. In short, as a country, we have never quite finished the Civil War, and that, in part, creates the divisions that now threaten any hope of bioregional accords across the Great American Divide. Yet, unlike the first American Civil War, the Great American Divide of today has no clear, singular geographical "Mason-Dixon" line. Instead, we manifest thousands of ideological and political cleavages across nearly every urban-rural boundary in the country. We are hard pressed to imagine ways of healing this urban-rural ideological rift; the problem breaks into ever more localized pieces, like a giant cultural fractal puzzle pattern. Instead of a civil war, we are starting to see increasingly violent skirmishes by various groups spread across the geography of the country. Yet a solution must be found; it is naïve to assume that either the cities or their regional countryside and wild lands could every really exist without each other.

7 Reversing the Flow of Value

The Great American Divide is not simply about rural white folk who are reluctant to share power and status with people of color. It is also about the withering urban comprehension of how life has been, and still is, lived in rural America. A critical lesson emerged from the 2016 election that urban liberal constituents must learn: a nation that divides its rural citizens philosophically and politically from its urban population cannot hold, and will eventually collapse upon itself.

Central to the dilemma is a simple fact: rural people, as inheritors of a long tradition of Jeffersonian agrarianism, must still make (or once made) their living off the land, while urban constituents often seem to forget that the land (and in our global economy, even American land) is the *basement* of the economy. It is true that economic studies point toward a declining contribution of the agricultural sector (even when multiplier effects are considered) toward total GDP. While California is the largest agricultural producer among the 50 US states, agricultural production contributes only 2% of the massive California economy, which is the fifth largest in the world, exceeding that of the United Kingdom. (https://www.usatoday.com/story/news/nation-now/2018/05/05/california-now-worlds-5th-largest-economy-beating-out-uk/583508002/)

However, as the economic calculus moves away from major metropolitan areas, the percentage that rural residents contribute to the economy through farming, ranching, mining, and logging, increases. Add in the loss of resource-dependent occupations that have gone offshore due to uncontrolled excesses of global economics or mechanization and the extreme dissatisfaction of a large percentage of mostly (but not exclusively) rural America comes into focus.

For a moment, let's set aside the obvious, nasty trick Trump pulled by scapegoating blacks, Hispanics, gays, immigrants, women, etc., such that rural constituents conflated this racism, sexism, misogyny, and xenophobia with their real concern: being left behind by the global economy, and discounted by their urban constituents. Indeed, it is hard for the liberal establishment to make this separation, but make it we must.

8 Technopoly

First, however, we must take a theoretical detour; there is another phenomenon at play here. There are those who believe (and I am one) that we now live in a "technopoly," and that the steamroller of technology, as Elon Musk says, will roll over us and our jobs will gradually be replaced by computers, algorithms, and robots. This seemingly unstoppable march of technology and its concurrent effects on the GDP has unfortunately hit the rural landscape and extractive industries first. But make no mistake, after decimating the rural landscape and its extractive or agrarian industries, it is coming for our suburban, then urban, jobs afterward. No one will be unaffected; it is merely a matter of time.

Some suggest (e.g., Elon Musk, Erik Brynolffson, Martin Ford, Jaron Lanier, the late Neil Postman, and others) that there will need to be a creative means of compensation to ordinary citizens for the loss of their ability to work. One such proposed solution is the Guaranteed Minimum Income, or GMI. This would be a kind of reverse taxation, and a form of unemployment compensation on a scale heretofore unheard of in the United States. It would also most likely be an anathema to the traditional rural employment based upon extracting a living by working in, or on, the land. Ultimately, the GMI would work its way up (or into) the urban economy, as medical professionals, attorneys, and other managerial employees are slowly replaced by informatics, algorithms, and robotic machines. In this future (which I believe is both inevitable and approaching fast), both rural and urban workers are similarly at risk. Technopoly is an equal-opportunity job killer: yesterday it was coal miners; today it is lawyers who are being replaced by algorithms and computing (Postman 1992; Lanier 2013; Ford 2015).

Let us now make the critical jump back to the survival of rural constituencies. We may start this by considering the situation of a hypothetical rice farmer in Colusa County in the central agricultural valley of California. What do urban communities seem to demand of this rice farmer and his rice-farming neighbors, besides the rice crop itself? We would like that farmer also to provide us with water conservation, water quality improvement of the run-off from the fields, wildlife habitat for waterfowl, clean air, habitat for spawning salmon in nearby streams, open space and aesthetic beauty, hunting and fishing opportunities, and access to land for recreation. And this farmer is currently expected to provide these benefits solely from the global price of rice received from a market controlled by a few gigantic corporations like Archer Daniels Midland, Monsanto, or Cargill. The expectation that rural communities should provide "us" (the urban majority) with the benefits we seem to demand, but are not willing to pay rural residents for, is a maladaptation of a global economy run amok. And this is not even considering that the real enemy of the rural American is the corporatization of agriculture and the epic, downward-squeezing of the price offered to farmers (or "growers," as the euphemism now goes) for their labors.

Consider a new idea: if the urban-centered majority actually wants these values from the rural landscape, then let us devise a way to return economic value to the rural environment via some kind of flow of money. If we value what we want rural landscapes to provide, let's pay them for providing it, even if that means payments for NOT taking certain actions. (There is plenty of precedent for this to occur in the United States' federal farm bills of the recent past.) These kinds of flows of monetary value toward rural land uses we expect have often been analyzed using willingness-to-pay methods, but these do not capture the entire spectrum of values implicit in rural landscapes. One essential component of a healthy bioregion, therefore, should be one where its rural residents can make a decent living and whose work is appreciated by the urban majority.

Metropolitan areas of the United States contain the vast majority of the population, yet much of this population has no connection to, decreasing experience with, and little knowledge of rural lifestyles or endeavors, such as agriculture, stock raising, forestry, or mining. This is merely a fault of ignorance due to diminishing exposure, not because of malicious intent on the part of city dwellers.

On the other hand, rural populations, once dependent on land-based livelihoods, have had to take second careers in nearby cities and towns. The amount of land necessary for an American family of four to survive has expanded exponentially, until only enormous ranches, vineyards, or farms can support their residents solely without secondary employment. Rural residents resent this trend and, in some cases, misplace the blame for their plight by scapegoating "illegal aliens" (whom they often must employ to work on their lands to make financial ends meet), or regulations that restrict their livelihoods without offering any compensation for that restriction.

9 A Model Bioregional Organization: The Center for Land-Based Learning

Located in rural agricultural lands in Solano County, California, there is a highly successful non-profit organization that I consider a model for the bioregional approach to bridging urban and rural philosophies for the benefit of the land and people themselves: The Center for Land-Based Learning, or CLBL, for short. CLBL was the brainchild of Craig McNamara, son of former US Secretary of Defense, Robert McNamara. Craig wanted to become a farmer, and subsequently moved to northern California and bought a walnut farm (about as far away from Washington politics as one could get!). He established the Center for Land-Based Learning in 1992, with the following mission:

> Our mission is to inspire and motivate people of all ages, especially youth, to promote a healthy interplay between agriculture, nature and society through their own actions and as leaders in their communities.
>
> The Center for Land-Based Learning envisions a world where there is meaningful appreciation and respect for our natural environment and for the land that produces our food and sustains our quality of life.

CLBL, then, was born out of joint respect for both environmental stewardship and local agriculture. There are a number of CLBL programs. One bears the acronym, SLEWS, which stands for "Student and Landowner Education and Watershed Stewardship." SLEWS engages California high school students in habitat restoration projects on farms, orchards, and ranches. Many of these high school students come from underprivileged urban areas, and many have never been on a farm or ranch before. They are invited at the behest of the orchard owners, farmers, and ranchers who volunteer their private lands for program. Under the guidance of mentors and instructors experienced in environmental restoration, the urban students plant native plants, hedgerows, and riparian trees on these private, rural lands. Aside from the obvious learning that goes on among the students, the program brings together urban youth and seasoned farmers and ranchers, and a mutual respect and understanding develops between the two groups. Other CLBL programs achieve similar interactions across the urban-rural divide. A program called "FARMS" (Farming, Agriculture, and Resource Management for Sustainability) provides innovative, hands-on experiences to urban, suburban, and rural youth at working farms, agri-businesses, and universities. The California Farm Academy is a 7-month internship program that provides an intensive overview of what it takes to succeed as a farmer or rancher.

Both FARMs and the California Farm Academy place 80% of their (often urban) graduates in farming careers and farm incubator programs, also often helping young farmers find land to farm and, eventually, to own. The Center for Land-Based Learning is perhaps the best contemporary example I know of a bioregionally-focused non-profit organization that connects urban and rural constituents together for the sake of both groups, and of the environment itself (https://landbasedlearning.org).

10 Conclusion

The genesis of the bioregion movement burst forth in the late 1960s and early 1970s in the United States, but reached its apogee during the 1990s, when governments like the states of California and Nebraska and the nation of New Zealand wrote into their laws participatory, adaptive management of regions defined by ecological rather than political dimensions. During post-2000 years, the political divisions already present in the American landscape were exacerbated by the ascendance of electronic communication, the division of the news media into partisanship, and self-reinforcing social media cliques, and the economic stagnation of the middle class (both rural white and urban mixed ethnicity), while wealth accumulated in the uppermost strata of society. Jobs, both rural and urban, have been permanently lost to off-shoring, mechanization, informatics, robotics, and algorithms. Conservative rural populations and urban progressives, while knowing less and less about what each other does for a living, form crude stereotypes of each other, and isolate themselves even further as part of what some commentators have called the "Big Sort" (Bishop 2008).

Yet we all occupy a bioregion, and wherever that is, it most likely extends from urban to suburban to rural to wild lands. Water, food, energy, habitat, raw materials, tourism, health care, and education, all flow between or span the breadth of a bioregion, which we, of course, share with manifold non-human species. It is an illusion to believe that the city could survive without the countryside and vice-versa.

In spite of the Great American Divide, I remain convinced that a bioregional approach to planning the American landscape is absolutely crucial to the future health and welfare of *all* Americans. But bridging that growing divide will now require even greater effort than ever before.

There is one idea that could be extrapolated as a necessary component of bioregional planning, and one that takes the Center for Land-Based Learning's approach one step further. Imagine that all across America (and, by extrapolation, the countries of the world) exchange programs for high school students were to be created, (with only willing participants, of course) that allowed rural students to live with urban families for 2 weeks, and urban students to live with rural families for 2 weeks. It may be necessary to reestablish this kind of real-space, real-time exposure between the various residents of a bioregion that have been eliminated by electronic communication "echo chambers," job-killing technologies, and crude stereotypes of those on the "other side." In the United States, as this urban-rural political and philosophical divide becomes a chasm, we urgently need a reconnection across it. I suspect that in the many countries represented by the authors of other chapters in this book, similar healing is urgently needed across urban-rural divides in their bioregions as well.

Current trends and political realities now place a very heavy burden on the realms of bioregional thought and practice. Yet that body of theory and practice itself may be the best bridge we can imagine across the growing cultural divide between urban and rural constituents.

References

Bishop, B. (2008). *The big Sort: Why the clustering of like-minded America is tearing us apart.* Boston: Houghton Mifflin Harcourt.

Ford, M. (2015). *The rise of the robots: Technology and the threat of a jobless future*. New York: Basic Books.

Kemmis, D. (1990). *Community and the politics of place*. Norman: University of Oklahoma Press.

Lanier, J. (2013). *Who owns the future?* New York: Simon & Schuster.

Piketty, T. (2014). *Capital in the twenty-first century*. Cambridge: The Belknap Press of Harvard University Press. Translated by Arthur Goldhammer.

Postman, N. (1992). *Technopoly: The surrender of culture to technology*. New York: Knopf.

Thayer, R. L., Jr. (2003). *LifePlace: Bioregional thought and practice*. Berkeley: University of California Press.

Part I
Rethinking Places for Community Life

The Territorialist Approach to Urban Bioregions

Alberto Magnaghi

1 From Contemporary Urbanisation to Urban Bioregion

The astounding dimensional growth of contemporary urbanisation—the UN estimates that, in 2050, some 6.4 billion people of the projected global population of 9 billion will be urbanised—threatens to definitively sever the territorial roots of urban areas: the very location of historic cities, at the confluence of waterways and roads or on strategic heights, has become incidental in a world increasingly dominated by overarching flows of goods, capital and people that reduce the places they reach to pure logistic ports, and those they do not reach to mere distances that can be overcome—possibly at the virtually infinite speed of global telematic networks. Such "pulverisation of places" (Becattini 2015), which has always accompanied phases of de-territorialisation (Magnaghi 2001), has become unprecedentedly pervasive, depositing seeds of de-contextualised modernity in every place on the planet, disfiguring urban and rural landscapes by forcibly inserting metropolitan functions in inner (rural, hilly or mountain) areas or condemning these areas to marginalisation, abandonment and degradation. Contemporary urbanisation, boundless, excessive and serial, is characterised by morphotypes which are totally incongruent with those that have stratified over time in historic cities: in fact we *live in vast post-urban areas* for work, training, communication, commerce, consumption and leisure. This means the spatial relationships which criss-cross these areas are multi-scalar, ranging from the proximity of local neighbourhoods, to the urban and

This chapter is the translation of a condensed and updated version of the chapter Professor Alberto Magnaghi wrote for *La Regola e il Progetto*, a collection of essays he edited, which was published in 2014 by Florence University Press. This is the first English translation to be published and, in accordance with the Open Access policy of Florence University Press, the Italian version is freely available on the internet.

A. Magnaghi (✉)
Architecture Department, Florence University, Florence, Italy
e-mail: alberto.magnaghi@unifi.it

D. Fanfani, A. Matarán Ruiz (eds.), *Bioregional Planning and Design: Volume I*,
https://doi.org/10.1007/978-3-030-45870-6_3

regional dimension of functional communities, to ethereal communications in cyber-space.

Such transformations entail an *anthropological mutation* in the relationship between human settlement and the environment, between functional geographies (flows) and places (funds),[1] and they increasingly reduce the reliability of the simple interpretive (and design) model based on *local* urban/rural polarisation.[2] This has led me to conclude that a possible "return to the city" (8), a restoration of the positive and liberating meaning of urban, requires *urbanity* to be comprehensively redesigned (Bonora and Cervellati 2009), because its value has been dramatically reduced to the *mort de la ville* envisaged by Françoise Choay (1994); such a redesign should take into account both the urban, *regional* scale of the new geographic dimension of living and the multi-scalar relationships generated by this new dimension, as well as the diverse relationships existing between the physical space of places (*limited, concrete, historic, local*) and the intangible space of networks (*unlimited, virtual, instantaneous, global*); the redesign should also attempt to redefine the relationships between historic (urban and rural) settlement systems and open spaces/built-up areas, and relationships between public spaces and their connective fabric; the redesign should also regenerate the city by facilitating the development of synergic relations with the surrounding territory and networks as well as multiplying its centralities. The starting point of any such redesign project will be to reinterpret the new forms of living that are incessantly generated by the diverse morphologies of regional urbanisation.

If the issues raised by the strategic perspective of "returning to territory"[3] are to be considered, answers to the problems of contemporary living must be sought in the relations generated by regional urbanisation *at the complex territorial systems scale,* and their critical issues, challenges and opportunities should be addressed through the concept of *urban bioregion.*

In this chapter, therefore, I have adopted the concept of *bioregion* to respond to the intrinsically *multi-scalar* issues posed by the need to (re)define a potential rebalancing of the relationship between human settlement and the environment, at the *geographical scale* of today's inhabiting territories, where it is possible to find technical solutions; I have introduced the adjective *urban* to take the challenge of global urbanisation to its home ground, proposing that it be reconverted by reconstructing the *urbanity* of places in a plural polycentric form, and by developing new synergic

[1] Here "flows" and "funds" terms are used according to the meaning introduced by Georgescu-Roegen (1976) referring to the explication and insights relating to the production process development.

[2] There have been several attempts to overcome this problem by redefining and vitalising mutual support relationships between city and countryside: see e.g. Fanfani (2009); Magnaghi and Fanfani (2010); Poli (2013, 2019); Ferraresi (2014).

[3] For more information on the "four moves" involved in this "return to territory" see Magnaghi (2013), § 4, and—more generally—the relevant issues of *Scienze del Territorio* (http://www.fupress.net/index.php/SdT), a journal published by the Territorialist Society: 1–2 "Back to earth" (2013–2014), 3 "Rebuilding the city" (2015), 4 "Reinhabiting the mountains" (2016), 6 "The new common property economies of the territory" (2018).

relations between the worlds of urban and rural life, starting with the denser fabrics of metropolitan areas and intermediate post-metropolitan territories, and continuing with the finer fabrics of hilly and mountainous areas. In other words, we need to design the *decomposition* of the *megacities* and *urban regions* being built today so they can be transformed *into urban places*, and to launch their *reticular and polycentric recomposition into bioregional systems*.

This process of re-conceptualising urban space in relation to its territory tends to overcome futile anti-urban positions or, even worse, approaches that reduce design action to spatial mitigation of contemporary urbanisation, intersecting the urban fabric with cycle paths and compensatory parks. The problem of "returning to the city" is, in fact, only partly a matter of morphological and environmental rebalancing; it is above all a matter of inhabitants reappropriating the power to determine their living environments (*polis*, public spaces), powers they have lost through the construction of increasingly global and a-spatial techno-financial machines, which have transformed inhabitants into users and consumers.

In this alternative vision, the dichotomy between historic cities and contemporary urbanisation can be addressed by using the paradigm of a self-governing urban bioregion and applying it to an entire regional territory; in this way, the paradigm becomes a conceptual tool that provides rules, methods and multidisciplinary techniques for tackling an (socially produced) inhabitant-focused territorial project[4] as a contextual, interactive redevelopment of rural, urban, central, peripheral and marginal territories.

2 Definition of Urban Bioregion

Urban bioregion is the appropriate conceptual reference for a territorial project which is designed to integrate the *economic* (referred to the local territorial system), *political* (self-government of inhabited areas and work places), *environmental* (territorial ecosystem) and *living* (functional and inhabited areas of a group of cities, towns and villages) components of a socio-territorial system that pursues a

[4]The three terms figuring in the Italian version of this expression, *progetto*, *abitanti* and *territorio*, present an intricate translation problem which is also a cultural and scientific issue: *progetto* covers the meaning of both the English words "project" and "design"; *abitanti* designates something halfway between "inhabitants", "residents", "citizens" and "dwellers"; *territorio* has virtually nothing to do with its "natural" translation "territory", since the latter indicates the extension of a domination or a species range, whereas the former—at least in its territorialist sense—is conceived as the result of the coevolutionary interactions between environmental frameworks and human actions in a long-term historical perspective. The choices here adopted try to roughly reproduce in English the same areas of determination and indeterminacy detectable in Italian; in particular: "design" prevails over "project" whenever a "draw" meaning is primarily involved; "dwellers" is always used as an abbreviation for "who lives there"; the plural form "territories", or the adjectival "territorial", replaces "territory" when a confusion with its other, ordinary sense may occur [*Translator's note*].

coevolutionary balance between human settlement and the environment, re-establishing new forms of the long-term relationships between city and countryside that tend "towards territorial fairness" (Madec 2012).

The territorial dimension of an urban bioregion is not pre-defined. Whatever the context, this dimension depends on what is required to develop the four components that identify the urban bioregion in question and on the complexity of the physical environments required to synergically integrate its functioning. Depending on which of the components is most dominant, an urban bioregion may be the size of a local territorial system (or SLoT, see Dematteis 2001), a district system (Becattini 2009), a water catchment (Nebbia 2012), a coastal system with its hinterland, an urban region (Dalmasso 1972), a landscape setting (Poli 2012) and so on; this demonstrates that characterising a bioregion's identity and landscape depends on several factors: accessibility; functional, urban and ecological complexity; the presence of distinct physiographical, hydrographical and landscape systems; the relationships between coastal and inland areas; the interactions between plains and hill or mountain valley systems; the presence of orographic nodes and river valleys, urban, infrastructural and rural systems and so on; this brings to mind the environmental and cultural complexity of Patrick Geddes' "valley section" (1915).

As part of territorial governance, each urban bioregion should develop an interpretive planning tool for *minimum spatial and landscape planning units* within a vast regional area (holistic criteria should be used to identify these units), so as to integrate the governance of housing, economic-productive, infrastructural, landscape, environmental and identity functions. The strategies of the regional spatial/landscape plan should, therefore, focus on enhancing the unique identities of every urban bioregion within the region.

This definition of bioregion represents a semantic and conceptual evolution from earlier definitions: when the term was first used, it had a definite *ecological* emphasis: this is particularly noticeable in the reflections, based on concrete experiments, made by the Todd and Todd (1984) and, in particular, by Kirkpatrick Sale (1985), who defined the deeper meaning of bioregionalism as referring to "a region governed by nature". The social dimension of the bioregion is already apparent in studies conducted by the American Peter Berg who, in his *Green City Program* (1987), wrote that cities were dominated by consumerism and needed to become more responsible and develop reciprocal relations with the rest of their bioregion, in order to create social units in which bioregional citizens would be able to understand and control decisions concerning their life.

A more socio-ecological and municipal view, put forward by Murray Bookchin (1989), focused on the problems of communities self-governing their living environment as essential to the very existence of the bioregion; this viewpoint was later developed by Serge Latouche (2006) who studied the bio-economy of degrowth, achieved by adopting different life, production and consumption styles.

In addition to these "humanistic" contributions, the "territorialist" sense of bioregion makes a direct reference to the *ecological geography* studies undertaken by Vidal De la Blache (2008) and to the work of the Regional Planning Association of America (MacKaye 1928); in particular, as already mentioned, it refers to Patrick

Geddes' *bio-anthropocentric* definition of "valley section" (1915), especially where he puts the peculiar features of the hydrogeomorphological structure of river basins in a *coevolutionary* relationship with specific productive cultures and lifestyles. Finally, the bioregion is also inspired by Lewis Mumford's "human region" (1961).

To ensure the territorial project is based on the concept of bioregion, we have reinterpreted the relevant Geddesian principles by:

- Reaffirming the principle of coevolution between *place*, *work* and inhabitants (*folk*)
- Promoting the specific and unique identity (*uniqueness*) of every region and each city
- Implementing long-term analyses (*reliefs and contours*) to discover the coevolutionary (natural and cultural) relations "at work" in each region
- Highlighting the long-lasting coevolutionary principles that emanate from these relationships (*regional origins*) as a guide to discovering the (genetic and transformation) invariant rules which, over time, make it possible to reproduce the bioregion's identity characteristics

The concept of "coevolution" (which refers to our methodological work on long-term territorialisation processes—see Magnaghi 2001) prevents the concept of bioregion from drifting towards determinism,[5] where human settlements are considered to be entirely dependent on their environmental framework (this tendency is present, for example, in the Chicago School's idea of the "city as an organism"); the coevolutionary process interprets the environmental rules using appropriate cultural mediation (Berque 2000, 2010), so a "place" is neither nature nor culture, but the fruit of a dynamic relationship between both components. Recent territorialist re-elaborations of these concepts, have provided an ecological slant to economic doctrines (Georgescu-Roegen 1966; Bonaiuti 2004); they also take into account Claudio Saragosa's definition of *territorial ecosystem*, which remodels the concept of "territory" so it is similar to the concept of "environment" (Saragosa 2005), and redefines the relational dynamics of human settlement, especially in cities, here reinterpreted as Biopolis, *the city of life* (Saragosa 2011).

These re-elaborations also refer to the theories of autopoiesis of living systems (Maturana and Varela 1984) and to the work of Christopher Alexander (2002) on the structures of living beings in an extensive sense, especially where he evaluates the quality of architecture, city and territories according to their "degree of life"; Alexander adopts the theory of expansion, recurrence, interaction and overlapping of "centres" and their properties ("field of organized forces"), to propose an optimisation of the settlement system as a deployment of the dynamic rules of life.

I have incorporated these conceptual advances in my detailed definition of an urban bioregion:

[5] See e.g. Berg (2002): "a bioregion is defined in terms of the unique overall pattern of natural characteristics that are found in a specific place. [...] People are also considered as an integral aspect of a place's life".

An urban bioregion is a local territorial system characterised by:

(a) the existence of a plurality of urban and rural centres, organised into reticular and non-hierarchical systems of small and medium-size cities; each city has a unique, synergic and multifunctional connection with its own rural territory for the production of ecosystem services;

(b) the existence of complex and differentiated hydrogeomorphological and environmental systems, related in coevolutionary and synergic forms with the urban settlement and the agro-forestry system. These coevolutionary relations, when related to the scale of a water catchment, a low-land system with its valleys, a coastal system with its hinterland and so on, characterise lifestyles and their quality, identity and heritage characteristics, sustainable ecosystem balances and the capacity of a place to self-reproduce.

An urban bioregion is a local territorial system equipped with forms of self-government that are designed to make the system self-sustainable and to promote the well-being of its inhabitants and, to this end, they activate local production systems based on the enhancement of long-lasting heritage resources (environmental, territorial, landscape, socio-cultural common goods) and encourage environmental policies aimed at the local closure of water, waste, food, and energy cycles.

An urban bioregion, in which every large city or "cluster" of small and medium cities is in ecological, productive and social equilibrium with its own territory, is an alternative to the strength and power of a metropolis: indeed urban bioregions are more powerful than metropolitan centre-periphery systems and diffused post-metropolitan systems because they produce more durable wealth by enhancing and networking their "peripheral" nodes in multi-polar exchanges; moreover, the creation of dimensional, relational and ecological balances within these polycentric territorial components, reduces congestion, environmental emergencies, pollution, external diseconomies, waste of energy and agricultural land, unnecessary mobility of people and goods; in this way bioregions help reduce the ecological footprint, namely the unsustainability caused by withdrawing resources from distant impoverished regions.

In this coevolutionary vision of the relationships between human settlement and the environment, bioregional territories assume the characteristics of a "highly complex living system" (Capra 1996; Magnaghi 2005) and, as such, are similar to autopoietic systems in which "environment and living organisms *coevolve*" (Maturana and Varela 1984) as part of a dynamic process, in which permanent features and structural changes induced by environmental perturbations ensure their self-reproduction as the autopoietic network "continuously reproduces itself".

In this sense, an urban bioregion is first and foremost an interpretative tool that can be used to evaluate, address and define the specific characteristics of degradation present in widely diffused post-urban urbanisation. The bioregional approach tackles these problems by assigning a central role in the territorial project, designed to promote self-sustainability, to the *multifunctional redesign of open spaces* (agro-forestry, riverside, natural areas) and by entrusting the *redesign of complex networks of urban centralities* with the all-important task of reshaping urbanity and self-government as they provide guidelines for differentiating territorial configurations and for retrieving the complexity and richness of their relations.

Indeed, a system of bioregions linked by supportive federal government networks facilitates the evolution of social-territorial relations, from the hierarchical systems typical of the globalisation paradigm, towards criteria of complementarity, synergy and cooperation among local self-determined systems (Thayer 2003); these local systems should produce a "competitive" advantage, not only in terms of environmental equilibrium and well-being, but also for the *long-lasting, self-sustainable* generation of wealth through forms of "grassroots" globalisation.

3 Designing the Urban Bioregion: A Glossary of "Construction Elements" and Their Rules at the Regional Scale

The methodological approach to urban bioregion requires the component sectorial elements to be recomposed in an integrated discipline that is suitable for redefining the basic elements of the territorial project, both in the elaboration of "treatise" rules which aim to ensure the reproduction and innovation of spatial structures, and in "modelling" design applications which exemplify their features. At both levels, it is *multi-sectoral integration* that ensures method effectiveness: each sectoral element of the territorial project must satisfy the treaty's multi-sectoral rules (e.g. those applicable to the hydrogeological, ecological, settlement and agro-forestry fields), and every sectoral rule has to be applied to all elements of the territorial project. As we have seen, these elements refer to both the needs and creative and operational fields of human activities (*necessitas*, *commoditas* and *concinnitas* for Alberti) and to built artefacts (the Vitruvian categories of *firmitas*, *utilitas* and *venustas*). In both cases, it is the relationship between the components that allows design visions and options to be consistent with each and every component and to also create synergies for the integrated project.[6]

The dialogic principle needs to be applied to ensure the components and their goals are properly embedded within the integrated project. This principle, which Françoise Choay (2004) ascribes to Leon Battista Alberti, affirms that buildings cannot be constructed without a dialogue with those for whom the building is intended, be they private individuals, communities of family members or members of the *res publica.* This principle becomes increasingly meaningful when it is updated to include not only buildings but also cities and territories as places of contemporary living, which assume the value of a common good to which the various forms of participatory active citizenship should be applied.

The inclusion of these new areas within the territorial project update and redefine the above-mentioned "classical" categories and connect them to issues related to

[6]An example: There are many possible solutions for reducing hydraulic risk in a river system section: some solutions such as collectors, river-bank rectification and artificial flood-expansion basins, are effective in that particular section, but they increase the run-off speed downstream, they do not fix the problem upstream, and, above all, they negatively impact other river system functions (e.g. riverside agriculture, river fruition, river landscape and the quality of ecological corridors); it is only by linking the objective of risk reduction with other objectives of the territorial project that it is possible to make sectorial choices (such as upstream water retention, rolling tanks, natural engineering works, etc.) that interact positively with other sectors, thereby raising the quality of life within the territory as a whole, as well as within that specific sector.

contemporary urbanisation such as: the hydro-geomorphological balance in water catchment areas and the quality of ecological networks within the regional territory as a whole, including the environmental quality of urban spaces (*firmitas*, *necessitas*); the regional re-balancing of settlement and urban systems, aimed at improving habitat, production and consumption quality, can be achieved by redefining the mutual relationships between city and countryside, by increasing the complexity and morpho-typological differentiation of city networks and by recreating urbanity within urban centres (*utilitas*, *commoditas*). Further improvements can be made by redefining landscape quality in relation to the inhabitants' living environments and to the recent heightened awareness of rural and urban landscapes (*venustas*, *concinnitas*).

The bioregion also has its generative rules and its basic elements—I call these "construction" elements, to use the metaphor of a building: foundations, walls, floors and a roof.[7] The *construction elements* of a bioregion have socio-cultural, political, environmental, productive, urban and landscape characteristics and they are inspired by the above-mentioned treatises and statutory rules. Rules, construction elements and their synergies (building methods and techniques, territorial and urban metabolism) represent the design guide, the "treatise" required to address territorial projects in bioregional terms. In this paragraph, I will extend the building metaphor as to include a "building-territory" which covers a vast area, in order to describe the main "construction elements" of urban bioregions, highlighting their role and the "compositional" rules of the design process. The construction elements are summarised in the "glossary" below.

3.1 Territorial and Landscape Cultures and Knowledge as "Cognitive Foundations" of the Bioregion

The bioregional design "lays" its foundation using local cultures as cognitive materials: long-lasting socio-cultural models, craftsmanship, artistic, environmental, territorial and landscape care expertise all provide tools for interpreting the relationships between nature and culture that are required to produce territory. The first "construction element" of a future bioregion is a multifaceted *corpus* of environmental and territorial knowledge emanating from the long historical development of that territory, which, over time, characterises its unique landscape and identity. The study of *territorialisation processes* (Raffestin 1980; Magnaghi 2001; Turco 2010; Fig. 1) identifies the *invariant* features of *environmental* and *building knowledge*

[7]The metaphor of building construction elements is useful, at the regional scale, for reframing relationships among the various design elements: very often, the territorial project underlying contemporary urbanisation, builds *walls and the roof* (diffuse and pervasive buildings, mega-infrastructures, etc.) but completely ignores the foundations (hydrogeomorphological and ecological balances) until it is too late, at which point emergency policies (usually extremely costly) are required.

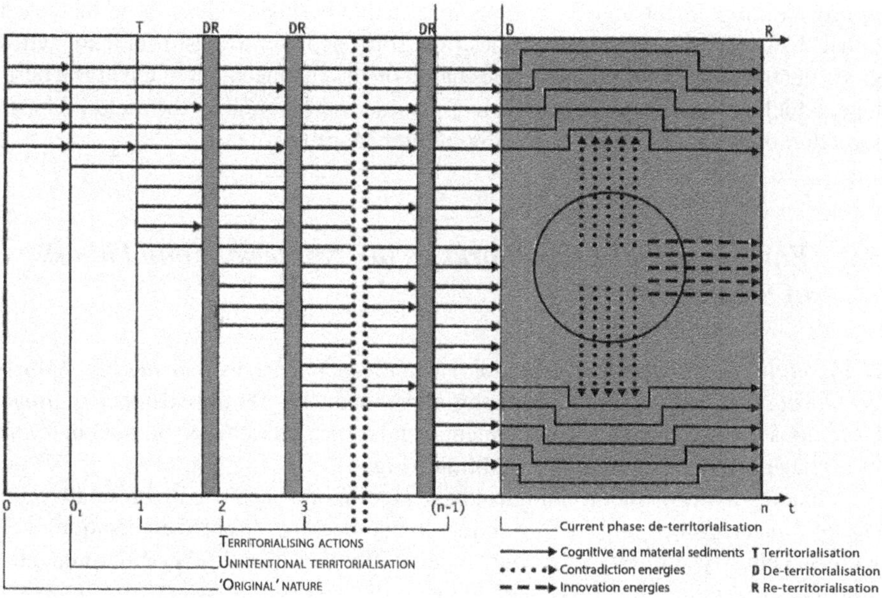

Fig. 1 Diagram of the "TDR" process: territorialisation – deterritorialisation – reterritorialisation. (Source: Magnaghi 2001)

and expertise that are laid down in cognitive and material sediments: territorial structures and landscapes that go beyond a single civilisation and represent the *long-term heritage of a place* (Marson 2016).

Recently developed disciplines can make important contributions to tracing *regional origins*: for instance, *global archaeology* (Brogiolo 2007, Volpe 2008), which shifts attention from single archaeological sites to historical territories and their stages of civilisation, and *historical geography and ecology* (Moreno 1990; Cevasco and Moreno 2013, Quaini 2011), which adopt local multi-disciplinary surveys to reconstruct the coevolutive relations between human settlement and systems that activate and use environmental resources.

Systematising the knowledge obtained from historical territorial projects helps select the rules and activities that, in the settlement models typical of each civilisation, produce an enhancement of territorial heritage in the bioregion, defining the development "style" and uniqueness of a place; evolutionary rules also guide us in the *quantitative and qualitative selection of which activities to introduce*: this is a chapter on the "statute of places" that highlights structural invariants and long-lasting reproductive rules (Magnaghi 2017), thereby making it possible to specify requirements for *production activities* (what, how and where to produce in order to increase soil fertility, social and human capital, local entrepreneurship, the self-reproductive ability of environmental systems and the heritage value of landscapes and built-up areas) and for *settlement models* (locations, dimensions, morphotypes, building materials and techniques, as well as environmental and energy balances), in order to implement transformations that enable heritage values to be increased rather than reduced; evolutionary rules [non sono sicura che questo sia il soggetto] guide the formulation of statutory rules based on the enhancement of territorial heritage, which is recognised as a collective good (common) and as the material basis for a durable production of wealth (Figs. 2 and 3a–c).

3.2 *Environmental Frameworks as the "Material Foundation" of Settlements*

High quality ecological networks and water catchments with a healthy hydrogeomorphological balance are the material preconditions for the existence of urban bioregions (*firmitas*), just as environmental and territorial knowledge, read in terms of heritage, are their *cultural* preconditions (Fig. 4).

A healthy hydro-geomorphological balance cannot be achieved with small-scale *end-of-pipe* projects (typical of the culture in our machine-oriented civilisation), nor with Sisyphus-type efforts of *ex post* repairs after floods and other environmental disasters; it requires the revival of a *hydraulic civilisation* which exerts cross-sectorial influence on the various actions of territory production, embedding the problem of hydraulic and water balance within the *ars aedificandi*. This methodology postulates that geo-pedological structures affect layout, location, the boundaries and forms of settlements and that water catchment areas represent the primary geographic environment in which to achieve a healthy production, conservation and balance of resources (especially water) essential for life reproduction. Recognising this primary function would restore strength to water catchment areas as physiographic entities with a housing, productive, administrative and political identity; it would also help to rebuild collective identities in valleys and coastal hinterlands, and to reconsider cities located on floodplains as "outposts" of the deep valley systems, of which they are an historical expression, "outposts" which reconnect the mountains to the plains and to the sea in a network of synergic relationships.

As regards our understanding of *ecological balances*, current ecological network designs mostly focus on protecting biodiversity in ecosystems (be they mountain, agro-pastoral, river, coastal, etc.), in order *to defend them* from settlement systems which tend to consume land, isolate open spaces, and fragment ecological networks and corridors. This repairing-compensating role of sectorial environmental design does nothing to undermine the generative rules of contemporary urbanisation which incessantly produce environmental degradation. This makes it necessary to include the design component of the ecological network *within* the generative design rules. A *regional ecological network* should therefore comprise a *corpus* of rules *internal* to bioregional design that ensure conditions of *ecosystem continuity* within the entire regional territory. The ecosystem should include agricultural land as a "secondary ecological network" with varying levels of ecological value, and urban areas

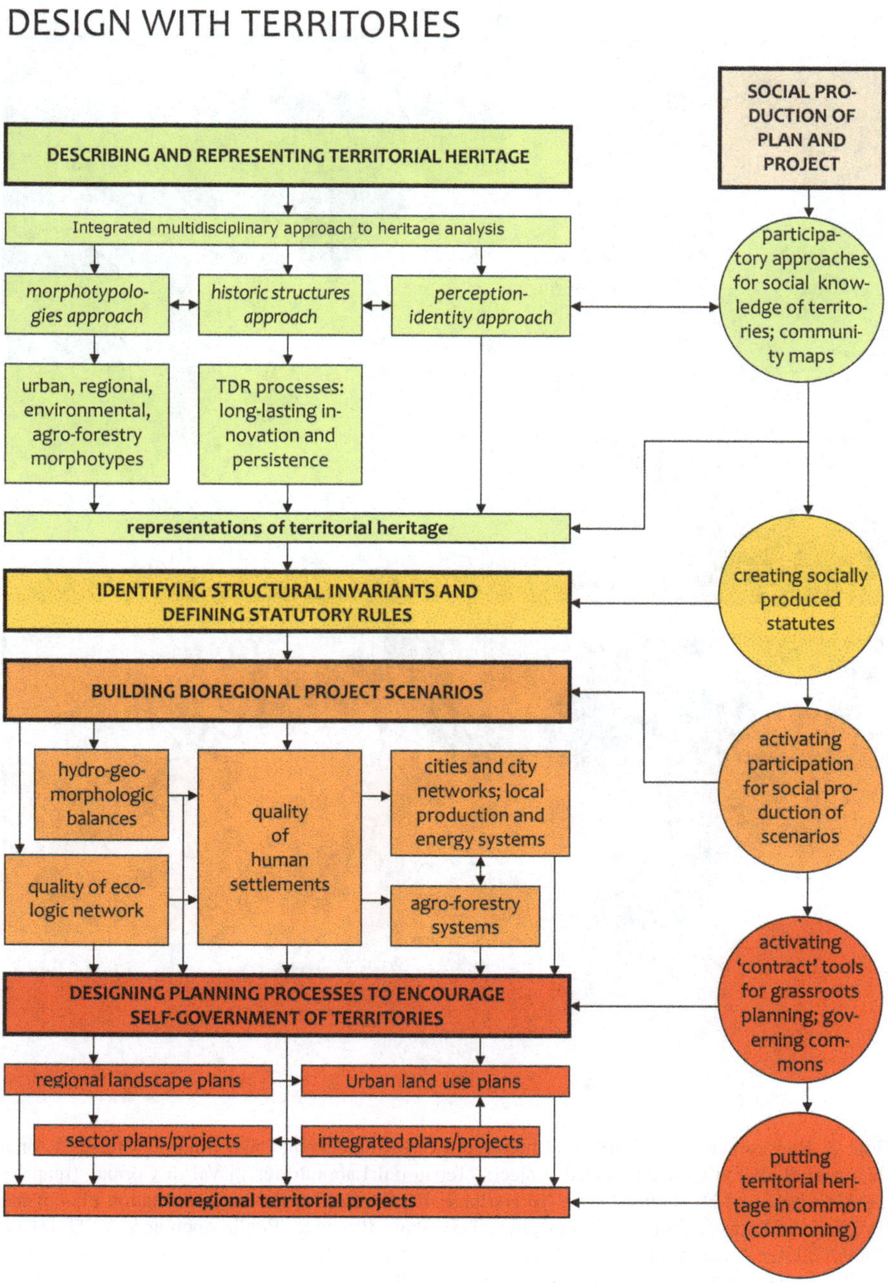

Fig. 2 Diagram of the bioregional design process. (Source: A. Magnaghi 2018 and author's elaboration)

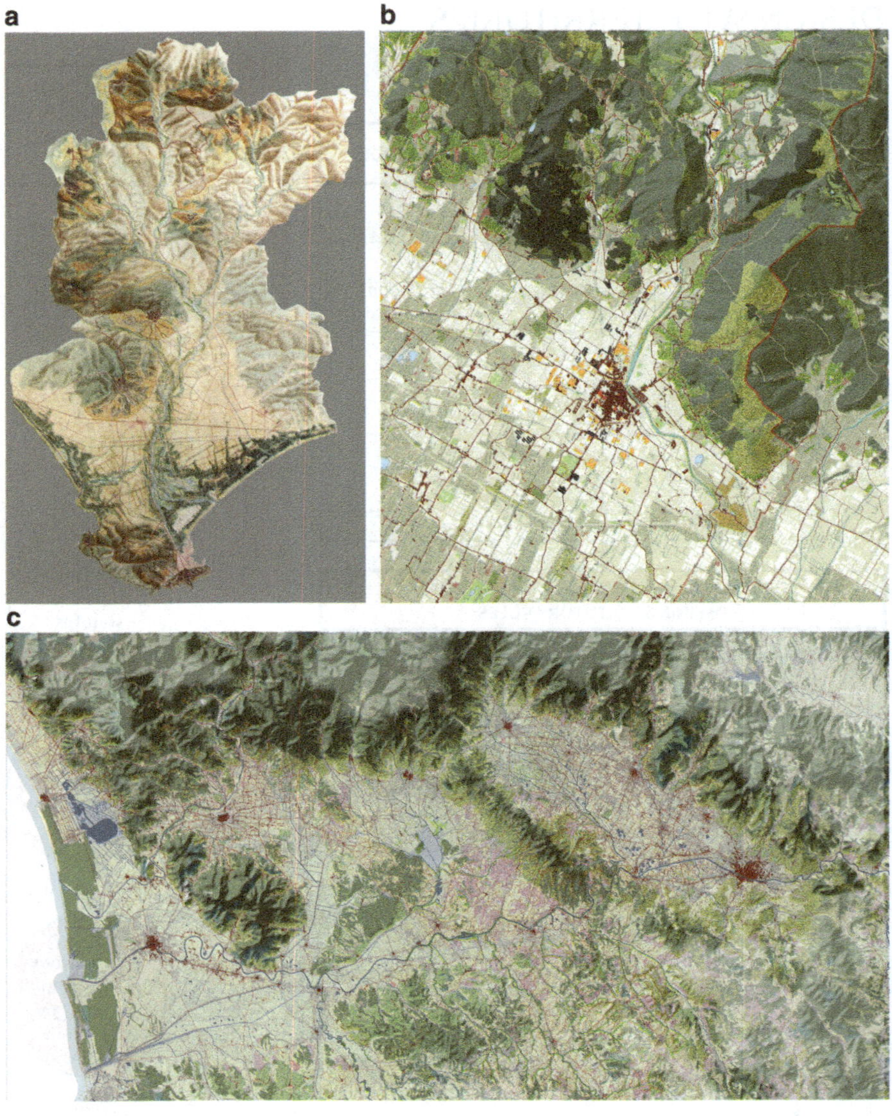

Fig. 3 Representations of territorial heritage: (**a**) Val di Cornia, Italy. Material prepared for a National Research Council funded project: "Territorial Laboratories in Val di Cornia" (map by A. Magnaghi and D. Fantini 1998). (**b**) Heritage map for the Territorial Coordination Plan of the Province of Prato (map by A. Magnaghi, 2003). Prato Province: Public open access SIT image file:///C:/Users/Acer/AppData/Local/Temp/Rar$DIa0.445/qc15b_a.pdf. Accessed 19 April 2019. (**c**) Territorial heritage of Central Tuscany. (Source: Magnaghi and Fanfani 2010)

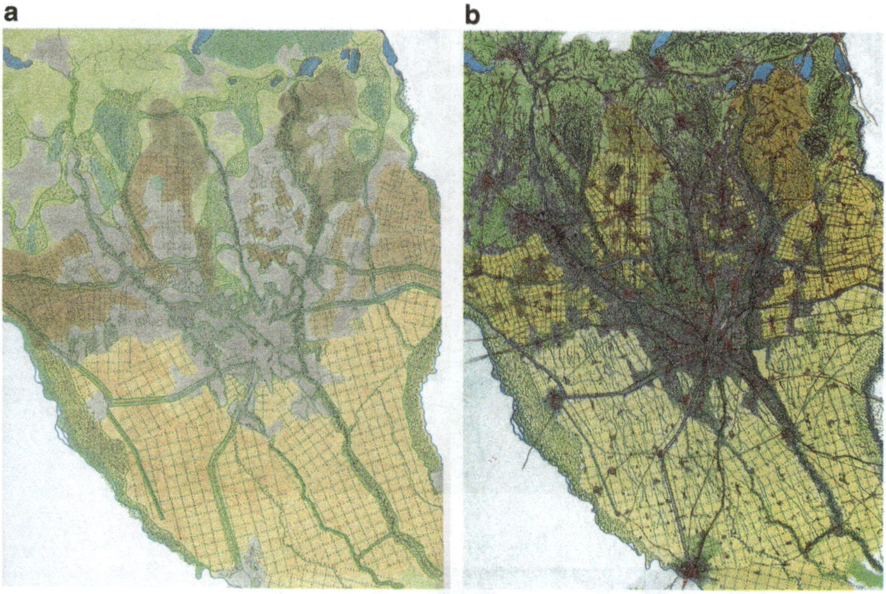

Fig. 4 The material foundations of the Milan urban bioregion: (**a**) an interpretive map of environmental systems; (**b**) a design synthesis map showing environmental systems and the pattern of reticular settlement. (Source: Magnaghi-IRER 1995)

as critical zones requiring treatment to ensure ecological corridor continuity and quality.

A precondition of settlement system quality in bioregional design is that the ecological quality of environmental systems must be raised *throughout the regional territory*; this is mostly achieved through multi-purpose *territorial eco-networks* (Malcevschi 2010; Fig. 5a, b) which ensure biodiversity, connectivity and complexity, multi-functionality of the ecological network and connecting corridors as well as bioregional metabolic recovery of water, waste, energy and food cycles.

3.3 Urban Centralities and Their Polycentric Settlement Systems

The *network of city constellations* is the morpho-typological element which generates urban bioregion settlement, the alternative to hierarchical centre-periphery models.

The growth of an urban bioregion, as a *highly complex living system*, depends largely on the structure and relational systems of its urban centres. In an interaction of multiscalar and polycentric relationships that revitalise the complexity of historic urban armours and their genetic, invariant, transformative rules, an urban bioregion

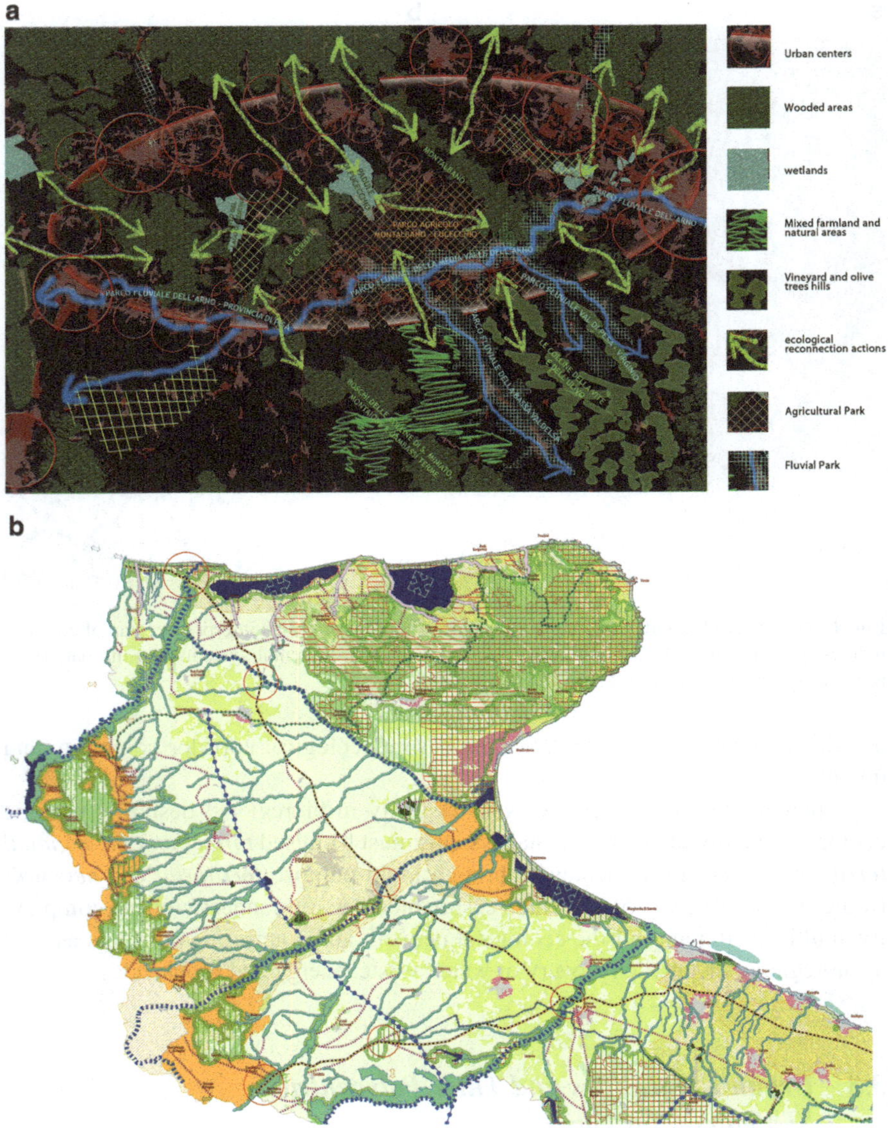

Fig. 5 Ecological networks: (**a**) Reconnecting the ecological network in Central Tuscany. (Source: Magnaghi and Fanfani 2010). (**b**) Master plan for the multipurpose ecological network in Puglia Region Landscape Plan. (Source: Magnaghi 2010). Puglia Region Territorial Landscape Plan (PPTR) Regione Puglia, Section Landscape Protection and Enhancement, (License Italian Open Data License-IODL). http://paesaggio.regione.puglia.it/PPTR_2015/4_Lo%20scenario%20strategico/4.2_Tavole/4.2.1_La%20Rete%20Ecologica_Regionale/4.2.1.2_Schema%20Direttore%20della%20Rete%20Ecologica%20Polivalente.jpg. Accessed April 19, 2019

consists of *inhabited countryside* (scattered rural buildings, hamlets, farms, farm-villa systems, farmhouses, rural ecovillages), *cities of villages* (eco-neighbourhoods) and *networks of cities* connected by complex grids of *infrastructural corridors* (roads, railways, rivers, paths, bridleways, bicycle tracks, telematic networks). The more the functions of each centre of this multipolar system have their own specific identity and differ from the other centres, and the more the mutual relations among the centres increase, the stronger each centre will become. Strengthening the polycentric system requires the identity, function and morphological differences of each centre to be reinforced; complementary relations among the centres also need to be reinforced. The system of centres with its rules of dynamic equilibrium becomes the ordering principle of the vitality of the bioregion in its appropriate relationships with the environment.

This means the design principles of a bioregional settlement system have to respond to two contrasting requirements: the need to strengthen the identity of each node in the network, without which multipolar relationships cannot develop, and the need to avoid this reinforcement disrupting the dynamic equilibrium between centres, so the system does not veer towards a hierarchical system of relations where dependency relationships develop between peripheral centres and the central city. Maintaining this delicate balance depends on rules that *control urban dimensions by qualifying urban growth*. The revision of the structural invariants of historic settlements allows urban scale and dimension to be defined in relation to: accessibility and proximity to public spaces; the minimum functional complexity required to guarantee a high ranking and exchanges with the regional network of cities; accessible services and temporal viability of soft mobility networks; reduction of functional mobility (jobs, consumption, goods, leisure); reproductive balance of the urban metabolism (water, food, waste, energy cycles); sustainability of the ecological footprint; multifunctional relations between city and countryside (balance and synergic exchange between open spaces and built-up areas, redefinition of urban fringes). These rules must be applied to both the level of the single urban node (cities of villages), and of the territorial network (cities of cities, networks of cities).

3.3.1 Cities of Villages (Ecopolis)

The metaphor of village (Magnaghi 1990; Kohr 1976; Krier 1984, Madec, *cit.* 2012; Friedman 1975, 2003) allows us to identify the minimum unit of aggregates that integrate social, community, economic and environmental elements. It is the system of these urban nuclei, connected in polycentric networks, which founds "Ecopolis" (Ferraresi 1992), "the urban village" (Friedman 1975; Magnaghi 2005), the *éco-quartier* (Madec, *cit.* 2012), the *bidonvillage* (Friedman, *cit.* 1975) and *Biopolis* (Saragosa, *cit.* 2011); once founded, each village is supported by a reconstruction of the network of public spaces as places of proximity and conviviality, fuelled by more participatory democratic forms (Magnaghi 2005); by the specialisation and complementarity of rare services and by housing typologies that define the functional, social and generational mix of each nucleus within the urban system, by implementing access to the distributive networks; by the reticular reorganisation of public transport with vast urban areas being reserved for pedestrians; by developing complex, interconnected local production activities; by adopting relative dense settlement morphotypes.

In contemporary urbanisation, the objective of the urban decomposition and reconstruction process is to recreate and rebuild public spaces by reconfiguring the role of *intermediate areas* between city and countryside through new agreements which implement the functions listed above.

3.3.2 Cities of Cities

At the bioregional scale, cities of villages make up the non-hierarchical mosaic of the cities of cities, founding the quality of city networks on the resistant pattern of historic settlement morphotypes.[8]

Interlocal networks (Camagni 1993; Bonavero et al. 1999; Davoudi 2003; Magnaghi and Marson 2004; Magnaghi 2017a) were developed with the strategic purpose of moving away from the centre-periphery model at the regional scale. This move enhances the uniqueness of the settlements within the territorial systems that make up the region and exalts their polycentric, federal, reticular vocation. The enhancement of the system's peripheral and marginal nodes (the multipolar distribution of network-connected rare services), so as to increase the relational, non-hierarchical complexity of the urban bioregional system, produces complexity, productive excellence and integrated supply chains in each territorial network node. The *functional polarisation* of diffuse peripheral conurbations identifies rules to prevent sprawl and the consumption of agricultural land: these rules make it possible to clearly define boundaries and to monitor the quality of urban fringes to safeguard the bioregional environmental balance (Fig. 6a, b).

3.4 *Production Systems That Enhance the Value of Bioregional Heritage*

The bioregional paradigm makes it possible to reframe the relationship between territorial heritage and the local production system in an innovative manner. In industrial districts, Marshall's concept of "industrial atmosphere" evokes the relationship between system productivity and local social and environmental endowments (natural and cultural resources, household structures, etc.). With the emergence of local development theories, though, the concept of territory (and

[8] In Italy and Europe, the historical urban *armour of* small and medium-sized cities has a generative force which is extraordinary for its quality and diffusion (Braudel 1979): in Italy, in particular, this makes it possible to largely found the settlement design of an urban bioregion by revitalising historical city morphotypes, the backbone of different civilisations over time (Bevilacqua 2017).

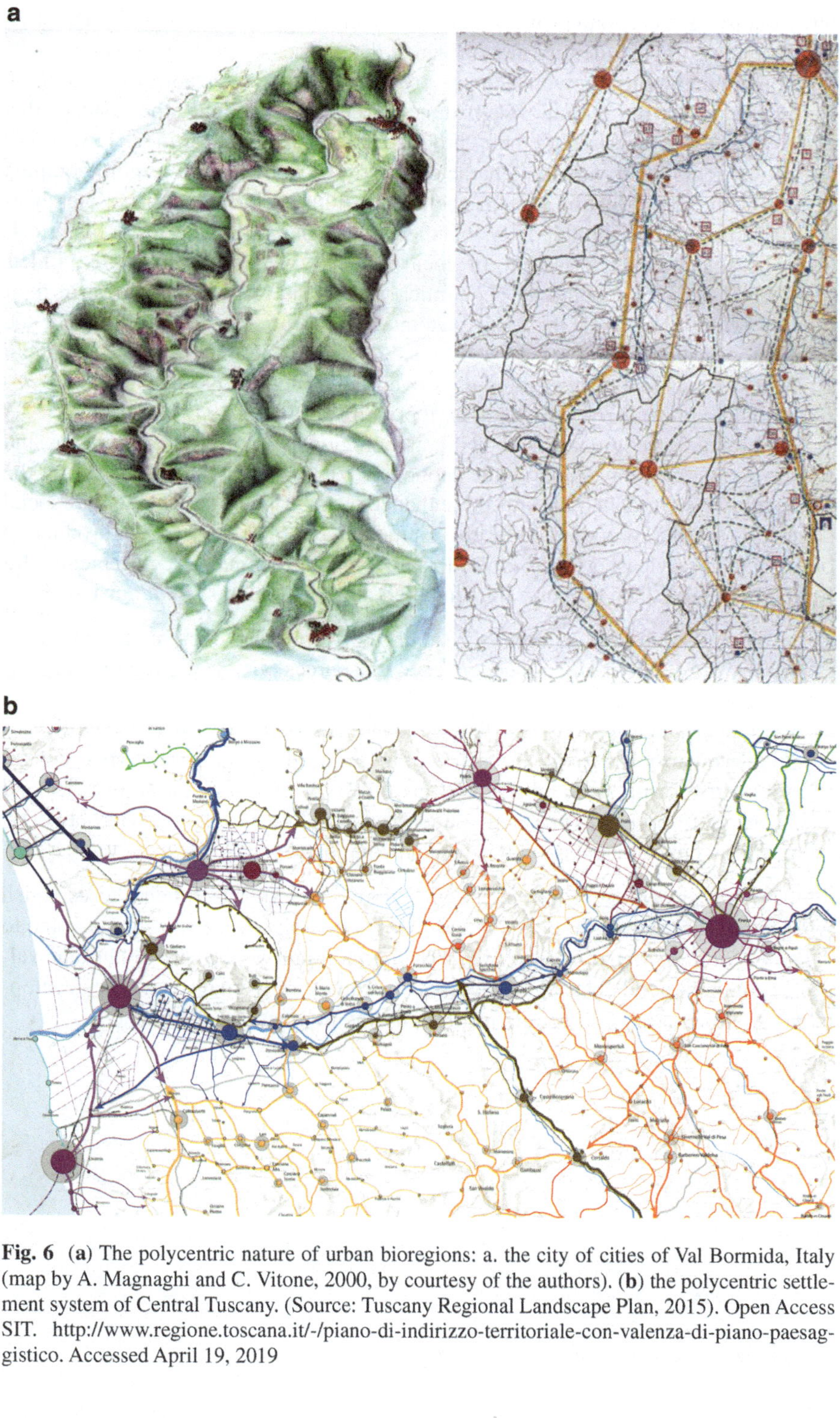

Fig. 6 (**a**) The polycentric nature of urban bioregions: a. the city of cities of Val Bormida, Italy (map by A. Magnaghi and C. Vitone, 2000, by courtesy of the authors). (**b**) the polycentric settlement system of Central Tuscany. (Source: Tuscany Regional Landscape Plan, 2015). Open Access SIT. http://www.regione.toscana.it/-/piano-di-indirizzo-territoriale-con-valenza-di-piano-paesaggistico. Accessed April 19, 2019

territoriality) goes beyond providing environmental support to industrial production to become a complex identity system which determines a two-way, dy*namic*, self-reproducing relationship with a local production system capable of generating "added value for the region" (Dematteis 2001). More recently, the concept that places can be characterised by their "productive chorality" (Becattini 2015a) allows territorial[9] socio-environmental characteristics to be integrated in a more complex fashion with the production system operating within territorial confines; merchandise specificity and productivity of the system is attributed to a historical-anthropological characterisation of local society, which, *as a whole*, affects "individual decisions including economic ones". This restores lifestyles, in their *identity relationship* with the local system, to the centre of the objectives of the production system. The "territory of inhabitants" (Le Lannou 1963; Magnaghi 1998) rises again and regains supremacy over the territory of producers; the *territorial* principle prevails over the *functional* principle (Olivetti 1945).

The production components of an urban bioregion also represent a testing ground for the ecological conversion of the economy (Viale 2011), which, in making the production system coherent with the enhancement of local knowledge and social contexts, with the reproduction of environmental systems and with the production of ecosystem services, brings it closer to satisfying bioregionalist requirements. But for the bioregion to be properly implemented, the production system must also:

- develop place-based economic systems that reproduce their own life cycle, thereby drastically reducing dependence on sources outside the region and their ecological footprint;
- develop production activities that enhance the value of specific qualities of unique territorial heritage in each bioregion, be they *material* (rivers, coasts, mountains, fertile soils, agricultural facilities, forests, infrastructure, cities and so on) or *immaterial* (productive and artistic cultures, *milieu*, civic networks, lifestyles, environmental knowledge and competence…).

In such a system of requirements, the bioregional approach helps to establish what to produce, how to produce it and in what quantity, thereby giving a voice to *economic and social actors who use innovation* to improve the care of heritage values as common goods, through processes of extended governance and the development of participatory democratic institutions and productive self-reliance.

[9] forse local oppure regional al posto di territorial?

3.5 Local Energy Resources for Bioregional Self-Reproduction

It is essential for local energy systems that settlement, urban and building systems are constructed in such a way as to ensure low energy consumption and high energy efficiency; furthermore, local energy needs to be produced from renewable sources that are consistent with the enhancement of bioregional and landscape heritage. This line of reasoning can be extended to urban morphotypes with low energy consumption and high-level climatic resilience (Fanfani and Fagarazzi 2012; Los, *cit.* 2007); in the presence of widely diffused production networks and a well-managed renewable sources mix, these urban morphotypes can revitalise the bioclimatic character of historical cities.

Developing an appropriate renewable energy mix requires careful analysis of local energy resource potential: every bioregion has its own particular energy potential associated with *natural* patrimonial assets (sun, tides, rivers, lakes, geothermal, wind energy) and local assets (canals, mills, artificial reservoirs, biomass from forests, cultivated fields and usable surfaces—roofs of industrial, residential and commercial buildings, car parks—urban waste, production waste, agricultural non-food production, etc.). Appropriate technological assistance and a precise combination of these resources provide a unique *bioregional energy mix* that makes *the entire bioregion* productive in a way that is consistent with the enhancement of territorial heritage (Van Dobbelsteen et al. 2008).

Local energy systems therefore, have the following objectives:

a. to switch from exogenous, centralised and privatised energy production to energy self-sufficiency and bioregional sovereignty by allowing local communities to valorise the widely diffused and integrated system of their local resources;
b. to remove the critical environmental, territorial and landscape issues arising from policies which deploy massive facilities to maximise the economic exploitation of single resources; to introduce dimensional, typological and technological standards appropriate to the particular mix of facilities used, to ensure long-lasting value enhancement of local assets; to increase the value of resources by blocking the consumption of agricultural land for new buildings and energy installations, by upgrading the energy efficiency of existing buildings and settlements and by reducing energy consumption;
c. to bring energy production sites closer to consumption sites so as to shorten supply chains, ensure highly reproducible energy supplies, reduce transport distances and minimise dispersion within the network; this will reduce the need for large distribution networks and the hierarchical systems, typical of large facilities, will be replaced by network systems (smart grids), better suited to the widely-diffused integrated systems of small and medium-sized facilities (Magnaghi and Sala 2013)
d. to recover/further develop urban metabolism and climate control qualities by designing bioclimatic cities".

3.6 *Agro-forestry Structures and Their Multifunctional Values*

The bioregional approach involves a radical change in how design methodologies consider the relationship between built-up areas and open spaces (agro-forestry systems, water catchments, fallow or abandoned areas, parks, biotopes); this approach defines new mutual relationships between urban and rural areas as a strength for redeveloping regional urban systems, and it uses the multifunctional values of open spaces (particularly agro-forestry areas) as a design base: the historical functions of hydrogeological protection, ecological balance, urban food supply, landscape fruition and hospitality production are thereby returned to these areas in an updated form. The bioregional approach also promotes new supply chains which work towards the local closure of food, water, energy and waste cycles. A new *agreement between city and countryside* (Magnaghi and Fanfani, *cit.* 2010) supports the reorganisation of contemporary urbanised areas, breaking down their urbanised continuum and re-aggregating their urban centralities with their agro-forestry areas using periurban agricultural areas as a filter. This process of urban decomposition and recomposition relocates and reorganises the fragments of metropolitan degrowth—from urban to rural villages and hamlets, to the inhabited countryside—within the bioregional paradigm (Fig. 7).

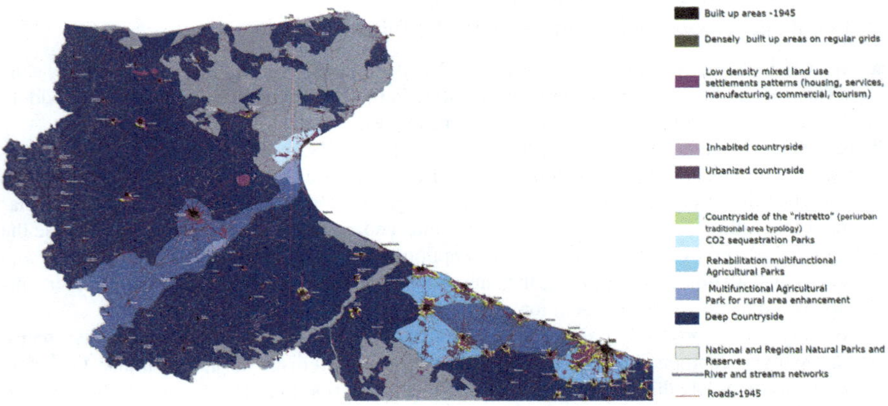

Fig. 7 Representation of the agreement between city and countryside in the Puglia Regional Landscape Plan. (Source: Magnaghi 2010). Puglia Region Territorial Landscape Plan PPTR), Landscape Protection and Enhancement Section (License Italian Open Data License-IODL). http://paesaggio.regione.puglia.it/PPTR_2015/4_Lo%20scenario%20strategico/4.2_Tavole/4.2.2_patto_citta'_campagna.jpg. Accessed April 19, 2019

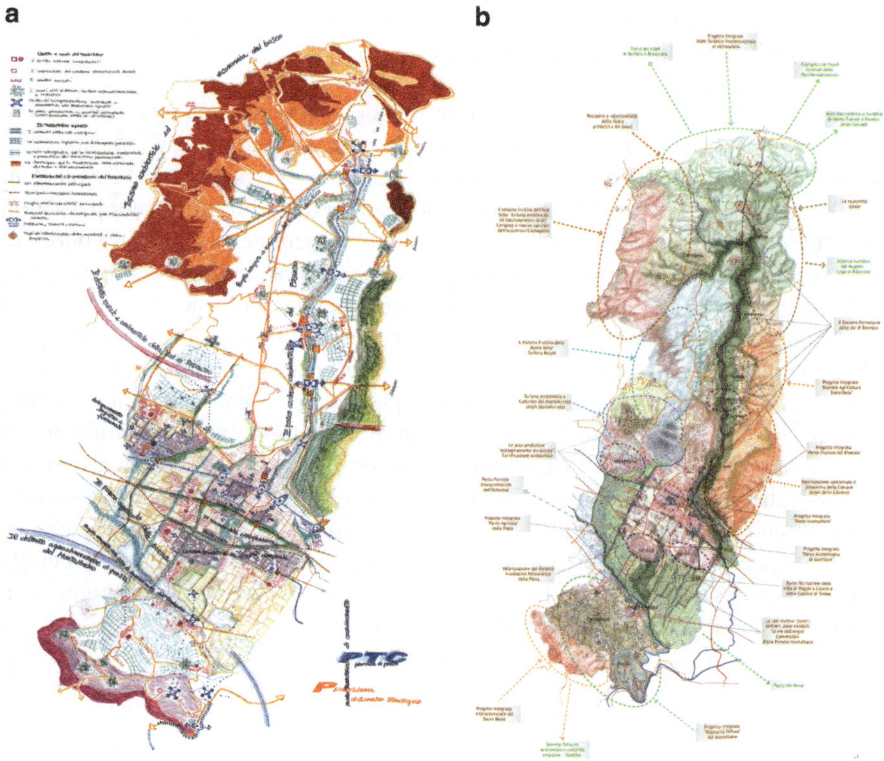

Fig. 8 Two shared bioregional scenarios for the Province of Prato: (**a**) Initial vision of the province's territorial systems and vocations. (**b**) "Integrated projects" for the Territorial coordination plan of the Province of Prato. (Source: Magnaghi 2003). Prato Province Public Open Access SIT image. file:///C:/Users/Acer/AppData/Local/Temp/Rar$DIa0.849/p02.pdf. Accessed 19 April, 2019

3.6.1 Producing Urban Quality: Urban and Periurban Agriculture

The number of urban and periurban gardens, orchards and vegetable gardens is rapidly increasing in metropolis, in areas that were once "awaiting urbanisation" or are now unexploited. The revival of these abandoned and degraded areas provides a buffer against expanding urbanisation and also defines *new standards* for *green agriculture* within urban suburbs. This agriculture has many functions: it provides food and leisure activities; it plays a role in environmental and microclimatic compensation and promotes high-quality redevelopment of the urban fringe; projects for reconnecting enclosed urban agricultural areas with the periurban agricultural belt adopt "blue and green threads"—cycle paths, tree-lined lanes and canals—to define city limits and reconnect urban public spaces with agricultural land ("green hands on the city", Donadieu 2012), thereby redefining the landscape quality of the latter (Poli 2013; Fig. 8).

3.6.2 Producing Environmental Balances and Ecosystem Services: Multifunctional Agricultural Parks

Multifunctional agricultural parks (or multifunctional agriculture *tout court*) restore the ecological functions of environmental protection and balance, historically assigned to agriculture, and they produce integrated *ecosystem services* (Rovai et al. 2010). These services provide *support* (reproduction of soil fertility, reorganisation of water distribution), *regulation* (conservation of agricultural land, water purification, natural habitat maintenance, hydrogeomorphological and microclimatic regulation), *supplies* (food production for bioregional cities with the development of local food-supply chains, biomass energy for the local energy mix), *cultural services* (maintenance and restoration of historical landscapes) and *production of common goods* (aesthetic quality of the landscape, access to and use of agricultural territory by city dwellers, multifunctional reuse of historic farm infrastructure for rural *tourism* and direct food and cultural exchanges). As a *secondary ecological network*, these multifunctional agricultural parks allow for the maintenance of *biodiversity* and ecological corridors; they also help mitigate climate change and reduce the ecological footprint (by facilitating a regional closure of water, waste, energy and food cycles); in fact these parks become the *ordering principle* of bioregional settlement and its infrastructure system (Ferraresi 2014; Fig. 9).

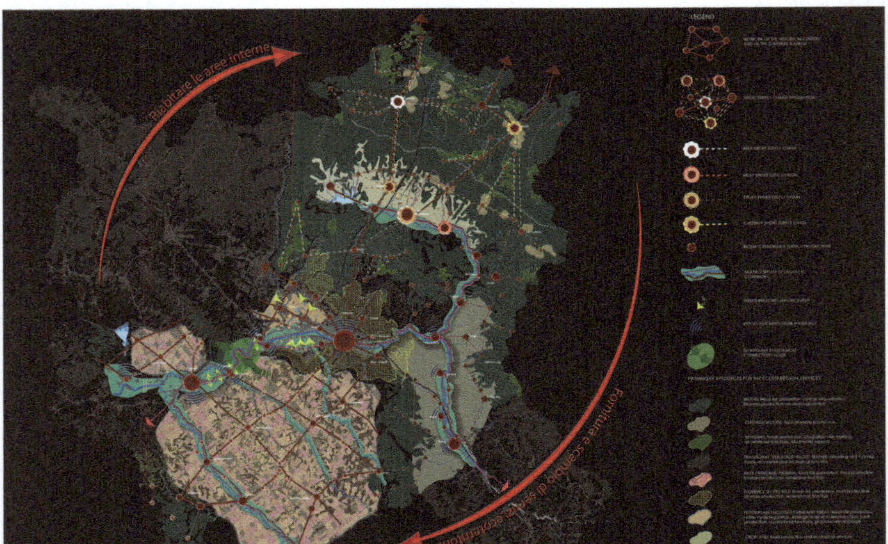

Fig. 9 An urban bioregion for the Florence Metropolitan Area (map by D. Poli and A. Magnaghi. 2018) (By courtesy of the authors. Unpublished research undertaken on behalf of the Metropolitan City of Florence)

3.6.3 Historic Rural Landscapes and Production of Knowledge for Climate Change

Historical rural landscapes represent a patrimonial concentrate of "wise" rules for producing and regenerating territories (Agnoletti 2013), and as such are able to contribute rules and knowledge to the drawing up of "territorial statutes" (or "territory statutes") and assist in overcoming the diseconomies of current agro-industrial models, help address climate change, the long-term environmental effects of which are currently operating, devastating and partially irreversible: desertification, violent floods, landslides, cyclones, melting of polar ice caps, rising seas, etc.; phenomena which are also accompanied by a growing scarcity of food and cultivable areas and by the exponential increase of environmental refugees. Historical rural landscapes can, therefore, represent the patrimonial nuclei which support retro-innovation processes (Stuiver 2006) aimed at addressing climate change issues by retrieving functions for enhancing valuable agricultural areas and redeveloping metropolitan areas and by mobilising the expertise of mountain communities (forest management, terracing techniques, water retention and regulation, etc.).

3.6.4 Revival of the Peasant Mode of Production and Rural Repopulation

The essential characteristics of traditional (Cevasco 2007) and *neo-peasant agriculture* present many of the elements required for bioregional design: production for personal use (not market dependent), of the system's reproductive resources ("peasant mode of production", van der Ploeg 2008); ecologically complex production; complex polyculture; hydrogeological protection; tendential local closure of environmental cycles; locally based economic production (local food-supply chains for food quality, forms of mutual aid and fair, non-monetary exchanges of produce); preservation of local identities and so on; when put into a system, these elements are the principles of agro-ecology (Gliessman 2014). The ongoing processes of revitalising peasant knowledge are already capable of triggering processes—weak, but qualitatively important—of rural repopulation (Canale and Ceriani 2013; Dematteis, *cit.* 2011) that contrast the long wave of planetary urbanisation processes; these processes should, therefore, be strengthened as an essential basis for the construction of urban bioregions.

3.7 *Structures for Self-Government and Social Production of Territory*

The "construction elements" of urban bioregion I have described cannot be deployed in territorial policies unless there is a definite transition towards forms of self-government: the very definition of a bioregion makes it impossible for production, culture, consumption and information to take place in a hetero-directed bioregion.

3.7.1 From Participation to Social Production of Territories

Throughout history, participation has resulted in technicians providing some sort of support to dwellers in developing claims, projects and forms of self-realisation and solidarity. Sometimes this participation has been negative: a mere creation of artificial consensus for pre-defined projects. In both cases, inhabitants are unable to master the cultures and means of production of their own neighbourhood, city, territory: they do not know where their light, water and food come from, or where their waste goes; in many cases, inhabitants no longer know who they work for. In the bioregion, the roles of inhabitant and producer merge together in urban and rural areas to outline a process which evolves from "participation" towards "social (co)production of territories" (in an economic system which reduces wage labour, enhances diffuse individual entrepreneurship and mutual relationships and expands the tertiary sector). This process also requires urban policies to evolve from *conservation* (of old towns, landscape, environment) to the activation of *reterritorialisation* processes: restrictions, rules and limits are still needed, but the most important requisite is the activation of inhabitants/producers (and of permanent institutions for consultation on shared projects) as the key actors in reconstructing territorial values.

3.7.2 Bioregional Self-Government Institutions

Urban bioregions require active citizen participation

(a) To reproduce life production factors (air, water, energy, health, ecosystem services…)
(b) To construct local socio-economic systems based on the enhancement of heritage resources

The merging together of inhabitants/producers takes place within decision-making institutions that decide what, where and how much can be produced without compromising the pursuit of public happiness and collective well-being. From this perspective, the *government of bioregional territory* no longer administers services in relation to exogenous and "global" economic choices, but, instead, it manages locally based economic systems and promotes unique "development styles" that help protect and enhance local identity; it establishes relationships—hopefully non-hierarchical and complementary (Thayer 2013)—with other bioregions and subsidiarity relations with higher government levels. The municipality, or rather the network of municipalities of an urban bioregion, becomes a promoter of local society, basing its development project on "pacts" agreed to by a plurality of actors who identified common interests when they deliberated their development objectives. This process strengthens the capacity of urban polycentric networks to tackle powerful (exogenous or endogenous) interest groups that, by simplifying the complexity of the decision-making system, tend to grab and exploit resources for their own profit, thereby damaging and consuming the commons.

4 Towards a Planet of Urban Bioregions

The territorialist paradigm of the urban bioregion, thus far outlined, clearly has both a *cognitive and* an *evaluative* value: it enables both unchanged and transformed areas of the region to be studied in an integrated and cohesive way, on the basis of their overall impact on long-term—material and immaterial—heritage assets that characterise identities and development styles that are unique to the particular region under consideration; it also has value as a *design* instrument: the consistent, coordinated use of the "construction elements" described above makes it possible to revitalise areas, transforming them into "highly complex living systems", whose self-government seeks to develop shared and locally self-sustainable projects for the future, and to achieve social well-being by caring for and enhancing commons heritage. On these two levels, there are future challenges which the adoption of the urban bioregion paradigm allows us to foresee:

- At the *conceptual* level, the ambit of the *Territorial sciences* needs to be expanded so they encompass the cross-disciplinarity (or more appropriately, the *transdisciplinarity*) required for a bioregional approach, where the expertise of individual disciplines is reinterpreted to reflect the view that the "territorial principle"—guided by a place-focused, participative, "reflexive approach" (Schön 1983)—prevails over the "functional" principle (Olivetti 1945)—even in the organisation of knowledge;
- At the *design* level, switching from developing individual bioregions to planning, predisposing and organising systems of "federal" relations that bioregions can or should establish with each other, so as to access the multi-scalar (better still, the *transcalar*) dimension of the "higher-order locale" (Giusti 1990), which appears to be the only plausible alternative to the eco-socio-catastrophic—and apparently unavoidable—destiny of planetary urbanisation/deterritorialisation.

In the overlap and probable integration of these two challenges, the vision of a planet swarming with urban bioregions advances; a planet made up of self-sustaining, self-determining territories which communicate with one another, which, instead of bowing to the war-like logic of violent, short-sighted dispossession (Kohr 2001), can once again become the unique habitat of human life on Earth:

the aware, conscious environment of the human species, their *home*. From awareness of place to awareness of species.

References

Agnoletti, M. (Ed.). (2013). *Italian historical rural landscapes. Cultural values for the environment and rural development*. New York: Springer.

Alexander, C. (2002). *The nature of order. An essay on the art of building and the nature of the universe*. Berkeley: The Center of Environmental Structure.

Becattini, G. (2009). *Ritorno al territorio*. Bologna: Il Mulino.

Becattini, G. (2015). *La coscienza dei luoghi. Il territorio come soggetto corale*. Roma: Donzelli.

Becattini, G. (2015a). Beyond geo-sectoriality: The productive chorality of places. *Investigationes Regionales/Journal of Regional Research, 32*, 31–41.

Berg, P. (1987). *A green city program for the San Francisco Bay area and beyond*. San Francisco: Planet Drum.

Berg, P. (2002). Bioregionalism (defined and updated). *Planet Drum*. http://www.planetdrum.org/shadow/bioregion_bioregionalism_defined.htm. Accessed 10 Jan 2020.

Berque, A. (2000). *Médiance de milieux en paysages*. Paris: Belin.

Berque, A. (2010). *Milieu et identité humaine*. Paris: Editions Donner Lieu.

Bevilacqua, P. (2017). *Felicità d'Italia. Paesaggio, arte, musica, cibo*. Bari: Laterza.

Bonaiuti, M. (2004). Relazioni e forme di una economia altra. Bioeconomia, decrescita conviviale, economia solidale. In A. Caillé & A. Salsano (Eds.), *Mauss 2: Quale 'altra mondializzazione'?* Bollati Boringhieri: Torino.

Bonavero, P., Dematteis, G., & Sforzi, F. (Eds.). (1999). *The Italian urban system: towards European integration*. London: Ashgate.

Bonora, P., & Cervellati, P. L. (2009). *Per una nuova urbanità dopo l'alluvione immobiliarista*. Reggio Emilia: Diabasis.

Bookchin, M. (1989). *Remaking society*. Montreal: Black Rose Books.

Braudel, F. (1979). *Civilisation matérielle, économie et capitalisme, XVe et XVIIIe siècles*. Paris: Armand Colin.

Brogiolo, P. G. (2007). Dall'Archeologia dell'architettura all'Archeologia della complessità. *Pyrenae, 38*(1), 7–38.

Camagni, R. (1993). From city hierarchy to city network: Reflections about an emerging paradigm. In T. R. Lakshmanan & P. Nijkamp (Eds.), *Structure and change in the space economy. Festschrift in honor of Martin J. Beckmann* (pp. 66–87). Berlin: Springer.

Canale, G., & Ceriani, M. (2013). Contadini per scelta. Esperienze e racconti di nuova agricoltura. *Scienze del Territorio, "Ritorno alla terra", 1*, 195–200.

Capra, F. (1996). *The web of life. A new scientific understanding of living systems*. New York: Doubleday.

Cevasco, R. (2007). *Memoria verde. Nuovi spazi per la geografia*. Reggio Emilia: Diabasis.

Cevasco, R., & Moreno, D. (2013). Rural landscapes: The historical roots of biodiversity. In M. Agnoletti (Ed.), *Italian historical rural landscapes. Cultural values for the environment and rural development* (pp. 141–152). New York: Springer.

Choay, F. (1994). Le règne de l'urbain et la mort de la ville. In J. Dethier & A. Guiheux (Eds.), *La ville, art et architecture en Europe, 1870–1993*. Paris: Centre Georges Pompidou.

Choay, F. (2004). Introduction. In L. B. Alberti (Ed.), *L'art d'édifier* (Translation from Latin, introduced and commented by P. Caye and F. Choay). Paris: Seuil.

Dalmasso, E. (1972). *Milano, capitale economica d'Italia*. Milano: Franco Angeli.

Davoudi, S. (2003). Polycentricity in European spatial planning: From an analytical tool to a normative agenda. *European Planning Studies, 11*(8), 979–999.

Dematteis, G. (2001). Per una geografia della territorialità attiva e dei valori territoriali. In P. Bonora (Ed.), *SLoT quaderno 1*. Bologna, Baskerville.

Dematteis, G. (2011). *Montanari per scelta*. Milano: Franco Angeli.

Donadieu, P. (2012). *Sciences du paysage. Entre théories et pratiques*. Cachan: Lavoisier.

Fanfani, D. (Ed.). (2009). *Pianificare tra città e campagna. Scenari, attori e progetti di nuova ruralità per il territorio di Prato*. Firenze: Firenze University Press.

Fanfani, D. & Fagarazzi, C. (Eds.). (2012). *Territori ad alta energia. Governo del territorio e pianificazione energetica sostenibile: metodi ed esperienze*. Firenze: Firenze University Press.

Ferraresi, G. (1992). Il progetto Ecopolis per Milano. In A. Magnaghi & R. Paloscia (Eds.), *Per una trasformazione ecologica degli insediamenti* (pp. 153–184). Franco Angeli: Milano.

Ferraresi, G. (Ed.). (2014). *Il progetto di territorio, oltre la città diffusa verso la bioregione*. Maggioli: Santarcangelo di Romagna.

Friedman, Y. (1975). *Utopies réalisables*. Paris: Union générale d'éditions.

Friedman, Y. (2003). *L'architecture de survie. Une philosophie de la pauvreté*. Paris: Editions de l'éclat.

Geddes, P. (1915). *Cities in evolution*. London: William & Norgate.

Georgescu-Roegen, N. (1966). *Analytical economics: Issues and problems*. Cambridge, MA: Harvard University Press.

Georgescu-Roegen, N. (1976). *Energy and economic myths*. New York: Pergamon Press.

Giusti, M. (1990). Locale, territorio, comunità, sviluppo. Appunti per un glossario. In A. Magnaghi (Ed.), *Il territorio dell'abitare. Lo sviluppo locale come alternativa strategica* (pp. 139–170). Milano: Franco Angeli.

Gliessman, S. (2014). *Agroecology: The ecology of sustainable food systems* (3rd ed.). Boca Raton: CRC Press.

Kohr, L. (1976). *The city of man (The Duke of Buen Consejo)*. Puerto Rico: University of Puerto Rico Press.

Kohr, L. (2001). *The breakdown of nations*. Cambridge: Green Books.

Krier, L. (1984). *Architectura Patriae*; or the destruction of Germany's architectural heritage. *Architectural Design, 54*, 101–102.

Latouche, S. (2006). *Le pari de la decroissance*. Paris: Fayard.

Le Lannou, M. (1963). *Le déménagement du territoire*. Paris/Seuil: Réveries d'un géographe.

MacKaye, B. (1928). *The new exploration. A philosophy of regional planning*. New York: Harcourt, Brace & Co.

Madec, P. (2012). Vers l'équité territoriale. In A. Masboungi (Ed.), *Projets urbains durables* (pp. 19–25). Paris: Le Moniteur.

Magnaghi, A. (Ed.). (1990). *Il territorio dell'abitare. Lo sviluppo locale come alternativa strategica*. Milano: Franco Angeli.

Magnaghi, A. (Ed.). (1998). *Il territorio degli abitanti: società locali e sostenibilità*. Milano: Dunod.

Magnaghi, A. (2001). Una metodologia analitica per la progettazione identitaria del territorio. In A. Magnaghi (Ed.), *Rappresentare i luoghi. Metodi e tecniche* (pp. 13–51). Firenze: Alinea.

Magnaghi, A. (2005). *The urban village. A charter for democracy and local self-sustainable development*. London: Zed Books.

Magnaghi, A. (2013). Riterritorializzare il mondo. In *Scienze del Territorio*: "Ritorno alla terra". *1*, 47–58. (theme issue).

Magnaghi, A. (2014). Il progetto della bioregione urbana. Regole statutarie e elementi costruttivi. In A. Magnaghi (Ed.), *La regola e il progetto. Un approccio bioregionalista alla pianificazione territoriale* (pp. 3–42). Firenze: Firenze University Press. (open access edition). http://www.fupress.com/catalogo/la-regola-e-il-progetto/2626. Accessed 25 April 2019.

Magnaghi, A. (2017). La storia del territorio nell'approccio territorialista all'urbanistica e alla pianificazione. In *Scienze del Territorio*, "Storia del territorio". *5*, 32–41. (theme Issue).

Magnaghi, A. (2017a). De la grande métropole à la biorégion urbaine. In A. Magnaghi (Ed.), *La conscience du lieu* (pp. 155–181). Paris: Eterotopia France.

Magnaghi, A., & Fanfani, D. (Eds.). (2010). *Patto città campagna. Un progetto di bioregione urbana per la Toscana centrale*. Firenze: Alinea.
Magnaghi, A., & IRER Lombardy Regional Institute for Research. (1995). Bonifica, Riconversione e Valorizzazione ambientale del bacino dei fiumi Lambro, Seveso, Olona. In *Urbanistica-Quaderni. 2*. Roma: INU Edizioni.
Magnaghi, A., & Marson, A. (2004). Verso nuovi modelli di città. In M. Carbognin, E. Turri, & G. M. Varanini (Eds.), *Una rete di città: Verona e l'area metropolitana Adige-Garda*. CiErre: Verona.
Magnaghi, A., & Sala, F. (Eds.). (2013). *Il territorio fabbrica di energia*. Milano: Wolters Kluwer Italia.
Malcevschi, S. (2010). *Reti ecologiche polivalenti. Infrastrutture e servizi ecosistemici per il governo del territorio*. Milano: Il Verde Editoriale.
Marson, A. (Ed.). (2016). *La struttura del paesaggio. Una sperimentazione multidisciplinare per il Piano della Toscana*. Bari: Laterza.
Maturana, H. R., & Varela, F. J. (1984). *El árbol del conocimiento: las bases biológicas del entendimiento humano*. Santiago de Chile: OEA Organización de Estados Americanos.
Moreno, D. (1990). *Dal documento al terreno. Storia e archeologia dei sistemi agro-silvo-pastorali*. Bologna: Il Mulino.
Mumford, L. (1961). *The city in history. Its origins, its transformations, its prospects*. New York: Harcourt, Brace & World.
Nebbia, G. (2012). Prefazione. In M. Ercolini (Ed.), *Acqua! Luoghi/paesaggio/territorio*. Aracne: Roma.
Olivetti, A. (1945). *L'ordine politico della comunità*. Ivrea: Nuove Edizioni Ivrea.
Poli, D. (Ed.). (2012). *Regole e progetti per il paesaggio. Verso il nuovo piano paesaggistico della Toscana*. Firenze: Firenze University Press.
Poli, D. (Ed.). (2013). *Agricoltura paesaggistica. Visioni, metodi, esperienze*. Firenze: Firenze University Press.
Poli, D. (2019). *Le comunità progettuali della bioregione urbana. Un Parco agricolo multifunzionale in riva sinistra d'Arno*. Macerata: Quodlibet.
Quaini, M. (2011). Fra territorio e paesaggio. Una terra di mezzo ancora da esplorare? In D. Poli (Ed.), *Contesti. Città, territori, progetti. Il progetto territorialista*. (Special issue), 2.
Raffestin, C. (1980). *Pour une géographie du pouvoir*. Paris: LITEC.
Rovai, M., Di Iacovo, F., & Orsini, S. (2010). Il ruolo degli Ecosystem Services nella pianificazione territoriale sostenibile. In C. Perrone & I. Zetti (Eds.), *Il valore della terra. Teoria e applicazioni per il dimensionamento della pianificazione territoriale* (pp. 135–162). Milano: Franco Angeli, Milano.
Sale, K. (1985). *Dwellers in the land: The bioregional vision*. San Francisco: Sierra Club Book.
Saragosa, C. (2005). *L'insediamento umano. Ecologia e sostenibilità*. Roma: Donzelli.
Saragosa, C. (2011). *La città tra passato e futuro. Un percorso critico sulla via di Biopoli*. Roma: Donzelli.
Schön, D. A. (1983). *The reflective practitioner: How professionals think in action*. Milton Park/Abingdon-Oxon: Routledge.
Stuiver, M. (2006). Highlighting the retro side of innovation and its potential for regime change in agriculture. In T. Marsden & J. Murdoch (Eds.), *Between the local and the global* (pp. 147–173). Bingley: Emerald.
Thayer, R. L. (2003). *Life place. Bioregional thought and practice*. Berkeley: University of California Press.
Thayer, R. L. (2013). The world shirks the world expands: Information, energy and relocalisation. In E. Cook & J. J. Lara (Eds.), *Remaking metropolis. Global challenges of the urban landscape* (pp. 39–59). London: Routledge.
Todd, J., & Todd, N. J. (1984). *Bioshelters, ocean arks, city farming: Ecology as the basis of design*. New York: Random House.
Turco, A. (2010). *Configurazioni della territorialità*. Milano: Franco Angeli.

van der Ploeg, J. D. (2008). *The new peasantries. Struggles for autonomy and sustainability in an era of empire and globalization*. London: Earthscan.

Van Dobbelsteen A, Gommans, L., & Roggema, R. (2008). Smart vernacular planning: sustainable regional design based on local potentials and optimal deployment of energy chain. In *Proceedings of the world conference SB08*, Melbourne, CSIRO – Commonwealth Scientific and Industrial Research Organisation, Australia. 967–74. http://www.irbnet.de/daten/iconda/CIB15946.pdf. Accessed 19 Jan 2020.

Viale, G. (2011). *La conversione ecologica. There is no alternative*. Rimini: NdA Press.

Vidal de la Blache, P. (2008). *Principes de géographie humaine*. Paris: L'Harmattan. (orig. ed. 1903).

Volpe, G. (2008). Per una 'archeologia globale dei paesaggi della Daunia. Tra archeologia, metodologia e politica dei beni culturali. In G. Volpe, M. J. Strazzulla, & D. Leone (Eds.), *Storia e archeologia della Daunia. In ricordo di Marina Mazzei*. Bari: EdiPuglia.

Rearticulating the Economy from the Local Level: Towards an Economy Rooted in Caring for Life

Marta Soler Montiel and Manuel Delgado Cabeza

1 Premise

Aristotle, in IV century BC, made a distinction between *oikonomia*, meaning the rules of the household, which provide "such things necessary to life, and useful for the community" and chrematistics, "originating in the use of coin" and "how they may be accumulated" (Politics, Book I, Chapter VIII and IX, 13–15). Based on this distinction, in the twentieth century, Karl Polanyi differentiated between a formal and a substantive economy. The first refers to the neoclassical idea that economy merely consists of individual choices within competitive markets, under the imperatives of maximum corporate profits and consumption. This business economy, a legacy of Aristotle's chrematistics, is responsible for the processes of deterritorialization that break the fragile socioecological equilibria at the local level (Magnaghi 2011). Conversely, Polanyi defined substantive economy as any social process aiming at satisfying human needs within its biophysical limits, socially embedded in territory, because every human being "survives in virtue of an institutionalized interaction between himself and his natural surroundings" (Polanyi 1977, p. 20). Polanyi's substantive economy recalls Aristotelian *oikonomia* and every territory-based economy which involves people's connections in their daily lives to provide what is necessary for life. Recently, feminist economics has pointed out historical responsibility of women in the economy that take care of life. This distinction between *oikonomia* and chrematistics, between substantive embedded economy and formal economy, between the economy that takes care of life and the one that destroys it is still nowadays at the core of current global crisis and its possible alternatives.

M. Soler Montiel (✉) · M. Delgado Cabeza
AREA Research Group, Department of Applied Economics II, University of Seville, Seville, Spain
e-mail: msoler@us.es; mdelgado@us.es

D. Fanfani, A. Matarán Ruiz (eds.), *Bioregional Planning and Design: Volume I*,
https://doi.org/10.1007/978-3-030-45870-6_4

This chapter is structured as follows. In the first heading, we analyse the main features of capitalist logic and dynamics in its current phase, and the evolution of the tensions associated with its reproduction. This dynamic is causing the existing socio-economic system to plunge into a deep crisis that calls for livelihood alternatives to the dominant forms. We are thus invited to rethink economy from a local standpoint by adopting a bioregional approach, where culture, nature and history are connected in the "territory" (Magnaghi 2011). The second heading contains a reflection on how territory-embedded substantive economies entail an economic alternative both at a material and at cultural and political levels. In it, social relations and relations with nature are reconstructed in the pursuit of sustainability of life through a bioregional approach. To that extent, changes are needed in at least four areas: the sustainable access and management of resources, the reorganization of production and labour, the questioning of consumption and its relation with production, and finally the logics and values that guide the territory-embedded economies which meet the criteria of social and environmental justice.

2 Modernity and Capitalism: The End of a Story

The evidence is growing that both modernity as a worldview and capitalism as a socioeconomic system that embodies it are reaching their limits and entering a period of slow decomposition or "terminal stage". Not only does this crisis question the management of the system but it also has broader consequences: it affects all the economic, social, political and cultural structures, together with the ethical and epistemological constructions that underlie the understanding and conception of life itself. This crisis is resulting in the collapse of the pillars underpinning the industrial civilization, so that dominant ways of thinking and living are at the core of the problems we face in this world-system (Wallerstein 2006). A system that follows the logic of monetary value—money is the measure of all things—and the accumulation of capital, wealth and power.

Therefore, the logic of profit needs and feeds a permanent expansion, driven by the imperative of converting money into more money. Various strategies are used to that purpose: the exploitation of wage labour, transformed into a commodity; the strengthening and rise of patriarchy as a form of domination and exploitation of women, who are made responsible for the indispensable work of material, emotional and affective care, but excluded from the commercial sphere; and the exploitation of nature through the appropriation of its resources on an industrial scale. The division of land use is the fourth capitalist way to foster the growth of capital accumulation and wealth appropriation and concentration. Territories are divided into peripheral areas and core areas. In the former, energy and materials are extracted and waste material is disposed of, whereas the latter attracts population, capital and resources. All these strategies represent the main sources of tension between accumulation of capital and sustainability of life (Pérez Orozco 2014).

The availability and use of the once-abundant fossil fuel energy are key in explaining the development and expansion of capitalism. They meant a radical change in the metabolism of the industrial society with respect to previous forms of social organisation, in quantitative and qualitative terms. Converting fossil fuels into mechanical energy entailed both a new dimension in material extraction and use and a more complex, dependent and specialized society. Moreover, it facilitated the concentration of power and higher levels of dominion and social control. As a result, the logic and functioning of the system spread globally (Fernández Durán y González Reyes 2014).

Some of the changes, obstacles and tensions that tend to be associated with the reproduction of capital have reached a peak stage within the system since the 1970s. Profit expectations, simulation of future benefits, and credit lie at the base of the prevailing regime of accumulation, due to the difficulties of converting money into more money in the sphere of production or *real economy*. They permit a *nonfactual creation of value* and currently set the pattern of modes and rhythms of growth and accumulation within the system (Chesnais 2003, p. 38). Confusion between wealth and debt is a key feature of this "paper economy" (Daly 1995). The sphere of production has thus largely become an excuse for capital revaluation.

In this way, accumulation in real economy is reaching its limits, since automation and productivity growth, produced by capital, parallel the shrinking of labour force needed and of unit profits. The global increase in the production of goods counterbalanced this shrinkage for over 150 years. The extraction and consumption of materials were boosted by the pressing need of permanent growth, to the extent that they led to the ecological crisis.

This compensatory mechanism has proven insufficient in fostering accumulation over the last four decades, even though the supply of goods has constantly increased. Conversely, financial capital "got off the ground" and let capitalism survive constantly basing on credit, that is to say through a sort of simulation (Jappe 2011: 53) based on the capitalization of future profits. Capital has fled "upwards" towards financial markets. Nonetheless, not only does this factor not interfere with a "healthy" economy: it has also created a fictitious prosperity and has made the processes of "accumulation by dispossession" (Harvey 2004) reach unprecedented limits over the last decades.

Dispossession can be obtained through a revaluation of assets or through big corporations issuing securities which serve the functions of money, creating bank and financial money out of nothing. These mechanisms allow financial capital to appropriate existing wealth. Moreover, they provide it with a tremendous purchasing power on the world market, letting it globally acquire properties of local capital, of the State and of the public administrations. As a result, financial capital holds increasingly high positions of power and privilege, in a context of growing unequal distribution of global wealth. In addition, these instruments promote the capture of rents, thanks to different strategies: the privilege over the control of public resources, the privatization, the priority over the use of utilities (water, electricity and gas), the management of transport as a private business, the housing regulation and finally the intertwined alliances known as private-public partnerships that are leading to the plunder of public resources. This path leads to the "dispossession of everyday life" (Taifa 2016), in a context where all areas of life are invaded by an increasing commodification.

Not only is life affected by commodification, when individuals sell working time for the production and its requirements or when using time for consumption, but also when an increasing amount of "time dedicated to the market-led construction of self" is spent creating a mode of existence obeying the rules of commodification (Baschet 2015, p. 44). Thus, people's relationships with themselves and the others are increasingly turning into relations between things in a scenario of deepening social degradation. The pressures of the global market and the value creation within financial markets result both in a deterioration of working conditions and in a growing gap between wage labour, which is seen as a sort of "deity" or the main "social intermediary", and its increasing scarcity. Competition for employment is exacerbated by wage labour shortage, and likewise the types of employment driven by the imperatives of value are becoming increasingly superfluous from the point of view of human needs (Baschet 2015). There has been an upward trend in social inequalities, which have reached unprecedented levels in this context (Informe sobre la riqueza global 2015; Oxfam 2014).

Political power is an accomplice of this situation, because it adapts to suit the requirements of the established power. "Laws and government may be considered in this and indeed in every case as a combination of the rich to oppress the poor, and preserving to themselves the inequality of the goods". Adam Smith's forceful statement (Aguilera 2016) clearly expresses the idea of politics at the service of economic power within capitalism. Regrettably, this trend is accelerating due to the consolidation of economic governance and to the fusion of wealth and power. Large corporate organizations hold the power to force the government in order to facilitate their business needs, in a context of a "community of interests" between the political and business elites increasingly intertwined.

In the industrial society, the imperatives of growth arose from capital accumulation and greater availability of energy and resulted in a transition from an economy of "production" to an economy based on the "purchase" or "extraction" of fuel and mineral sources. The monetary reductionism facilitated this process, concealing the physical costs of economic processes (Naredo 2015). As a consequence, we may depict massive extraction as a key element of modern society and capitalist system (Bednik 2016) insomuch that the industrial system currently moves more tonnage than any geological force. Some authors point out that the human species has produced a new geological era, the Anthropocene, in which the separation between nature and human beings is emphasized and their interaction is of increasing importance (Naredo 2016).

Since the beginning of capitalism, the quantity of materials used has increased steadily, accelerating since 1950 (Schaffartzik et al. 2014) and with a further intensification over the last decades (WU Material Flow 2017). The use of materials was ten times higher at the beginning of the twenty-first century than 100 years ago. The use of abiotic resources has greatly increased, considering that they have multiplied more than 25 times (Krausmann et al. 2009). Global extraction has more than doubled over the last 30 years, and it has grown yearly, from 36 billion metric tons in 1980 to 85 billion metric tons in 2013 (WU Material Flow 2017). In that period, the proportion of mineral and fossil fuel extraction is trending upwards compared to biomass extraction, which has diminished from 1/3 to 1/4 of the total. The gap between the behaviour of the contemporary industrial civilization and those of other cultures and previous ages in human history is thus widening. Human beings have changed from an organization based on the photosynthesis and its by-products to another sustained by the extraction of *resources* from the Earth.

In this way, planet Earth is increasingly turning into a great mine. Even agriculture has become an extractive activity, since it demands the injection of large amounts of fossil energy, water, fertilizers, pesticides, etc. (Naredo 1999). It is a sort of constant "re-materialization" in terms of volume of material and energy used (Infante 2014). Besides fostering unsustainable waste production, resource-use intensification is constantly degrading planet Earth and resulting in the rapid depletion of the resources themselves. Many researchers agree on this point and claim that our planet is turning into a "*Thanatia*" (Valero y Valero 2015). If this trend continues, it is estimated that, by 2050, the levels of consumption of the Earth's natural resources will be five times higher than now. In such a scenario, the demand of some important ones (gold, silver, copper, nickel, tin, zinc, lead, antimony) would exceed the reserves currently known. As a consequence, humanity might have to deal with a mineral crisis in a few decades, since substitution of minerals might not be viable due to global shortage. In this respect, peak oil was reached in 2008, while peak natural gas is expected in 2023. The depletion of these resources is expected to occur by the end of the twenty-first century (Valero y Valero 2009; Prats et al. 2016).

Moreover, due to falling EROEI (energy returned on energy invested), very high investments will be required in order to meet energy demand in the coming years. As an example, petroleum EROEI has fallen from 100:1 in 1900 to 18:1 at present. In this situation, the prices of fossil fuels are likely to steadily rise, which will lead to major socioeconomic consequences (Prats et al. 2016). Conversely, renewable energy is a negligible percentage (around 2%) of the total energy consumption, and has low EROEI rates. As Jorge Riechmann (2009) points out, every day we consume the same amount of fossil fuels as the amount of plant material growing in more than one year on the Earth and in the oceans (p. 144). Replacing fossil energy thus appears to be impossible.

The ecological footprint analysis also confirms that the current use of resources is becoming increasingly unsustainable. Since approximately 1975, global consumption of resources exceeds our planet's biocapacity to regenerate them. In 2010, 150% of Earth's biocapacity was used, and the quantity is expected to reach the equivalent of two planets (280%) by 2050 (WWF 2011). In the words of the Stockholm Memorandum, developed and signed during the Nobel Laureate Symposium on Global Sustainability (2011): "Science indicates that we are transgressing planetary boundaries", and "we cannot continue on our current path".

The unsustainable consumption of resources is responsible for climate change. In 2016, carbon monoxide emissions into the atmosphere exceeded 400 ppm. This amount is considered to be the limit beyond which global temperature may rise more than 2 °C compared to the pre-industrial era. If these levels were reached, global damages would be serious, irreparable and out of control. Lately, this limit has been lowered to 1.5 °C (Prats et al. 2016). Accordingly, 2016 proved to be the hottest year in history, with a 1.1 °C rise compared to the pre-industrial era (OMM 2016). The Fifth Assessment Report on Climate Change in 2014 warned that, compared to 1850, "global surface temperature change for the end of the 21st century (….) is projected to likely exceed 1.5 °C" for all possible scenarios (IPPC 2014).

A radical transformation in industrial society's metabolism is thus a primary condition for the reduction of emissions in order to help reduce climate change. This transformation will only be technically viable with reliable technology and materials, which can provide enough energy for a sustainable society. However, in Riechmann's words (2015), this will only be possible if the investment effort is deeply reoriented, which is incompatible with private priorities of investment under capitalism and with the perpetuation of the exponential economic growth over the last decades (p. 33).

Given this situation, how can we start a transition into a sustainable society, fitting the current context of socio-ecological crisis?

3 Towards an Economy Rooted in Caring for Life

Degrowth and alternatives are inevitable, as indicated by the ecological deterioration, the depletion of resources and the social degradation. There are many examples of emerging or resisting alternatives stemming from bioregional roots. Some of them are: peasant and agroecological farming supported by the community and integrated in short distribution channels ensuring local food sovereignty; small scale systems of manufacturing production—i.e. textile and timber—connected to local markets; housing cooperatives; small-scale decentralized production of renewable energy, which is essential for energy sovereignty; local currencies, barter trade markets and credit unions for financial sovereignty; time banks, parenting groups, health and education cooperatives and so forth. Although, in the present article, we cannot perform a detailed analysis of each proposal, we can characterize four areas of economic deconstruction and reconstruction. In them, both social relations and relations with nature are reformulated on a local basis in order to nourish and support life. The confluence of these four areas implies the interaction between alternative socio-cultural rationalities and ecological rationalities, which enables the construction of new bioregional economic processes based on diversity.

3.1 Sustainable Access and Management of Resources: Enhancing Commons

Economic alternatives require constant access to material and immaterial resources, so as to provide all that is necessary for life. Privatization and commodification of fundamental resources, such as water, soil fertility, energy, housing, health, education, result in processes of physical destruction and social exclusion. These are all increasingly creating socio-environmental conflicts in the whole world, including Europe[1] (Martínez Alier 2002; Temper et al. 2015). Against this backdrop, the debate and defence of commons revive. In the present discourse, commons are understood as communitarian forms of resource and territory management beyond the market and the state. They are able to ensure their conservation and equal access to all that is necessary to provide sustenance to who takes care of them (Ostrom 2005).

In order to reverse the commodification of the access to resources and to democratize it, both natural and immaterial commons, such as knowledge and health, must be defended and enhanced. It is a tangible matter and it is also closely related to politics, which defines the conditions for access. Private property dominates as a mechanism of exclusion in capitalism, while what is public and common prevails as a strategy of inclusion in the world of economic alternatives. Moreover, cultural aspects also define this matter, taking into account that alternatives to the market are given shape by the forms of organization, collective practices and underlying values. All these, in the words of decolonial theorist Arturo Escobar, come from a cultural plurality, with diverse ways of "feeling and thinking" the world (Escobar 2014). Substantive economies seek to ensure constant forms of resource access and management through a variety of strategies suited to local circumstances. Materiality is indeed a necessary yet not sufficient condition for alternatives. Even when private property prevails, as is the case with most peasant agroecological farming, resource management is aimed at ensuring cooperation, reciprocity and care in order to provide sustenance and all that is necessary for life. It is not merely a matter of access, although it is fundamental, but it is also about the way in which obtained resources are used.

These alternative strategies for the defence and access to necessary resources can only be developed through a bioregional approach. As a matter of fact, local contexts are the place where these resources are managed democratically, according with the use rooted in people's real needs. Moreover, traditional knowledge and institutions for a sustainable management of resources resist in these contexts, as both Alberto Magnaghi (2011) and Eleonor Ostrom (2005) remark.

---

[1] See the Environmental Justice Atlas https://ejatlas.org/ and Temper et al. (2015).

3.2 *About the Social Reorganization of the Activity for Caring Life*

In market economy, the concept of "production" is mainly connected to wage labour in companies, which transforms nature making intensive use of capital, machinery and tools. Its purpose is to create monetary "value", since the production outcomes (goods or services) are exchanged for money within the market. This definition of "production", frequently reduced to buying and selling at a profit, is an anthropocentric and Eurocentric idea. Although historically recent, this concept is currently predominant (Naredo 2015). Ecological economic warns that this metaphor of "production" conceals essentially destructive processes not only in biophysical terms (Naredo and Valero 1999) but also in social terms, because "our technics has become compulsive and tyrannical, since it is not treated as a subordinate instrument of life" (Mumford 1952, p. 137).

At present, no long-term viable economic activity can be conceived of without taking into account the ecological limits of the biosphere where life develops. This implies that we have to quit the world of "production" and approach "biomimicry", which is a way of meeting human needs through processes stemming from a conscious and innovative emulation of nature (Benyus 2002). Biomimicry is a strategy of ecological reconstruction of economy based on a quest for coherence between human systems and ecosystems[2] (Riechmann 2006, p. 194). It is necessary that we "produce" fewer things, using less energy and materials. For this reason, economic alternatives must necessarily be ecological at present. Human sustenance must be re-thought of in biomimetic and bioregional terms, recovering the ecological rationality of local knowledge.

The advance in biomimetic processes implies a reduction in the contributions of capital and natural resources in order to progress towards a life-centred economy, as has been claimed by solidary economy[3] (Coraggio 2007) and feminist economics (Pérez Orozco 2014). Handcraft Manufacturing and knowledge from experience are at the centre of economic alternatives, mainly as a result of the necessity derived from exclusion (Quijano 2007). But they are as well, often and increasingly, a

[2] "Nature runs on sunlight, (…) only uses the energy it needs, (…) fits form to function, (…) recycles everything, (…) rewards cooperation, "banks on diversity, (….) demands local expertise, (...) curbs excesses from within, (...) taps the power of limits" (Benyus 2002: 7). Jorge Riechmann (2006) identifies six principles of biomimicry: (1) Stable state (homeostasis) in biophysical terms; (2) The sun as source of energy for life; (3) Close material cycles; (4) Do not transport materials for long distances; (5) Avoid xenobiotics as POPs (Persistent Organic Pollutant), GMO (Genetically Modified organisms), etc.; (6) Respect biodiversity (p. 233, 234).

[3] José Luis Coraggio (2007) claims a work-centred economy, with a new definition of work which refers to all the different human activities, mainly manual, aimed at meeting human needs. This meaning goes beyond the traditional definitions of "productive" work and, although not explicitly stated, it approximates to the care-centred proposals of the feminist economy. In accordance with Coraggio's text, we used the word "activities" instead of work, reflecting the basic ideas of the author. A similar reflection can be made on Quijano's cited text (2007), where the author considers the limits of alternative ways of doing things based on necessity without any political awareness.

conscious and political process aimed at bringing back "that respect for the essential attributes of personality, its creativity and autonomy, which Western man lost at the moment he displaced his own life in order to concentrate on the improvement of the machine" (Mumford 1952: 11).

It is not about reviving Luddism, but it is a matter of rebalancing social relations using the tools of artisan activities and their pragmatist view: "the craft of making physical things provides insight into the techniques of experience that can shape our dealings with others. Both the difficulties and the possibilities of making things well apply to making human relationships" (Sennet 2008: 289). As Richard Sennet argues, craftsmanship is closely linked not only to manual skills, but also to slowness, to commitment to doing things well, to lack of self-conceit towards the outcome and pride in one's work, to playfulness, to creativity and a sense of freedom rooted in the community. Consequently, it implies a new temporality which is able to respect both nature and the rhythm of life of the community (Riechmann 2004; Baschet 2015). Moreover, it is thoroughly democratic, since it is not restricted to an elite only; it is essentially a cooperative organizational structure oriented towards "learning by doing". Artisan activity is also helpful in the necessary de-specialization required by economic alternatives in order to break the hierarchies (Baschet 2015). As a matter of fact, "the whole of our civilization is founded on specialization, which implies the enslavement of those who execute to those who co-ordinate; and on such a basis one can only organize and perfect oppression" (Weil 2013, p. 41).

We therefore need to exit the world of production and enter artisan biomimicry, at the same time as we exit the world of work in order to enter the world of doing, especially the world of care. The current notion of work is a historical construction inherent to capitalism, which has ended up praising the relationships of dependency and subordination that lie at the basis of paid work, which is necessary in "production" and acquisition processes (Naredo 2001). As feminist economy points out, in this androcentric-biased vision, the concept of work is reduced to employment, with the result that housework and care work, mostly carried out by women, are ignored and devalued. These activities are in fact essential for life, but the monetary economic process in the market system takes them for free (Picchio 1992), and exacerbates the conflict between capital and life (Pérez Orozco 2014).

The exit from the world of production and work in order to enter the care world for life's sustainability[4] (Carrasco Bengoa 2001, 2014), all forms of life (Puleo 2011; Pérez Orozco 2014), entails breaking the oppressive dualisms of patriarchy (Puleo 2005). These dualisms hierarchically oppose "male" and "female", and thus organize binary opposition between the "public" and the "private", the "productive" and the "unproductive or reproductive", reason and emotions, culture and nature, etc. Embracing the care world and life's sustainability implies that the centrality of

[4] In the first stage, this proposal of Feminist Economy had an anthropocentric bias, since it defended a reorientation of economy towards care and sustainability of human life. Nevertheless, together with ecofeminism, the proposal progresses towards the aim of sustainability of human and non-human life forms (Pérez Orozco 2014).

markets is displaced and that we enter the feminized world of cooperative activity and of life-centred available time.

3.3 Critical Consumption and a Stable Connection with the Needs of a Committed Community

We live in a dual society: a part of it is characterized by the extreme shortage of resources and the other by wastefulness. This duality must be doubly broken. In the current ecological crisis, the necessary social redistribution of material resources is only possible in a dematerialization context that goes beyond a biomimetic change in the organization of the supply system. On the one hand, people who lack the necessary means try to obtain them, which is directly linked to the access to resources. On the other hand, the ones who have too much need to practice degrowth and conscious self-restraint (Riechmann 2004). This is the way in which material justice can be reached among all social classes, between rural and urban worlds, between men and women or any possible sexual identity, between ethnic groups and territories, between global North and South, all this respecting the existing multiple worlds in the cultural diversity of the "pluriverse"[5] (Escobar 2014). It is not merely an individual matter, but it is mainly a political and civilizing one.

A new, deeply-felt cultural conception of what is necessary is essential for a change towards material distribution and reduction. In order to achieve this, the first step is to reject the concept of consumption as a symbol of status and social power in a hierarchical class system (Veblen 1899; Bourdieu 1979 [2000]), and to start considering it as a driving force of social and ecological destruction. The imaginary of the Western urban-industrial way of life of middle and high class, violently proposed by culture, must be displaced from being the universal standard of social desirability in consumerism (Latouche 2008). At present, this imaginary produces contempt for traditional ways of life and their ethics of frugality in daily life, whereas these are at the core of the process of critical and solidarity-based consumption in progress (Ariztia et al. 2016). Furthermore, we must break the Western confusion between potentially infinite desires and limited needs (Doyal and Gough 1994) and its hierarchized conception. Starting from a concept of human need as universal and non-hierarchical (Max-Neef 1994), material and political debate must focus on the redefinition of the ways of satisfying these needs, meeting social and ecological justice criteria. These are the socio-cultural means to reach material and psycho-emotional fulfilment. It is thus necessary to exit the world of "having" and progress towards the world of "being". Only within this new imaginary the necessary and urgent redistribution of resources will take place non-traumatically, so that we can reach that de-materialized abundance we need.

---

[5] It is that "world where many worlds fit" and where "we are equal because we are different" as claimed by the Zapatista movement.

As a first step, the concept of individual subjectivities must be broken, since the addiction to consumption and extreme commodification of Western market society life are deeply rooted in individualistic, hypercompetitive and narcissistic ways of feeling the world (Baschet 2015). These ways are painful but also indifferent to other people's pain and to ecological destruction (Shaw and Bonnett 2016). Moreover, they are rooted in a profound feeling of fear of being excluded or uprooted (Bauman 2015). But individual change can only be promoted by collective action, since it requires a sense of belonging, social ties and responsibility, in a community built on non-sectarian and non-essentialist principles of social justice (Bauman 2009). As communitarian feminism claims, the change towards responsibility and care for self and other's wellness must exceed the restricted realm of the family and the emotional boundaries of the private space of the house: on the contrary, it must pervade all spheres of life (Paredes 2010). The change, in essence, is a civilizational one. It rejects the logic of Western development and can only be practically achieved starting from the diversity of the territories and the multiplicity of people and identities in them. Direct social relationships are only possible in local territories, where they generate deeply-felt and embodied connections within the community. Therefore this civilizational change is in essence and by definition a bioregional one. Yet it carries a potential risk of ethnic essentialism and of dynamics of exclusion which might result in oppressive local communities. To avert this risk, we should not abandon the construction of new bioregional communities. Conversely, the alternative is to promote local political processes in order to break Western cultural bias of developmental ethnocentrism (Escobar 2014) and of androcentrism (Pérez Orozco 2014), so to build a community life with a "global sense of place" where diversity is welcome (Massey 1991). The bioregional project will avert the risk of producing essentialist and sectarian exclusion only through a "global sense of place". That would generate a multiplicity of local worlds, open and inclusive to cultural diversity: a necessary feature, given the migratory connections typical of our interconnected world.

In order to practically reconstruct economic life, almost all alternatives are rooted in the local domain. Nevertheless, a bioregional perspective is fundamental as a means to question consumption and combine it with new forms of artisanal activity. The main aim is to find access strategies in which exchange becomes separated from selfish commodified relationships and progresses towards a communitarian conception, within the frame of material possibilities of agroecosystems and ecosystems. Local markets become then a meeting point where necessities are satisfied beyond exchange. In doing that, the duality between production and consumption is broken by daily connections of care among neighbours in squares, parks, studios, vegetable gardens, homes, neighbourhood associations, fields, community centres, *etcetera*. Provided that as individual sustenance is rooted in cooperative relationships, new processes of individual self-construction will be activated, along with new subjectivities with a sense of proportion.[6] In this process we break and exit economy, we go beyond reciprocity and we reach the generosity that support connections[7] (Graeber 2012). In such a way, collective individualism and essentialism break down, so that the bodies and territories are combined into a single entity, in the way pointed out by communitarian feminism[8] (Cabnal 2010).

3.4 Beyond the Material Question: Epistemology of the South and Relational Ontologies

Taking care of necessities and caring life as a goal is diametrically opposed to the aim of market economy, which is pursuing profit and accumulation. Economic goals are linked to socio-cultural processes. Therefore, they are rooted in the worldviews, which is in the ethical, epistemological and ontological matrix of the people who give life to these economic relations.

Bioregional-coherent economic alternatives are rooted in a moral economy, historically linked to the peasantry (Thompson 1995; Scott 1976) and now acquiring new practices and values regarding socio-economic justice (Lechat 2009). They tend to generate new cooperative subjectivities in which "*I is we*, because each one weaves the bonds that link themselves to their fellow people" (Baschet 2015, p. 103), as communitarian feminism also asserts. When sustenance directly depends

[6] "The notion of proportion, better than the one of limit, allows for rejecting the ghost of unlimitedness, typical of the commodity society (…). Proportion entails posing the problem in terms of relationships. The sense of proportion is one of fair relationships. In it, self-consciousness is the prerequisite for respecting others, while the concern for others is the prerequisite for widespread beneficial cooperative relationships. Proportionality should not be intended as an obligation that limits each person's freedom (…). Conversely, it means being aware of the consequences that unlimitedness and forgetfulness can entail in terms of well-being, peace, available time, friendship, etcetera". (Baschet 2015, p. 101, footnote 19).

[7] David Graeber (2012) argues that the connections derived from gift and not from reciprocity are the foundation of all societies. He contends that when, in a quantified exchange, the goods given and received are equal, even though they are non-material, the connection is broken, being the connection a relationship of commitment among the people in a community who share a "debt". Market economy is based on quantified exchanges, where supply equals demand. These kinds of exchanges free from the connections and combine individualism, lack of solidarity and affective indifference towards others. As Polanyi claims in The Great Transformation, this economy destroys the community and solidarity.

[8] Communitarian feminism, a proposal led by Latin-American indigenous women, combines a call for gender equality in the community (for "us") with the defence of the community in the territory. Some of its fundamental teachings are as follows: "When I defend my territory or land it is not just because I need natural resources for living and for allowing other generations to live a dignified life. In a view of recovery and defence of my body-land territory, I assume the recovery of my expropriated body, in order to generate life in it, happiness, vitality, pleasures and the construction of liberating knowledge for decision taking. I join this power with the defence of my land territory, because I can't conceive this woman body without a place on the earth that dignifies my existence and promotes my life's fulfilment" (Cabnal 2010).

on natural resources, it generates an ecological rationality that tends to take care of them (Toledo, 1993). Joan Martínez Alier (2002) defined it as the "ecologism of the poor". Conversely, self-restraint and self-construction, both individual and collective, are the protagonists of the construction of ecologically and socially ethical alternatives, when alternatives come from will rather than from a pressing material need (Riechmann 2000). At any rate, bioregional economic alternatives are built around ecological and biocentric ethics that break Western anthropocentrism. Moreover, these economic alternatives are rooted in the ethics of care promoted by feminism, in order to break patriarchal dualities and to place life sustainability at the centre (Pérez Orozco 2014).

Bioregional economic alternatives defy the three basic axes of oppression of Western economistic culture, namely, anthropocentrism, ethnocentrism and androcentrism, which underlie the current conflict between capital and life.[9] Bioregional economic alternatives entails a new materiality, which can only stem from new conceptions of the world, from new knowledge alternative to Western epistemology (Sousa Santos 2009), and from new forms of being and feeling the world. We need relational ontologies where territories are vital times and places interconnected with the natural world (Escobar 2014, pp. 58–59). From this standpoint, the respect for cultural diversity as a basis for local economic alternatives implies the challenge of explicitly linking the bioregional project to the decolonial and ecofeminist critique. This would direct the practical construction of economic alternatives towards sustainability and care of all forms of life.

4 Conclusions

The ongoing ecological degradation, along with the socio-cultural conflicts, creates a pressing need for economic alternatives. The bioregionalist approach requires the construction of a balanced territorial dynamic of human activity, which must harmoniously fit in the biosphere. Therefore, it is necessary to exit the market economy, or even to exit the world of economy and enter the world of caring for life. This difficult and slow transition can only be initiated from the "local" by combining change processes in the four strategic areas previously analysed: sustainable access

[9] The first axis of oppression is against nature. In anthropocentrism, nature is despised and it is seen as freely accessible, in such a way that the ecological destruction resulting from economic growth is endorsed for the sake of growth. The second axis is ethnocentrism, which has generated a *series* of hierarchized cultural "alterities". They are the basis for socio-economic and ethnic inequalities rooted in classism and racism. The urban-industrial way of life of white middle-upper class is considered the main model of socio-cultural desirability. Thus, commodification of life is promoted, while disdain is directed at popular and working-class ways of life, together with rural and peasant's ones and all non-Western indigenous people's ones. The third axis of cultural oppression is androcentrism, which implies the contempt for anything feminine identifying it with nature, and promote a patriarchal culture. Within this culture, the economic system takes advantage of unpaid housework and domestic care work (Pérez Neira and Montiel 2013).

and management of resources through the enhancement of commons; the reorganization of sustenance based on artisanal activity for care; leaving the world of consumption and entering the one of life-caring, and the redefinition of our worldviews and social imaginaries.

In this transition process, Polanyi's distinction between formal economy and substantive economy remains fully valid, although an ecofeminist approach should be incorporated. It is both a material distinction and a conceptual one. On the one hand, it is related to the social organization of tasks, their results and the exchanges within the markets. On the other hand, it concerns the rationalities, aims and values that differentiate the dominant utilitarian economy from the multiple substantive economies stemming from the "local". These necessity-oriented economies entail materialities, activities and relationships that are different from what is currently dominant. Furthermore, they imply different forms of conceiving and understanding reality, different worldviews, epistemologies and ontologies. In Arturo Escobar's words (2014), we need different forms of "feeling and thinking" the life of territories and their people, combining new different ethics: ecological, feminist and postcolonial ones.

These different economies continuously emerge and endure, despite the growing oppression of formal economy. They have been called different names, they defend different practical proposals and are visibilized through different theories, which are not always mutually consistent and that are always under debate and in progress. Some expressions of the different substantive economies are: solidary economy (Coraggio 2007), degrowth (Latouche 2008), well living ("buen vivir") inspired by Latin American indigenous worldviews (Acosta 2013), indigenous communitarian feminism (Cabnal 2010), some theoretical proposals like the ecological economics (Martínez-Alier 1987; Naredo 2015) and feminist economics (Carrasco Bengoa 2014; Pérez Orozco 2014) and other practical proposals as Towns in Transition (Hopkins, 2008) and food sovereignty (Desmarais 2007; McMichael 2014). These "other economies", often excluded and removed by dominant views, are creating fair and sustainable ways of providing what is necessary for sustenance starting from the territories, in accordance with bioregional principles (Magnaghi 2011; McGinnis 1999).

References

Acosta, A. (2013). *El Buen Vivir: Sumak Kawsay, una oportunidad para imaginar otros mundos*. Editorial Icaria: Barcelona.

Aguilera, F. (2016). *Naturaleza humana, economía y cultura. Hábitos de pensamiento y reglas del juego*. Ediciones del Genal y El Acebuche Libertario.

Aristotle. (IV century BC). *Politics Batoche Books Kilchener* 1999 https://socialsciences.mcmaster.ca/econ/ugcm/3ll3/aristotle/Politics.pdf

Ariztia, T., Kleine, D., Bartholo, R., & Brightwell, G. (2016). Beyond the "deficit discourse": Mapping ethical consumption discourses in Chile and Brazil. *Environmental and Planning A, 0*(0), 1–19.

Baschet, J. (2015). Adiós al Capitalismo. Autonomía, sociedad del buen vivir y multiplicidad de mundos, Ned Ediciones (2014 Adieux au capitalisme. Autonomie, societé du bien vivre et multiplicité des mondes, La Découverte, París).

Bauman, Z. (2009). *Comunidad. En busca de seguridad en un mundo hostil*. Madrid: Siglo XXI de España Editores. (2001 Community, Seeking Safety in an Insecure World).

Bauman, Z. (2015). *Miedo líquido. La sociedad contemporánea y sus temores*. Barcelona: Paidós. (2006 Liquid fear, Polity Press, Cambridge, RU).

Bednik, A. (2016). *Extractivisme. Explotation industrielle de la nature: logiques, conséquences, résistences*. Ed. Le passager clandestin.

Benyus, J. M. (2002). *Biomimicry. Innovation Inspired by nature*. New York: HarperCollins Publishers.

Bourdieu, P. (2000). *La distinción. Criterio y bases sociales del gusto*. Madrid: Editorial Taurus. (1979 La distinction Les Éditions de Minuit).

Cabnal, L. (2010). *Acercamiento a la construcción de la propuesta de pensamiento epistémico de las mujeres indígenas feministas comunitarias de Abya Yala* (pp. 11–25) en Feminismos diversos: el feminismo comunitario. Madrid: ACSUR Las Segovias.

Carrasco Bengoa, C. (2001). La sostenibilidad de la vida humana: ¿un asunto de mujeres? *Mientras Tanto* nª 82 p. 43–70.

Carrasco Bengoa, C. (2014). La economía feminista: rupturas teóricas y propuesta política. en C. Carrasco Bengoa (Ed.), *Con voz propia. La economía feminista como apuesta teórica y política* (pp. 25–48). Madrid, y la Oveja Roja, colección libros de Viento Sur.

Chesnais, F. (2003). La teoría del régimen de acumulación financiarizado: contenido, alcance e interrogantes *Revista de Economía Crítica*. n°1.

Coraggio, J. L. (2007). Una perspectiva alternativa para la economía social: de la economía popular a la economía del trabajo. en J. L. Coraggio (organizador). *La Economía Social desde la Periferia. Contribuciones Latinoamericanas* (pp. 165–194). Buenos Aires, Editorial Altamira y Universidad Nacional de General Sarmiento.

Daly, H. (1995). "Dinero, deuda y riqueza virtual" en *Ecología Política*, n° 9 *El Memorando de Estocolmo* (2011). http://www.nobel-cause.de/stockholm-2011/download/Memorandum_ES.pdf

Desmarais, A. A. (2007). *La Vía Campesina. La globalización y el poder del campesinado*. Madrid: Editorial Popular.

Doyal, L., & Gough, I. (1994). *Teoría de las necesidades*. Editorial Icaria: Barcelona.

Escobar, A. (2014). Sentipensar con la Tierra. Nuevas lecturas sobre desarrollo, territorio y diferencia, Medellín, Ediciones UNAULA, Colección Pensamiento Vivo. https://mundoroto.files.wordpress.com/2015/03/sentipensar-con-la-tierra.pdf

Fernández Durán, R., & González Reyes, L. (2014). *En la espiral de la energía. Historia de la humanidad desde el papel de la energía (pero no sólo)*. Ed. Libros en Acción/Baladre.

Graeber, D. (2012). *En deuda. Una historia alternativa de la economía*. Barcelona: Ariel Editorial Planeta. (2011 Debt: the first 5.000 years Melville House Publishing NY).

Harvey, D. (2004). *El nuevo imperialismo*. Barcelona: Akal.

Hopkins, R. (2008). *The transition handbook: From oil dependency to local resilience*. Cambridge: Green Books.

Infante, J. (2014). La desmaterialización de la economía mundial a debate. Consumo de recursos y crecimiento económico. (1980–2008). en *Revista de Economía Crítica*, n°18.

Informe sobre la riqueza global. (2015). Credit Suisse.

IPPC Intergovernmental Panel of Climate Change 5° Informe. (2014). http://www.ipcc.ch/pdf/assessment-report/ar5/wg1/WG1AR5_ALL_FINAL.pdf

Jappe, A. (2011). *Crédito a muerte. La descomposición del capitalismo y sus críticos*. Ed. Pepitas de calabaza.

Krausmann, F., Gingrich, S., Eisenmenger, N., Erb, K., Haberl, H., & Fisher-Kovalski, M. (2009). Growth in global material use, GPD and population during the 20th century. *Ecologial Economic, 68*(10), 2696–2705.

Latouche, S. (2008). *La apuesta por el decrecimiento ¿cómo salir del imaginario dominante?* Barcelona: Editorial Icaria. (2006 Le pari de la décroissance Librairie Arthème Fayard).

Lechat, N. M. P. (2009). Economía Moral. en A. D. Cattani, J. L. Coraggio y J. L. Laville (org.). *Diccionario de la otra economía* (pp. 144–149). Buenos Aires: Universidad Nacional de General Sarmiento, Editorial Altamira, CLACSO.

Magnaghi, A. (2011). *El proyecto local. Hacia una conciencia del lugar*. Barcelona: Universitat Politécncica de Catalunya.

Martínez Alier, J. (1987). *Ecological economics: energy, environment and society*. Basil Blackwell: Oxford.

Martínez Alier, J. (2002). *The environmentalism of the poor: A study of ecological conflicts and valuation*. Cheltenham: Edward Elgar.

Massey, D. (1991). A global sense of place. *Marxism Today*, pp. 24–29.

Max-Neef, M. (1994). *Desarrollo a Escala Humana. Conceptos, aplicaciones y algunas reflexiones*. Barcelona: Editorial Icaria.

McGinnis, M. V. (1999). *Bioregionalism*. London/New York: Routledge.

McMichael, P. (2014). Historicizing food sovereignty. *The Journal of Peasants Studies, 41*(6), 933–957.

Mumford, L. (1952). *Art and technics*. New York: Columbia University Press.

Naredo, J. M. (1999). Síntesis de la intervención de la especie humana sobre la Tierra. en J. M. Naredo, y A. Valero (coord.). *Desarrollo económico y deterioro ecológico*. Ed. Fundación Argentaria y Visor.

Naredo, J. M. (2001). Configuración y crisis del mito del trabajo Archipiélago. *Cuadernos de Crítica de la Cultura, 48*, 13–23.

Naredo, J. M. (2015). *La economía en evolución*. Ed. Siglo XXI. 4ªedición.

Naredo, J. M. (2016). La ideología económica en la historia y el medio ambiente. en OMM Organización Meteológica Mundial (2016). https://public.wmo.int/en/media/press-release/wmo-confirms-2016-hottest-year-record-about-11%C2%B0c-above-pre-industrial-era

Naredo, J. M., & Valero, A. (1999). *Desarrollo Económico y deterioro ecológico n° 11 Colección Economía y Naturaleza*. Madrid: Fundación Argentaria y Visor.

OMM. (2016). Organización Meteorológica Mundial. *WMO News*. Comunicado de prensa 18 enero 2017.

Ostrom, E. (2005). *Understanding institutional diversity*. Oxford: Princeton University Press.

Oxfam Intermon. (2014) *Gobernar para las élites: secuestro democrático y desigualdad económica*. http://www.oxfamintermon.org/sites/default/files/documentos/files/bp-working-for-few-political-capture-economic-inequality-200114-es.pdf

Paredes, J. (2010). *Hilando fino desde el feminismo comunitario la Paz: Ded*.

Pérez Neira, D., Soler Montiel, M. (2013). Agroecología y ecofeminismo para descolonizar y despatriarcalizar la alimentación globalizada *Revista Internacional de Pensamiento Político* n° 8 pp. 95-113.

Pérez Orozco, A. (2014). *Subversión feminista de la economía. Aportes para un debate sobre el conflicto capital-vida*. Madrid: Traficantes de Sueños.

Picchio, A. (1992). *Social reproduction: the political economy of the labour markets*. Cambridge: Cambridge University Press.

Polanyi, K. (1977, 1994). *El sustento del hombre*. Barcelona: Mondadori (1977, *The livelihood on man*. New York: Academic).

Prats, F., Herrero, Y., & Torrego, A. (2016). *La gran encrucijada. Sobre la crisis ecosocial y el cambio de ciclo histórico*. Ed. Libros en acción.

Puleo, A. (2005). Los dualismos opresivos y la educación ambiental. *Isegoría, 32*, 201–214.

Puleo, A. (2011). *Ecofeminismo para otro mundo posible*. Madrid: Ediciones Ca.

Quijano, A. (2007). ¿Sistemas alternativos de producción? en J. L Coraggio (organizador). La *Economía Social desde la Periferia. Contribuciones Latinoamericanas* (pp. 145–164). Buenos Aires: Editorial Altamira y Universidad Nacional de General Sarmiento.

Riechmann, J. (2000). *Un mundo vulnerable: ensayos sobre ecología, ética y tecnociencia*. Madrid: Los libros de la catarata.
Riechmann, J. (2004). *Gente que no quiere viajar a Marte: Ensayos sobre ecología, ética y autolimitación*. Madrid: Los Libros de La Catarata.
Riechmann, J. (2006). *Biomímesis. Ensayos sobre imitación de la naturaleza, ecosocialismo y autocontención*. Madrid: Los libros de la Catarata.
Riechmann, J. (2009). *La habitación de Pascal. Ensayos para fundamentar éticas de suficiencia y políticas de autocontención*. Ed. Catarata.
Riechmann, J. (2015). *Autoconstrucción. La transformación cultural que necesitamos*. Ed. catarata.
Schaffartzik, A., Mayer, A., Gingrich, S., Eisenmenger, N., Loy, C., & Krausmann, F. (2014). The global metabolic transition: Regional patterns and trends of global material flows, 1950–2010. *Global Environmental Change, 26*, 87–97.
Scott, J. C. (1976). *The moral economy of the peasants: Rebellion and subsistence in Southeast Asia*. New Haven: Yale University Press.
Sennet, R. (2008). *The craftsman*. New Haven: Yale University Press.
Shaw, W. S., & Bonnett, W. (2016). Environmental crisis, narcisissm and the work of grief. *Cultural Geographies, 23*(4), 565–579. https://doi.org/10.1177%2F1474474016638042.
Sousa Santos, B. (2009). *Una epistemología del Sur* México: Siglo XXI CLACSO.
Taifa. (2016). *La desposesión de la vida cotidiana*. Informes de economía crítica n° 11. Barcelona. http://informes.seminaritaifa.org/informe-11/
Temper, L., del Bene, D., & Martínez Alier, J. (2015). Mapping the frontiers and front lines of global environmental justice: The EJAtlas. *Journal of Political Ecology, 22*, 255–278.
Thompson, E. P. (1995). *Costumbres en Común*. Barcelona: Editorial Crítica. (1991 Customs in common The Merlin Press Ltd Londres).
Toledo, V. M. (1993). La racionalidad ecológica de la producción campesina. en E. Sevilla Guzmán y M. González de Molina (Eds.), *Ecología, Campesinado e Historia* (pp. 197–218). Madrid: La Piqueta.
Valero, A., Valero, A. (2009): El agotamiento de la ´gran mina Tierra. La valoración exergética, una forma de medir la disponibilidad de recursos minerales *El Ecologista* n° 63 pp. 18–21.
Valero, A., & Valero, A. (2015). *Thanatia: The destiny of the Earth's mineral resources*. Londres: World Scientific Publishing.
Veblen, T. (1899). *The theory of the leisure class*. New York: Macmillan.
Wallerstein, I. (2006). *Análisis de sistemas-mundo* Volumen I Editorial Xiglo XXI.
Weil, S. (2013). *Oppression and liberty*. London: Routledge.
WU Material Flow. (2017). www.materialflow.net
WWF. (2011). *Planeta Vivo. Informe 2010. Biodiversidad, biocapacidad y desarrollo.*

Bioregion and *Spatial Configurations*. The Co-evolutionary Nature of the Urban Ecosystem

Claudio Saragosa and Michela Chiti

1 The Concept of Ecosystem and the Human Settlement

The concept of urban ecosystem began to be addressed in the 1960s. There have been several experiences on the topic (Douglas 1983; Bettini 1990) and, over time, the definition of it as *territorial ecosystem* (Saragosa 2001, 2005) has taken shape. I will briefly describe the concept of *territorial ecosystem*. Its conceptual model is well defined by Eugene Odum (1988, p. 13) when he speaks about the ecosystem: *an ecosystem is given by the entry environment, the system considered, the exit environment* (E = EE + CS + EE). Since I deal with human settlement, the system considered is to be identified in the settlement and the environments of entry and exit are to be recognized, respectively, in the areas of the open territory from which the settlement draws the basic resources for living and in those where it expels its waste.

According to Odum, the *territorial ecosystem* has to be studied as a system related to its own entry and exit environments: this also means that we can connect it to another very productive research path, the territorialized *ecological footprint* (Rees and Wackernagel 1996). Therefore, it is possible to think of a system—the human settlement—that is strongly correlated to the environments of both the origin of its vital resources and the destination of its waste; thus, a settlement that produces a footprint on an area of the earth. This footprint may be abstract, but, most of the time, it has an exquisitely spatial dimension, i.e. territorialized.

By adopting the conceptual tool of *territorial ecosystem*, it is useful to connect the problem of self-sustainability of the human settlement to the management of the

The chapter is the result of a common work of the authors. However, paragraphs 1 and 2 should be attributed to Michela Chiti, whereas paragraphs 3,4 and 5 have been written by Claudio Saragosa.

C. Saragosa (✉) · M. Chiti (✉)
Architecture Department, Florence University, Florence, Italy
e-mail: claudio.saragosa@unifi.it

D. Fanfani, A. Matarán Ruiz (eds.), *Bioregional Planning and Design: Volume I*,
https://doi.org/10.1007/978-3-030-45870-6_5

environments of origin-destination (therefore of the ecological footprint) of the observed settlement.

Again, from a conceptual point of view, it is possible to create a process of analysis of the self-sustainable human settlement produced by the *territorial ecosystem*. A sustainable settlement can be seen as a *living system*. For Fritjof Capra, living systems are identified by the "three conceptual dimensions of scheme, structure and process" (Capra 1997, p. 180). In synthesis, what Capra proposes is to interpret *autopoiesis*, defined by Maturana and Varela (1980, 1987), as the scheme of life (i.e. as the organization scheme of living systems); the dissipative structure, defined by Prigogine, as the structure of living systems; and cognition, initially defined by Bateson and more comprehensively by Maturana and Varela, as the process of life.

The self-sustainable human settlement, which I am conceptually outlining, has its own internal organization scheme of an *autopoietic* type, too. Each sustainable settlement, inserted in its own environment, has its own internal configuration that continuously reproduces itself in a continuous process (if, of course, mechanisms of necrosis do not arise).

Autopoietic processes evoke an internal organizational closure, while every living system (and metaphorically the settlement I am observing) is an open system continuously crossed by flows of matter-energy. The characteristic of a living system, as we know, is to be both open and closed at the same time: a living system "is structurally open, but organically closed. Matter flows continuously through the system and yet it maintains a stable form, doing so autonomously by means of self-organization" (Capra 1997, p. 115).

The self-sustainable settlement can only be an open system, continuously crossed by flows of matter-energy and information. To maintain its internal organization and its configuration, as to preserve its identity and vital characteristics, it must also ensure the continuous regeneration of the network of *autopoietic* processes.

In other texts, I realized how to use some concepts developed by ecology also for our settlement issues.

According to Ilya Prigogine, «*dissipative structures* are islands of order in a sea of disorder and they maintain and even increase their order at the expense of greater disorder of the environment. For example, living organisms take structures with an order (i.e. food) from the environment, use them as resources for their metabolism and eliminate structures with lower order (i.e. waste). This means that the order "floats in the disorder", to use the words of Prigogine, while total entropy continues to increase in harmony with the second law"» (Capra 1997, p. 210).

It is evident that the concepts of *autopoietic scheme* and *dissipative structure* are closely interrelated: in synthesis, autopoiesis is a set of relationships among production *processes*; a dissipative structure is a combination of metabolic and developmental *processes*. However, according to Capra, both the previous two definitions of vital processes must be correlated with another interpretative principle, that of cognitive processes: "in the emerging theory of living systems, the process of life – the continuous materialization of an autopoietic scheme into a dissipative structure – is identified with cognition, the process of knowledge [...]. The interactions of a living organism – vegetal, animal or human – with its environment are cognitive, i.e.

mental interactions" (Capra 1997, p. 192). It must be pointed out again how, for Humberto Maturana and Francisco Varela, every living system interacts with its environment through a *structural coupling*, "that is, through recurrent interactions, each of which triggers structural changes in the system" (Capra 1997, p. 243).

Within this concise reconstruction of the conceptual model, in the phase of defining this analysis of the settlement systems as *living systems*, it is fundamental to underline the importance of the cognitive process previously indicated. In this context, the identity configuration of a settlement can be defined as the *physiognomy* of the settlement and the dissipative structure as the *physiology* of the settlement. Therefore, it becomes crucial to also define the learning process that each settlement experience produces in its complex interrelation with its reference environment.

We all know that every living organism responds to environmental influences with structural changes that will lead to changes in the organism's behaviour in the future. In other words, a *structurally* coupled system is a learning system: structural changes in response to the environment (adaptation, learning and development) allow us to define its behaviour as intelligent.

According to Maturana and Varela, "the environment can be seen as a continuous "selector" of the structural changes that the organism undergoes in its ontogenesis" (Maturana and Varela 1987, p. 97). Hence the consequence that adaptation is reciprocal: environment and living organisms *coevolve*. As James Lovelock states: "the evolution of organisms is so closely coupled with the evolution of their environment that together they constitute a single evolutionary process" (Lovelock 1991, 99).

According to Maturana and Varela, as already observed, an *autopoietic* system preserves at the same time its own networked organizational scheme and its own identity, even if it undergoes continuous structural changes. As a result, living systems specify *which perturbations* from the environment trigger their own structural changes. Since, according to Santiago's theory, such changes consist of cognitive acts, by specifying which *perturbations* from the environment trigger changes, the system "generates a world" (Capra 1997, p. 295).

In other words, Santiago's theory states that the organism does not react to environmental stimuli by means of a linear chain of cause and effect but responds with structural changes in its non-linear *autopoietic* network, which is closed from an organizational point of view. This allows the organism to continue to live in its environment, while preserving its own organization. The consequence of this is that cognition is not a representation of an independent world, but rather the *generation of a world*. "What is generated by a particular organism in the process of life is not the *world* but a *world*, a world that always depends on the structure of the organism" (Capra 1997, p. 298).

To give a simplified, but hopefully effective, example, let us imagine a settlement system immersed in its own environment. The system has its own internal *configuration* produced by the continuous work of *dissipative structure* connected to an environment from which it draws the neg-entropic resources to be able to perform its vital functions. In a human settlement, the external environment is originally given. The settlement system develops in *structural coupling* with this environment, producing a complex system of rules for utilizing of the original nature. Therefore, the system generates a complex process of *learning* of adaptation methods and use of the neighbouring environment that evolves with the system itself over time.

If all this makes sense in the conceptual sphere, what happens empirically? If we shift from the sphere of the generalization of phenomena to the sphere of the observation of the empirical world, we know that, within settlement systems, we must consider that each experience is a unique case: a configuration, a special *dissipative* structure, a singular *structural coupling* that produces a special *learning* process.

As a matter of fact, every settlement experience is produced starting at least from an original nature that, in every point of the earth sphere, is different from the others. If we think of a settlement that proceeds throwing *roots* in a reference environment, we must consider that this environment is endowed with a specific and unique structure and functioning.

2 The Generation of a Bioregional World

The generation of a world, as mentioned earlier, involves both a metabolic structure that manages to build its own dynamic balances and a structuring of the physical space able to activate emotionally positive perceptual processes.

It is no longer an ideological or spiritual choice, but a necessity. Taking care of the city and the territory, which are common goods (Magnaghi 2010), means taking care of the community in which it develops, looking for a space as an *environmental therapy* for the healthiness of living, a space as a device that nourishes the *desire for sociality*, a space as the essence of its being for others pursuing a public objective aimed at the *welfare of the inhabitants*. In this sense, a new perspective of research opened, outlining a code of ethics of design control for the building of living spaces, based on a new physiocracy, towards the city of life, "a *Biopoli*, what it has always been until recently, when it got sick." (Saragosa 2016)

When space is generated, it needs both an ecological and a perceptive verification; in the latter case, it must meet the deep feeling of the human psyche. To give quality to the life it welcomes, the urban and territorial space must be in harmony with a sense that characterizes the way men feel spiritually fulfilled. At the same time, the forms of the anthropic space must not only satisfy the sensual feeling: they also have to resist (and feed themselves) to the flows of matter and energy that naturally characterize the world. In the management of flows, space seeks a dynamic balance with the forms that can give an empathic satisfaction when they are perceived. Therefore, the correct management of flows must consider the forms. It is necessary to identify that plot that connects us, as inhabitants, to the world in which we are immersed in and that it is characterized by those forms that manage the flows (Figs. 1 and 2).

Then, the city and the territory are always shapes that support flows and always flows that generate shapes: it is this unity, this fundamental plot that constitutes the world in which our bodies are surrounded. The city and the territory exist because we are immersed in and moving within them, we are swimming in their forms and

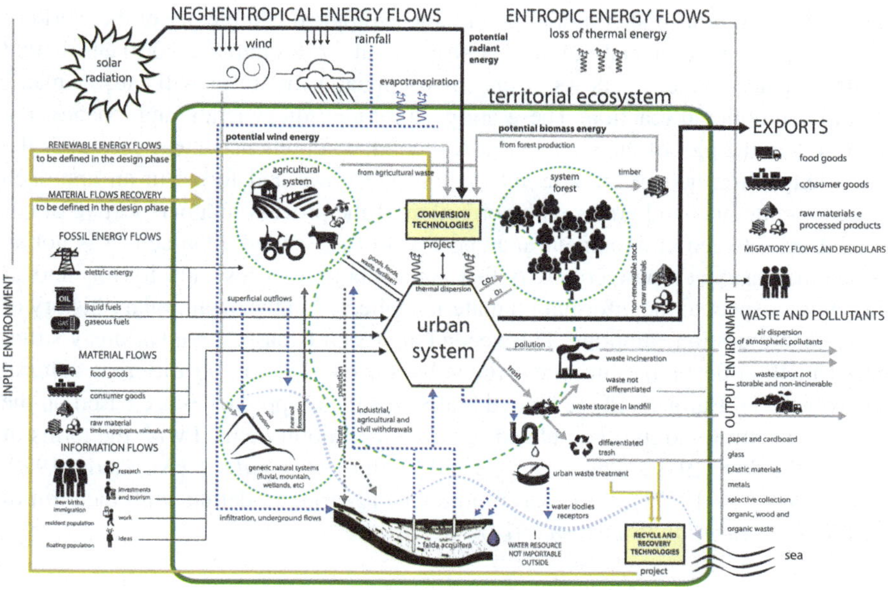

Fig. 1 Flow management scheme in the territorial ecosystem. (Source: Authors' and Rossi elaboration)

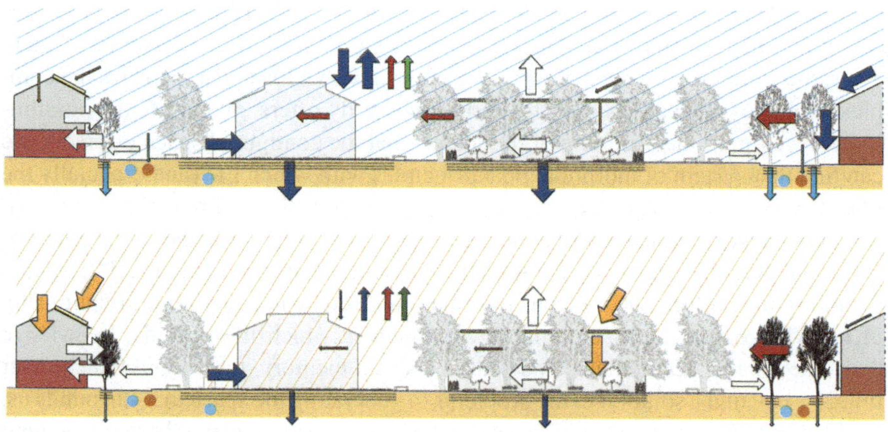

Fig. 2 The dynamics of energy-material flows in the morphogenetic process of the shape of an urban square in the alternation of seasonal winter-summer cycles. (Source: Chiti M., "From growth to degrowth: theories, measures, flows and rules for the regeneration of the urban bioregion", PhD thesis, 2014)

flows, we are moving through an atmospheric cauldron of changing stimuli, involving or comparing multiple sensations (Mallgrave 2015).

There are different ways to build a project, in the sense of generating the world that is not yet manifest in front of us. A first, mechanical method consists in proposing solutions that do not fit in with the ecological complexity of the world or with the perceptive capacity of men. A project that throws into the world a form that badly manages either the flows of the environment or the forms will cause a man's negative emotional reaction. These are gestural and idiosyncratic approaches that tend to tear the plot of the vital world. A second, comprehensive way preserves the knowledge stratified in the attempts to manage flows and forms in an approach based on attempts and errors with correction of the process in a perspective of co-evolution between environment and species. In this second approach, it is not so much the designer's pure creativity that counts, but rather his capacity for innovation with respect to the information material collected in the evolutionary history of space configuration solutions. This second approach is based on a variously structured method developed in recent times by various scholars in different cultural areas between Europe and the United States. All these approaches are based on the concept of information accumulated in an abstract point defined with the terms of *meme* (Dawkins 1979), *type* (Caniggia and Maffei 1979), *pattern* (Alexander 1979; Alexander et al. 1977), or, as I have more recently tried to define, with the term of *spatial configuration* (Saragosa 2014).

3 Spatial Configuration and World Generation

The concept of spatial configuration is to be related to that of *configured space*. The configured space is the one that stretches in front of us, the result of long processes of structuring that have transformed the original nature into the territory of men. Thus, this configured space has its own identity, its own form that manages the complex ecologies that each part of the Earth necessarily offers, giving life the possibility to develop. In the decoding of the secrets that the configured space offers us, we can find that system of morphological principles with which life (and especially the life of men) can manage the necessary matter-energy flows. From the configured space we can extrapolate those characters of the form that, unfolded in the environment, support the organic generation of the space that surrounds us. The spatial configuration collects the precious information given by the continuous relationship of knowledge with the fluctuating environment in which life unfolds; knowledge that, like a gene, accumulates and sediments as a memory, the way in which, over time, we can find a solution to the problems of generating the space that surrounds us.

The *spatial configuration* is an accumulator of information and therefore a *memory*. It accumulates the solutions that, once tried and tested and in relation to specific context, are selected in the fluid process that gives rise to a configuration. In the long period, the *spatial configuration* learns to both solve the problems of spatial organization and manage the flows, checking which decision seems to solve the coupling between the subject and the reference environment in the best way. A process that we could define as *Darwinian*, a process with testing and error correction, a process of selecting configurations that, at that time and in that place, seems to be the most appropriate, discarding configurations that do not solve any of the emerging problems. This continuous process of selection of forms through the generation and re-elaboration of formal material is never stopping and concerns both the correction of the management of the metabolic flow and the correction of the principle that underlies the perceptive evaluation of the form. In this case, it is clear how the processes of defining the result by activating the chain sensation-perception-emotion are necessary: the formal representation is always produced carefully, contextualizing the formal adjustments that are under continuous evaluation by the operator. This is a complex operation not only because is it necessary to identify a form that satisfies the sensation-perception-emotion chain, but also because this form must be able to manage the flows of matter-energy. This complexity requires a long preparation phase in the process of test and error, to accumulate those spatial configurations that can solve perceptual problems in a space to be used in its multiverse aspects in which men must move within. Any form of life works in the same way. DNA accumulates information that can generate a new person as it unfolds.

This metaphorical approach between spatial configurations and DNA has appeared possible to many. If we consider the *spatial configurations* as an entity capable of accumulating a memory, able to generate new configurations, the metaphor seems even more pertinent. Moreover, the *archetype*, as Jung would like it to be (Jung 1968), seems to have its own genetic origin, an instinctual way, an inner instinct, a deep drive to organize the world that derives not much from the information accumulated by the individuals, but from those accumulated during the evolution of the species to which it belongs. A way of organizing the world that Kandel (2012) would say to be *wired*, inscribed in the genetic organization of the nervous system as a result of the accumulation of nerve bundles to other nerve bundles, of memories to memories, during the long evolution of species. This deep interiority is what probably gives us the sense of some things as we perceive them, as perceiving is also due to this hidden nervousness. As Maurice Merleau-Ponty (2012) said, it is due to tensions that, like lines of force, *cross the visual field and the system own body-world and that animate it with a deaf and magical life, imposing here and there twists, contractions and swellings*.

Although the way we relate to the world derives largely from individual experiences, the experiential memories, some behaviours and the way we build a sense of the world clearly derives from our *wiring*, from the way our interface with the environment has been built over time to help with survival in the tumultuous cosmos that surrounds us. Our *wiring*, in short, depends on the way we evolved over time, but our *wiring* is also the way we organize many factors with whom we perceive and organize the world; the way we instinctively feel the things that surround our body. And despite the structural differences of individuals, these emersions from the deep appear as collectively similar ways of floating in the fluid world that surrounds us. The *archetypes* that emerge are produced by this complex management of the genetic memory sedimented in the *collective unconscious* of Jung, in the collective feeling-perception. In the configuration of space, the *archetype* cannot be denied (and we could not do so, it being a deep part of our way of being), the *archetype* can only be discovered and managed to make even more effective the activation of processes of meaning, including, perhaps, beauty.

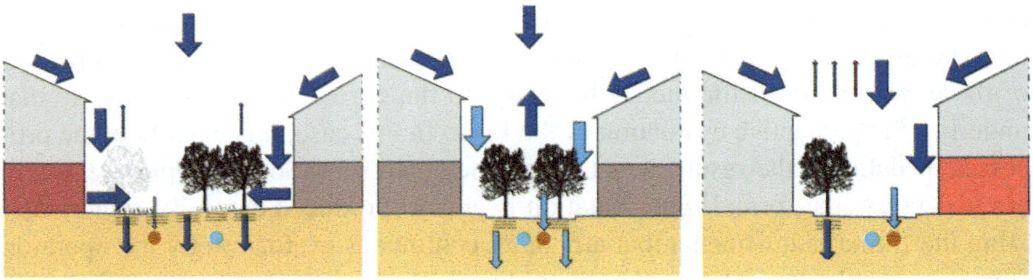

Fig. 3 The road *type*: some spatial configurations in the management of form and flows. (Source: Chiti M., "From growth to degrowth: theories, measures, flows and rules for the regeneration of the urban bioregion", PhD thesis)

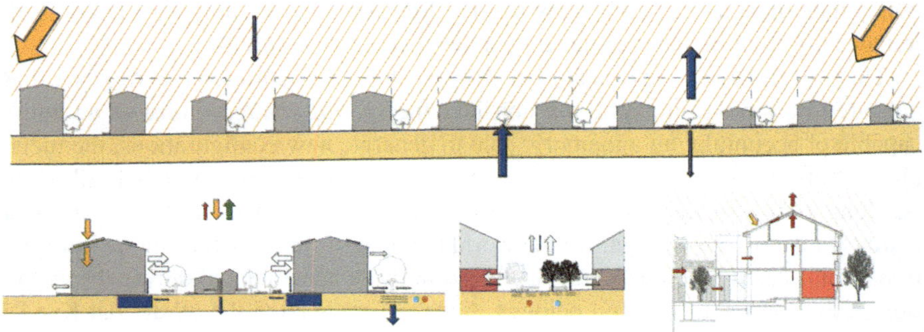

Fig. 4 The transcalarity of relationships in *spatial configurations* and in managed flows: the *type* of neighbourhood unit, the block *type*, the road *type*, the building *type*. (Source: Chiti M., "From growth to degrowth: theories, measures, flows and rules for the regeneration of the urban bioregion", PhD thesis)

But it is with the *spatial configurations* that the issue becomes even more interesting. Through the *spatial configurations*, the memory collected is in finding a solution in close confrontation with the reference environment, in seeking the space-matter configuration that solves the problems of form and flow (Figs. 3 and 4). The solution to an emerging problem, the solution to a problem of *coupling* an organism with its environment can never be extemporary. Obviously, in this process of attempts and errors, stochastic methods play a fundamental role. We throw many arrows, but only some of them hit the target. Chance plays a key role, but it is not just chance that drives the process: the dart thrown hits the target and the target is the selective criterion. Perhaps the trajectory of the darts is random, but only the darts that hit the target are selected as entities that can last to give substance to the complex relationship between creatures and the environment. A *spatial configuration,* born to solve some facts of spatial configuration, collects, in a memory, a thousand attempts made to solve the problem and especially collects those attempts that increase the degree of complexity of the configuration to manage form and flow. At each attempt, the mistakes made, if corrected step by step, accumulate an information system that will lead to a correct deployment of the *spatial configuration*. This (a *priori synthesis, heuristic principle, operating gene*) is the knowledge of the correct relations accumulated after the experimental path of contact between the operating creature and the surrounding world.

When we talk about the configuration of the structures of the anthropic space, we refer to problems of collective order: a road must *mean* road not for a single individual but for all the individuals in a community. Therefore, the selection process does not only select those configurations that respond to perceptual-emotional criteria (and to the ways of managing the flows) of the individual but, above all, select those solutions that respond to the feeling that matures within an entire community, which, in that configured world, must recognize itself and live. The *type* accumulates the correct solutions that are then submitted to the scrutiny of the entire community living in a place. It forms, in fact, a common language capable of activating precisely *those* deep meanings, which can be understood by *this very* community.

Spatial configurations are subjected to continuous updating, just as a genetic pool or a living language evolves continuously. It is in the continuous relationship between the memory deposited in the *type* and the comparison with the reference environment, fluid and changeable, that the information set is updated, responds to the *becoming* adapting itself. The *spatial configuration* unfolds contextually and, in becoming matter-space, it is measured with the complexity of the environment. It updates itself and learns from the relationship with the surrounding becoming, more capable of responding to the changed world even only by its presence. Bowing to the impending future, the past sedimented in the *spatial configurations* offers all its *wisdom* to the present that flows in its becoming an elusive world. The *spatial configuration* is not a static entity, it evolves; it continuously modifies the *information* that composes it. When it comes into contact with new situations that need to be solved, it deploys all the accumulated knowledge and, in this unfolding (in this contact with the chaotic world), it learns new ways of solving problems of form and flow. The community that uses it evaluates its application and corrects any errors that emerge in its deployment. The community associates the *spatial configuration* that belongs to a scale level with the *spatial configurations* that act at the other levels (it unites the unfolding of the *spatial configuration* house, the *type* of building, with the unfolding of the *spatial configuration* at a larger scale, for instance, the *type* of road, the urban-*type*), correcting any elements of disorder that occur in the relationship of the *types* to the different scales.

The analysis of configurations is multi-scalar, as are the flows that pass through them. The scalar factor is not a quantitative territorial measure, but rather a correlation of relationships between the sequence of single urban events (the *type* of neighbourhood unit, the block *type*, the road *type*, the building *type*) until it recomposes the global unit in the passage between the different dimensional thresholds. The complexity of the system lies in the continuous verification of the genetic code with which it was generated; as a consequence of the reconstruction of the individual elements, the complexity of the urban bioregion recomposes itself.

It is a long learning process that takes place over time. This learning process is governed by the information accumulated in history and continuously updated when organizing matter-space, according to both the perceived forms that activate emotions and the management of the flows that the changing environment presents at that point of the universe.

4 A Generation Method That Has Its Roots in Life and Rules the Bioregion

It is in this process that a rich and shared *information* is collected, a memory that is accumulated in the stones (arranged according to relations obtained in the long process of selecting forms and flows); a memory that is accumulated in the extra-somatic physical memories (books, manuals, photos, paintings, etc.); a memory that is accumulated in the collective memories of the *civitas* that inhabit the *urbs* (Romano 2010) and that produce the sense of belonging to the places because men know how to decode the hidden meanings in the forms and flows generated by the place itself; a memory that is accumulated in the synaptic-genetic processes of the brain when we were born in a place where the first relationship with the environment occurs and produces the first *dispositional representations* (Damasio 2003) that will go with us perpetually during the course of our life; a memory that is accumulated in the brain memory, in the form of acquired functions, when our body distils information in the continuous experience of matter-space that surrounds it in its specific organization produced over time. The culture of generation of matter-space (the information accumulated in memories by the *spatial configurations* in the making of the world) influences the way of operating that will take place starting precisely from that accumulation of solutions verified over time and subjected to the long process of evaluation by attempts and errors. We do not start over again and again, we only correct that construct that must be organized differently because the world has varied even from this unfolding of accumulated information; we do not start over, but we implement our memory when new qualities of matter-space, not previously read in their possible usefulness, come out. This process of accumulation is obviously the one that verifies the information (tests and errors, tests and errors, tests and errors, …), but it is also the one that allows us to select *a way* (the *italics* are necessary since infinite ways, as the possible species, in the evolution of species, are infinite, and perhaps those now unimaginable will soon be around us) in the fluctuating complexity of the world.

Our *spatial configurations* (like language or the genome that stores information for the development of life) collect and petrify the information that produces the spatial solutions that organize matter-space in the world (Fig. 5). And this system of *spatial configurations* would be negative if it were a very rigid system that does not evolve together with the community in the world. A language would be only negative if it was failing in inventing new symbols able to interpret a world that necessarily evolves, if it was not able to describe the changing world of becoming with new words, if it was not suitable for evolving in the definition of the new qualities that are discovered in the experiential study of matter-space. If life were not given

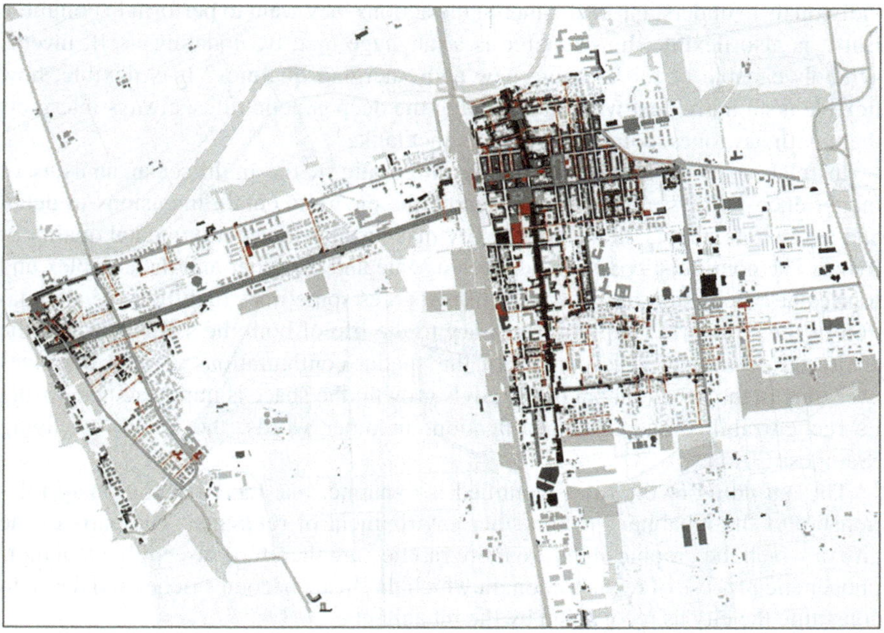

Fig. 5 The dense places of the spatial configurations of the city. In the figure, the areas of the existing city, in which the spatial configurations identified in the urban code recur, are identified (the brightest colours highlight the accumulation of spatial configurations; the dullest colours detect the rarefaction of the spatial configurations). (Source: Research project "Activities of technical-scientific collaboration to support the Revision of the Urban Regulations of the City of Cecina", Prof. C. Saragosa, coordinator)

by a continuous updating of the information contained in the genetic memory, it would be a continuous reappearance of an organism that, if placed in the changing world, would soon be suppressed. In the selection method, which is hidden in the selective process of a language and of life, there is something powerful; even though the selection method tends to store and use the information that has been laboriously collected in a rigid way, it is a method open to the future and is able to update itself continuously with the changing environment to which it is *ecologically* and *empathically* linked. If the language or the code were abandoned, it would always be necessary to re-start from the beginning, losing that precious information accumulated over time that allows us to build those bodies capable of deploying without making evident mistakes.

A *set* of *spatial configurations* that organizes matter-space works in the same way: it is powerful because it acts as a memory that collects information, experienced over time, that helps to solve the problems of living; it is powerful because it is open to the future by continuously updating itself according to the needs that arise in the becoming of the fluent world. It is rigid, just like the compendium of genetic information that generates an individual according to the rules of its species; it is rigid, just like a language that, being a set of shared symbols, allows more individuals to understand each other in the actions they want to perform in common. But it is also flexible; how flexible is a language that, by updating itself, invents symbols capable of representing new and emerging qualities? It is flexible; how flexible is an individual who, in unfolding the deep genetic rules, always intersects them with new ones, combining two distinct tanks?

In relation to the decoded spatial configurations, the multi-scalar analysis of matter-energy flows allows us to examine the environmental dimensions in detail and as a whole, that is, in the complexity that sustains the environmental quality of living. The continuous passage between a scale and the other and the complex and transcalar articulation of the system of resources sometimes highlight the attenuation of the structural coupling necessary to the life of both the settlement and the territorial ecosystem. The density of the spatial configurations created dissolves over time in the development of the city's growth; the space is impoverished, losing its recognizability and self-identification; in other words, the quality of living (Saragosa 2011).

The unfolding of the rules identified is dynamic, like the co-evolutionary relationship of the inhabitant with his/her environment of reference. The parts of the city in which the graphic signs are more rarefied are therefore susceptible to a morphogenetic process of regeneration, in which the space becomes richer and dense to constitute the city as recognized by the inhabitants.

In this process that unfolds slowly and collects solutions verified with the method of attempts and correction of errors, each increase in information is therefore a verified, rare, precious information. Every attempt considered correct is collected, memorized and made available to the following situations. In language, signs or symbols that do not come from this long and slow process of synthesis have labile meanings; in the biological genetic sets, information that has not been subjected to this long screening process is even harmful, with the risk of tearing apart the organic tissues that are trans-scalarly bound to each other and that result from the slow deployment of the information sedimented in the genetic memory. Mutated genetic material produces the cancerous tissues, lacerating the organic unity.

There are *archetypes* that operate on the information accumulated thanks to which, man, over time, has evolved, has wired up. There are *types* (*spatial configurations*) that are cultural constructs created by the slow evolution of the solutions of the organization of matter-space that have been screened, for form and flow, in the long application period of a community to the solution of the problem of living in a place of the Earth. And this selection takes place through continuous experimentation, with continuous hybridization of the coded material selected elsewhere, with evaluations of the continuous fluctuation of the world that welcomes us. Between the diversity of matter-space and selection guided by chance and between successful attempts and correct errors (stochastic processes), in the relationship with the places of the Earth and in relation to the processes of selection, a culture of settlement is born that helps man to distil those configurations that give existential meaning to the word living.

It is precisely at the point of the cosmos where the evolutionary process is born, characterized by properties of matter-space to which we recognize some utility and on which lies the material to which we already assign some value (from the forms that excite us, to the flows that feed us), that the life of a settlement is born.

5 Form (Morphology) and Flow (Ecology), Empathy and Entropy in the Morphogenetic Processes of Space

As we have mentioned, *spatial configurations* are *types*, *memes*, which have a shape and manage a flow. The way in which they develop over time is linked to a long process of testing and correction of errors similar to what happens when the genetic heritage of various species in the world of life is formed. While in genetics, the bonds of informational structures are rigid, in *memes*, which collect the basic information for generating space, the bonds are much weaker. While in the gene the information is collected in a long theory of tests and errors within the changing environment with a system of continuous mixing of information supported by stochastic processes, in the *memes*, the selective process is linked both to the ecological relationship with the world of flows and to the perceptual evaluation of the species that produces structural changes in the geometry of physical space. This variation must be produced considering the relationship between perceptual capacity and produced forms. Obviously, not all forms produce the same emotional effects in the presence of complex evaluation systems. There are forms of fear and forms that make us feel like we belong to a world that welcomes us and produces a sense of fulfilment. The accumulation in the *spatial configuration* (this somewhat special meme) of rare information capable of leading to a more correct and profitable management of the metabolic flows of the environment and capable of producing the emotional forms that support a living rich from an emotional point of view is what gives substance to the very concept of configuration. Therefore, the configuration contains selected information that guarantees a more correct coupling with the environment (in the management of the flow) and with the mind (in the definition of the emotional forms). Information is accumulated in these *memes* that help us to manage the *continuous morphogenetic process* in which our existence in the world necessarily invites us to participate.

If one type of evaluation concerns the quality of the flows, or rather the state variations between matter and flowing energy in the metabolic processes, then to evaluate it is possible to approach the very complex concept of *entropy*. Every organism needs to metabolize flows of matter-energy for living, optimizing the processes of entropic degradation. If another evaluation concerns the psychic processes, considering that the *spatial configuration* collects the information generated in the long processes of testing and error in the evaluation of the perceptive correctness of the forms, then we can use the equally complex concept of *empathy*.

In conclusion, the way we use to shape the space in front of us is the result of a long series of assessments of the ecological and perceptual rightness of the *meme* that will then allow us to operate. We collect and send information that is increasingly rare because it is more and more elaborate. And just as *genetic heritages* always unfold new life from time to time, updating themselves with respect to the ever-changing environment where they operate, so *Memic heritages* deal with their ability to solve the relationships between life and the environment by transmitting the knowledge accumulated in previous procedures of ecological and perceptual adjustment. It is a transfer, it is a making available to the future that is about to come the wisdom of a past in which the relationship of a changing world has been experienced. It is a *tradition* that generates a world.

Two words, then, *entropy* and *empathy*, can guide us in a dynamic process in which the genesis of forms occurs, avoiding the trivial errors given by gestural, idiosyncratic, mechanical approaches. Evaluating flows, using forms through the change in the quality of matter-energy (entropic evaluations), allow us to find more effective ways to synchronize ourselves with the environment in which we are immersed. With the evaluation of forms and of one's own perceptive rightness (empathic evaluations), we can identify those configurations that produce spaces capable of activating that emotion that makes the world so precious, at least for men. Indeed, perceiving means enriching the sensation we get from that world in front of us with memories sometimes unconsciously preserved in our mind. The perception creates the meaning we give to the things when we wrap those things with the mnemonic veils hidden in our own, and sometimes impenetrable, *Ego*. And when this process of dressing of the sensation releases internal reactions, we call these reactions emotions. When a bond is created between my *Ego* and the forms that appear before me, I will call this bond *empathy*, a concept on which we have been working for years.

References

Alexander, C. (1979). *The timeless way of building*. New York: Oxford University Press.

Alexander, C., Ishikawa, S., & Silverstein, M. (1977). *A pattern language*. New York: Oxford University Press.

Bettini, V. (1990). *L'analisi ambientale*. Milano: Clup.

Caniggia, G., & Maffei, G. L. (1979). *Composizione architettonica e tipologia edilizia. 1. Lettura dell'edilizia di base*. Venezia: Marsilio Editori.

Capra, F. (1997). *La rete della vita. Una nuova visione della natura e della scienza*. Milano: Rizzoli. (orig. tit. Capra F. (1996). *The web of life. A new scientific understanding of living systems*. New York: Anchor Books).

Damasio, R. A. (2003). *Alla ricerca di Spinoza. Emozioni, sentimenti e cervello*. Milano: Adelphi.

Dawkins, R. (1979). *Il gene egoista*. Bologna: Zanichelli. (orig. tit. Dawkins, R. (1976). *The selfish gene*. Oxford: Oxford University Press).

Douglas, I. (1983). *The urban environment*. London: Edward Arnold.

Jung, C. G. (1968). *The archetypes and the collective unconscious*. Princeton University Press: Princeton.

Kandel, E. R. (2012). *L'età dell'inconscio. Arte, mente e cervello dalla grande Vienna ai nostri giorni*. Milano: Raffaello Cortina Editore. orig. tit. Kandel, E. R. (2012). *The age of insight. The quest to understand the unconscious in art, mind, and brain, from Vienna 1900 to the present*. New York: Penguin-Random House).

Lovelock, J. E. (1991). *Healing Gaia*. New York: Harmont Books.

Magnaghi, A. (2010). *Il progetto locale. Verso la coscienza di luogo*. Torino: Bollati Boringhieri.

Mallgrave, H. F. (2015). *L'empatia degli spazi. Architettura e neuroscienze*. Milano: Raffaello Cortina Editore.

Maturana, H. R., & Varela, F. J. (1980). *Autopoiesis and cognition: The realization of the living*. Dordrecht: Reidel Publishing Company.

Maturana, H. R., & Varela, F. J. (1987). *The tree of knowledge: The biological roots of human understanding*. Boston: Shambhala.

Merleau-Ponty, M. (2012). *Fenomenologia della percezione*. Milano: Bompiani.

Odum, E. P. (1988). *Basi di ecologia*. Padova: Piccin. (orig. tit. Odum, E. P. (1983). *Basic ecology: Fundamentals of ecology*. Philadelphia/London: Holt-Saunders International).

Rees, E. W., & Wackernagel, M. (1996). *L'impronta ecologica. Come ridurre l'impatto dell'uomo sulla terra*. Milano: Edizioni Ambiente. (orig. tit. Wackernagel, M., & Rees, W. (1996). *Our ecological footprint: Reducing human impact on the earth*. New Society Publishers).

Romano, M. (2010). *Ascesa e declino della città europea*. Milano: Raffaello Cortina Editore.

Saragosa, C. (2001). L'Ecosistema Territoriale e la sua base ambientale. In A. Magnaghi (a cura di). *Rappresentare i luoghi. Metodi e tecniche*. Firenze: Alinea Editrice.

Saragosa, C. (2005). *L'insediamento umano. Ecologia e sostenibilità*. Roma: Donzelli.

Saragosa, C. (2011). *La città tra passato e futuro. Un percorso critico sulla via di biopoli*. Roma: Donzelli.

Saragosa, C. (2014). Bioregione e identità urbane: le configurazioni spaziali di Cecina (LI). In A. Magnaghi (a cura di). *La regola e il progetto. Un approccio bioregionalista alla pianificazione territoriale*. Firenze: Firenze University Press.

Saragosa, C. (2016). *Il sentiero di Biopoli. L'empatia nella generazione della città*. Roma: Donzelli.

Social Justice in Spatial Planning: How Does Bioregionalism Contribute?

Coline Perrin

1 Introduction

Spatial planning aims at coordinating different public policies affecting spatial organization (such as land use, transport, and environment). By influencing the distribution of people and activities in space, it has social impacts. Many European cities still use traditional land-use planning based on comprehensive statutory spatial plans but have also developed in the last 20 years a new type of "strategic planning" aimed at social, economic, and cultural development in a context of both competition and co-operation between city regions (Booth et al. 2007). Together, this evolution of planning practices and the large scale of metropolitan planning projects stimulate new interest in the question of how planning takes into account social justice.

Since David Harvey wrote *Social Justice and the City* (1973), the scientific literature has regularly addressed questions of justice and its manifestations in the city, at the intersection of critical urban geography and urban policy or planning. This chapter intends to clarify what can be considered fair planning, in relation to the bioregional approach. In contrast to current planning and development practices, which are often extractive and can exacerbate socio-spatial inequalities (Anguelovski et al. 2016), many components of the bioregional approach contribute to more fair and inclusive planning. However, some dimensions of social and spatial justice may be overlooked and need specific attention in the planning process, even within a bioregional approach. In this short essay, we explain the complementary dimensions of social justice, the scientific controversies over how to promote socially just planning, and we ultimately discuss the impact of the bioregional approach on the fairness and inclusiveness of planning practices.

C. Perrin (✉)
UMR INNOVATION, Univ Montpellier, CIRAD, INRAE, Institut Agro, Montpellier, France
e-mail: coline.perrin@inrae.fr

D. Fanfani, A. Matarán Ruiz (eds.), *Bioregional Planning and Design: Volume I*,
https://doi.org/10.1007/978-3-030-45870-6_6

2 Diverse Approaches to Social Justice and Their Use in Geography

The definition of social justice, as well as the means to achieve it, has been widely debated in political philosophy (Kymlicka 1992; Smith 1994). These debates are beyond the scope of this paper. It is however useful to be aware of the diversity of (sometimes competing) theoretical approaches to social justice.

A first distinction is often made between approaches focusing on the issue of *distribution* of rights or resources and approaches focusing on the decision-making *processes*. Distributive (or structuralist) approaches (Rawls 1971; Walzer 1983) define principles of (re)distribution of resources among individuals. Several "just" distributions (in the sense of morally preferable) can be envisaged. While equality gives individuals the same compensation for the same task, fairness gives to each individual according to his/her needs. For example, Rawls (1971), the most famous proponent of the "liberal" approach to justice, bases his "justice as fairness" on two principles: the first states that every individual has an equal right to basic liberties (freedom of thought, of speech, of press, of assembly and association, etc.). The second principle gives the rule of distribution. It states that every individual should have the same opportunities (an equal chance to access offices or positions) and therefore that the only inequalities allowed are those favoring the least advantaged.

In contrast to distributive approaches, procedural (or post-structuralist) approaches focus on the fairness of the procedures and the processes by which decisions are made. They are based on the idea that "a fair procedure transmits its character to the result" (Rawls 1971, p. 118). So an unequal distribution can be just if it results from a fair procedure. What is considered a fair procedure depends on the authors (transparency, democracy, participation, hearing of multiple voices, recognition of differences and of minorities). A major author within these post-structuralist approaches is the Marxist and feminist theorist Iris M. Young. In *Justice and the Politics of Difference* (1990), she stresses the need to recognize the differences between social groups and to ensure their meaningful participation in decisions that affect them. Justice is thus achieved through negotiation between social groups.

A second useful distinction can be made between conceptions of justice that provide a *universal framework*, an abstract definition of social justice and of the means to achieve it – like Rawls' principles – and *pluralistic conceptions* that are concerned with concrete situations of inequality or injustices and not only with the conditions of possibility and the properties of just institutions. In these pluralistic conceptions, justice becomes relative, depending on the groups and individuals considered: "In the same place and at the same time there are actors who have different, often contradictory, even conflicting, conceptions of what isjust" and "unjust" (Gervais-Lambony and Dufaux 2009). For Walzer (1983), one of the leading proponents of the "communitarian" approach, justice is not objective; there are no principles valid for all on all goods in a universalized abstraction. Justice is rather a relative moral standard, defined within communities according to shared meanings. According to Walzer, there are different "spheres of justice," each having a particular way of distributing social goods. A feeling of injustice can emerge when one sphere dominates another (e.g., when money gives political power). Young (1990) maintains that the recognition of social groups (not conceived as communities, but as affinity groups) is essential to redressing structural inequalities, because we often compare classes of people rather than individuals in our evaluations of inequality and injustice. She thus proposes to identify concrete situations provoking a feeling of injustice, distinguishing five forms of injustice or "faces of oppression": exploitation, marginalization, powerlessness, cultural domination, and violence. Her theory has had a great impact on contemporaneous geographers working on spatial justice (Gervais-Lambony and Dufaux 2009), environmental justice (Blanchon et al. 2009), or planning (Fainstein 2010).

Geographers refer alternatively to various theoretical perspectives on social justice. The concept of social justice is more a theoretical lens for geographical issues (especially related to public policies) than a research question in itself, as it is in political philosophy. Soja forged the concept of spatial justice (2010): it "is not a substitute or alternative to social, economic, or other forms of justice but rather a way of looking at justice from a critical spatial perspective. From this viewpoint, there is always a relevant spatial dimension to justice while at the same time all geographies have expressions of justice and injustice built into them" (Soja 2009). Following Soja, but also the cornerstone works of Henri Lefebvre (1974), Michel Foucault, and David Harvey (1973), geographers developed a spatial perspective on justice aimed at describing inequalities (the distribution in space of socially valued resources and the opportunities to use them) and at identifying and understanding the underlying processes that produce these unjust outcomes.

3 Social Justice: A Challenge for Spatial Planning?

Many scholars denounce planning as unjust. Winkler (2012) points out that the modernist planning project, dominant since the Second World War, is grounded in an unquestioned liberal ethic, aimed at economic efficacy rather than social justice. This liberal ethic is entrenched in the norms of planning and remains unchallenged by most planners. Marxian geographers have deeply influenced critical perspectives on planning up until now. In *Social Justice and the City*, Harvey (1973) documented urban injustice in spatial processes and planning action. He sought to understand and address the issue of urban poverty and inequality and showed how the production of urban space contributes to the reproduction of capitalism. More recently, scholars of environmental justice have also shown that the "sustainability" principle is not a guarantee of social justice (Agyeman and Evans 2004). In this line of research, Anguelovski et al. (2016) reveal how planning can exacerbate socio-spatial inequalities. They denounce the negative impacts in terms of social equity of urban land-use planning for climate adaptation, bringing to light "unjust" public interventions, which "negatively affect or displace poor communities" (such as mega-projects for flood mitigation) and/or "protect and prioritize elite groups at the expense of the urban poor" under the legitimating banner of climate change mitigation.

The question is how to improve current planning practices, using contributions from political philosophy on social justice and the findings of concrete case studies highlighting current injustices. For Campbell and Marshall (2006), there is a kind of misunderstanding: the philosophical "conceptualizations were never intended to be applied to the task of situated judgment associated with the highly contested decisions at the heart of the planning activity. Consequently, the issue for the planning community is not so much 'can the concepts of justice embodied in Rawls' "justice as fairness" or Habermas' "discourse ethics" be found in practice but could they ever'." Fincher and Iveson (2012) also stress this frequent problematic relationship in geographic analyses between philosophical principles and the application of such ideas to actual circumstances and contexts, outcomes "on the ground."

A first recommendation is thus to adapt the social justice perspective to each local context. There cannot be one fit-for-all definition of principles of justice for more fair and inclusive planning. Justice is context-sensitive. For example, many researchers have denounced the social issues surrounding urban planning in post-apartheid South Africa. Visser (2001) argues that "if geographical social justice discourse is to be useful or relevant to urban planning practice in South Africa, new theoretical frameworks, sensitive to the geographically and historically located interpretations of this concept need to be developed." In particular, his case study illustrates that "social justice encompasses multiple, diverse and even theoretically incompatible distributive ideals" (p. 31). He thus advocates better taking into account what ordinary urban citizens consider as socially just, even if their liberal understanding of social justice does not fit within the current structuralist/poststructuralist scientific debates. In accordance with this, Barnett (2011) suggests that justice norms be considered in conjunction with social practices, "emerging from situated conflicts," from "widely shared intuitions of *injustice*." The best progress toward justice is made through actions, in actual social movements in situations. This is also emphasized by theorists of the right to the city and by the environmental and food justice movements. Scholar-activists involved in such movements thus propose to focus on solutions-oriented policy and planning initiatives that specifically address issues of equity and justice (Agyeman 2013; Reynolds and Cohen 2016). In this line of research, normative concepts are less important, or they are generated in response to real-world instances of injustice.

Other scholars prefer to specify justice norms in advance of empirical analysis in order to connect social justice theory and planning practice. In *The Just City*, Fainstein (2010) develops an urban theory of justice and "uses it to evaluate existing and potential institutions and programs" (p. 5). She not only specifies the three norms of justice that she will use in her assessment – equity, democracy, and diversity – but even lists criteria of justice by which to formulate and judge planning initiatives at the urban level. For instance, in order to achieve more material equality, "no household or business should be involuntarily relocated for the purpose of obtaining economic development or community balance" or "transit fares should be kept low" (Fainstein 2009). To this end, she discusses the antagonist models of communicative planning (influenced by Habermas' deliberative democracy) vs. the just city (Marcuse et al. 2009; focusing on the equity of outcomes). She highlights the potential contradictions between participation and just outcomes but retains the two principles of democracy and equity as major components of her just city. Then, drawing on the work of Young (1990) and Fraser (1997), she adds diversity as a third component, acknowledging the potential tension between diversity (or recognition, in Fraser's words) and equality or democracy. Thus, her three normative categories combine the core principles of recent theories on social justice, but they are not universal rules for social justice, as they may clash in particular situations or require trade-offs. They are more an analytical device, three useful categories with which to evaluate actual planning initiatives.

Fainstein's effort to connect social justice theory and planning practice has been widely praised. Fincher and Iveson (2008) similarly tried to look beyond inclusionary planning processes to consider outcomes too. However, they criticize the way Fainstein applies top-down normative categories to analyze and interpret actual situations (Fincher and Iveson 2012). In response to that criticism, they promote a continuous "dialog between foundational norms and analysis of situations and actions in the world": "justice norms and unjust practices have to be held in tension, in conversation, in an analysis." This may "involve the specification of justice norms in advance of analysis, but in a manner that is more tentative and suggestive rather than dogmatic and final" (p. 237). In fact, their three key principles – redistribution, recognition, and encounter – are similar to Fainstein's three categories and influenced by them. However, they not only reveal unjust planning practices but also try to promote more just practices by highlighting through examples the efforts to shape cities according to such principles. They identify general "decision rules" and emphasize the significance of context and local specificity in determining what generates greater equity and justice in urban life.

4 How Bioregionalism Contributes to Socially Just Planning

Bioregionalism is connected to anarchist, utopian socialist, and regional planning traditions (Sale 1985). It gestated in the 1960s' counterculture of interrelated social change movements within activist communities fighting against capitalism. It was first conceived as the interaction of concern for place, politics, and ecology in order to balance machine-driven economic progress with cultural and ecological sustainability. It aims at reconnecting "socially-just human cultures in sustainable manner to the region-scale ecosystems in which they are irrevocably embedded" (Aberley 1999, p. 13). Hence, even if most bioregionalist approaches do not explicitly aim at improving social justice, several core principles of this social movement and action-oriented field of research embrace the values of social justice and can contribute to fairer and more inclusive planning.

First, bioregionalism implies concern for distributive justice, as it highlights the connection (and promotes a reconnection) between human cultures and region-scale ecosystems. For Aberley (1993), "the promise is that these bioregions will be inhabited in a manner that respects ecological carrying capacity, engenders social justice, uses appropriate technology creatively, and allows for a rich interconnection between regionalized cultures." Hence a bioregional approach should engender social justice. Place is considered as a community of beings, human and nonhuman. In addition to enhancing justice among human beings, such an approach will even contribute to a better balance (and justice?) between human and nonhuman beings.

Then, bioregionalism promotes context-based or life-place planning. Place – or life-place to use bioregionalist words – is produced or co-constituted by the long-term interaction between nature and culture (Alexander 1990). A bioregional planning initiative will thus always take into account specific local features and the context in all its dimensions (physical, cultural, etc.). It won't apply top-down universal rules: it will, on the contrary, integrate different physical sciences (biogeography, climatology, geomorphology) with other forms of knowledge (natural history, indigenous knowledge). It aims at articulating the economic, political, and sociocultural spheres according to the norms of ecological sustainability, social justice, and human well-being through the concept of place (Evanoff 2011). Such an eco-systemic multidisciplinary context-based approach will thus avoid extractive planning practices, mega-projects prioritizing urban and economic development, which have proved to have a negative impact on social equity. Instead, it will promote projects that recognize and take into account the diversity of local communities and the heritage of the place. For Thayer (2003), what will in practice drive toward bioregional or life-place planning are the limitations of conventional planning approaches (often involving a lack of regional plans and a top-down expert or engineer approach to planning) and "a growing demand for comprehensive, ecosystemic social and physical planning" (p. 146), i.e., the recognition by the civil society and more and more experts of the validity of this comprehensive approach to planning.

Such life-place planning needs to be adapted to every single context: "The practical bioregional hypothesis, then, is simply that for every bioregion there is a unique *method* or *set of practices* of planning, design, and management of the land and that this approach will result in a bioregionally unique set of *landscape patterns*" (Thayer 2003, p. 162). How can this be put into practice?

Practically, the reinhabitation of place promoted by bioregionalism implies increased procedural justice in planning because it relies on wide and open participation in decision-making processes. It promotes more face-to-face voluntary, affinity-based, horizontal interactions between local economic, political, and social actors. This empowerment of inhabitants requires a shifting of power to the more local level. For Thayer (2003), "in the case of life-place planning, there is no boundary between planning, education, and participation: all are subsumed into a general, reinhabitory culture. Bioregional education, in fact, is likely to be a many-sided dialogue, with local residents teaching experts as well as vice versa, and the whole gamut of stakeholders exchanging views on many interrelated subjects" (p. 175). In this paradigm shift, he mentions the role of unofficial civic planning organizations "to counterbalance the incremental and unsustainable 'business-as-usual' planning and development demonstrated by most city governments" (p. 170).

Aberley (1993) underlines the useful and empowering role that locally made maps can play in building a common vision for the future, in depicting strategies of resistance, and in opening up the possibility of actually building an alternative. The Italian territorialist scholars have shown in the region of central Tuscany how to involve the inhabitants at various stages of the planning processes, in order to combine expert knowledge with social production of plan, territory, and landscape (Magnaghi 2014). Innovative methods such as participatory mapping (community maps) actually contributed to a co-building of the territorial project. This requirement for participation and social production of planning is consistent with Fainstein's principles of democracy and diversity, as well as with Fincher and Iveson's principle of encounter: bioregionalism implies not only communicative and inclusive planning but also a community-building process (including community power/capabilities) and more egalitarian forms of power. Thayer (2003) concludes that "ultimately, a bioregenerative pattern language is a manifestation of a smaller-scaled, finer-grained, more participatory, democratic approach to land planning and management."

Moreover, the bioregionalist approach includes principles of spatial justice in its promotion of a decentralized structure of governance that promotes autonomy, subsidiarity, and diversity (Sale 1985). The conception of the bioregion as a territory, possibly a federation of autonomous communities, contrasts with the overarching schematic opposition between a center (main city) and periurban/rural peripheries under its influence and domination. Interactions between the communities are conceived as horizontal, without hierarchical relations of power. For instance, Magnaghi and Fanfani (2010) promote a renewed social contract (pact) between cities and countryside in the long term as a way to achieve the objective of reconnection and balance between human and physical systems. They recognize the multifunctional role of open space within regional planning: forest and farmland are not only productive for one sectorial industry; natural spaces are not only to be "protected" via restrictive regulations. Such renewed urban-rural relations can contribute to more territorial equity.

Hence, the bioregionalist approach shows interconnections between ecological restoration and social justice. The conception of place as a unique community of human and nonhuman beings, the promotion of more equal urban-rural relations and of inclusive decentralized governance, like the social production of planning/mapping, all promote more fair and inclusive planning.

5 Contemporary Challenges for Bioregional Planning

Despite these essential contributions, the bioregional project for reinhabitation has been criticized as utopian and ecologically deterministic. Moreover, some initiatives inspired by bioregionalism do not actually include the "redistribution of decision-making power to semi-autonomous territories who can adopt ecological sustainable *and* socially-just policies" desired by Aberley (1999, p. 35). Such criticisms should be put into context: bioregionalism is "a story of many voices" (ibid.), a body of thought and related decentralized practice that has evolved both as a body of teaching and as a social movement change. "There are, as yet, no professional schools of 'bioregional planning.' There is no professional society and no coherent body of theory (…), only scattered examples of such planning might be construed as success stories" (Thayer 2003, p. 144).

Concerning its consideration of social justice, a first criticism levied at bioregionalism is that it does not make it a priority to combat existing structural patterns of inequalities: "In its desire to forge a community that can reinhabit a bioregion, bioregionalism has a dangerous tendency to ignore the differential structural positions of present groups" (Menser 2013). According to Young (1990), it is essential to understand how groups have been structurally disadvantaged and then to develop a specific policy that integrates these groups, in order to compensate for such inequalities. That is why activist-scholars maintain that projects led by these groups and "projects focused explicitly on dismantling oppressive systems have the greatest potential to achieve substantive social change (…) and disrupt the dynamics of power and privilege that perpetuate inequity" (Reynolds and Cohen 2016). This issue is relevant at the scale of individuals or social groups *within* a community. For instance, how does bioregionalism address the integration of waves of culturally diverse and socially deprived migrants within the reinhabitation project? What happens if the projects of some native individuals or groups undermine the pursuit of the ecological good or of local community-building?

A first reply to this criticism is through the connections needed between diverse movements opposed to a resource-intensive global economy. In his bioregionalist alternative of place-based, socially just, and ecologically sustainable human cultures, Aberley mentions the challenge of integrating this with other social change movements (such as the environmental justice movements): "the bioregion could become the political arena within which resistance against ecological and social exploitation could be produced" (Aberley 1999, p. 34). Thayer (2003) too notes how the environmental justice movements have shown "the futility implicit in any separation between environmental and social planning" (p. 164). According to him, advocates for responsible land patterns and planning practices "have come to realize that their interconnections are more important than their distinction."

Pezzoli et al. (2014) go further by defining bioregional justice as a concept pertinent to reinventing place-based planning:

> The concept of bioregional justice shares the concerns of environmental justice, but does so in a way that also highlights ecosystems as common good assets, and human–nature relations as manifest in human settlement patterns at a regional scale. Bioregional justice integrates multiple layers of justice (e.g., social, economic, environmental, global) by advancing a unifying place-based approach to improving the land, ecosystems and urban–rural relationships in a particular bioregion. Bioregional justice ensures that the benefits, opportunities and risks arising from creating, operating and living in a territorially bounded network of human settlements (i.e. a bioregion where urban–rural–wild- land spaces co-evolve socially, culturally and ecologically) are shared equitably through healthy relationships and secure place-based attachments. Bioregional justice seeks equity and fairness in how a bioregion's assets—including nature's sources, sinks and ecosystems needed for life and

living—are accessed, utilized and sustainably conserved for current and future generations.

For such authors, social justice is hence at the center of the bioregionalist approach.

Second, this issue of structural patterns of inequalities may also be relevant *between* the various communities belonging to a bioregion or between bioregions, with a negative impact on territorial equity or spatial justice. As Menser (2013) points out, "because of spatial segregation within the region in terms of income and assets and burdens and benefits, bioregionalism could decentralize power in a way that reinforces existing inequalities." To illustrate this, the author takes the example of the New York City metropolitan region: if it was a federation of autonomous communities, the Hudson River north and the Bronx could be two good candidate communities, small enough to promote a "*Gemeinschaft* culture" based on personal relations (Evanoff 2011), sharing a sense of place, a territorial identity. However, such decentralization of power "would further promote inequality and injustice by releasing better-off communities from any obligation to assist worse-off ones" (Menser 2013). Thus, "the bioregional program to dismantle urban megaregions and forge a federation of autonomous communities could exacerbate socioeconomic and racial inequalities" (*ibid.*). Spatial justice would require that the communities that have benefitted from all the polluting facilities located in the Bronx (power and sewage sludge treatment plants, agribusiness infrastructure, waste transfer stations and incinerators) today jointly deal with the associated environmental burdens. For Menser (2013), this cannot be achieved within a federation of autonomous communities: it would take a confederation in which the Hudson River north and the Bronx "would be non-autonomous sections within, and subordinate to, the larger polity of the New York City metropolitan region" (p. 457). Because of such interdependencies between neighborhoods, Young also argues that the right level for the polity should be the metropolitan region (1990). Hence, Church (2014) notes several critiques of the bioregionalist assumption that decentralized, self-ruled communities would be altruistic (collaborative and not competitive, ignoring power relations).

In fact, such risks of socio-spatial segregation depend on the articulation of power between scales of governance and especially on how the principle of subsidiarity is applied. This raises the question of the scale/political organization of the bioregional project. Scale still plays a central role in debates on sustainability (Sonnino 2010). For some authors, the local level is the site of resistance to the destructive neoliberal rationales of globalization: equitable forms of economic development, environmental integrity, and social justice cannot be achieved without community control and shared access to resources, ideas of decentralization, self-sufficiency, and subsidiarity (Feagan 2007). However, other scholars show the inherent contradictions in such a relocalization project, considering, for instance, local food initiatives (Born and Purcell 2006; Guthman 2008).

The reinhabitation objective of bioregionalism entails this kind of local pitfall, since it considers that "the road to environmental sustainability lies in the creation of eco-local economies, which are place-specific and bounded in space by limits of community, geography and the stewardship of nature" (Curtis 2003, p. 83). However, Sale avoided this local pitfall by dividing the earth into "nested scales of natural regions" (1985), and Thayer was in favor of a trans-scalar planning approach, even though he conceived a bioregion as "a reasonably scaled, naturally bounded, ecologically defined territory, or life-place" (2003, p. 6). For Magnaghi (2014), the scale of the bioregion varies according to the local context. A bioregion may be a watershed, a city region, and a coastal region with its hinterland. It depends on the scale needed to articulate environmental, economic, political, and sociocultural spheres and achieve the objectives of reconnection and reinhabitation. Pezzoli and Leiter (2016) stress that although problems often occur at a localized scale, they often cut across scales and the urban-rural divide and "create cumulative impacts that can have deleterious effects on bioregional and even global environmental systems" (2016). Hence they advocate, like Thayer, an *Integrated Planning Framework* (IPF) combining horizontal integration (across topical areas) and vertical integration (across scales) of plans and policies, as defined by Godschalk and Rouse (2012). In his bioregional agenda, Pezzoli also underlines the need for "global trans-bioregional alliances and knowledge networks" as well as for a "global commons stewardship" (2013).

Finally, these potential risks of social and/or spatial segregation raise the question of the way bioregionalists consider cities. The bioregional project is not meant for megacities: it is not anti-urban, but it aims at finding new forms of urbanity (like polycentric urban centers or networks of cities), as "an alternative to the catastrophic future of megacities and urban regions" (Magnaghi 2014, p. 76). Early bioregional thinkers even regarded the city primarily as a site of ecological and social degradation; some were back-to-the-lander enthusiasts (Carr 2004). Sale advocated the integration of urban, rural, and wild environments (1985). Although, until recently, little attention has been paid to the implementation of bioregional principles in urban areas, cities are now at the center of some bioregional projects. For instance, Fanfani (2018) calls for a "re-embedding" of cities in their surrounding regions and a return to, "in planning practices, the 'urban bioregion' concept, as key feature for balanced and co-evolutionary polycentric urban regions." Advocating an "urban bioregionalism model," Church (2014) explains how to implement incrementally bioregionalist principles into existing urban areas, combining municipal policies and individual actions to improve the physical environment, with concurrent promotion of environmental education and neighborhood-oriented stewardship opportunities, to foster a reconnection between urban dwellers and natural processes.

Nevertheless, the bioregionalist emphasis on carrying capacity, designing with nature, may take precedence over the social/political aspects of the city. A future challenge could be for the bioregionalist movement to also acknowledge the potential positive moral and political values of cities for social justice. For Young (1990), the city provides opportunities for freedom and self-development not found in other living places (rural, village, suburban). In contrast to the communitarianism underlined by some bioregional thinkers, she values the dynamics of multiplicity and even anonymity of the modern city, the social relations that she defines as "being together of strangers", which enable religious, sexual, and cultural differences to flourish and coexist. Preserving this capacity of the modern city to recognize differences would be an important component of a just planning approach.

6 Conclusion

The spirit and the core components of bioregionalism contribute to more fair and inclusive planning. Conceiving of place as a unique community of human and non-human beings should help to avoid extractive planning practices and promote projects that recognize and take into account the diversity of local communities. The promotion of more equal urban-rural relations within a bioregion should create more egalitarian relations between communities and territories. The social production of planning should imply not only communicative and inclusive planning but also a community-building process. Bioregionalism will thus have positive impacts on social justice, as assessed in terms of democracy, diversity, and more egalitarian forms of power.

However, the bioregional project of reinhabitation was not built on social justice principles. It did not make it a priority to combat existing structural patterns of inequalities and exclusion, neither between individuals nor between communities or territories. Its communitarianism may represent a threat to improved social justice, assessed in terms of the recognition of difference, more material equality and territorial equity. Nevertheless, in the last decades, bioregionalism has expanded to encompass globally minded trans-scalar approaches, avoiding the local trap and connecting with environmental justice movements. Going beyond the initial project of reinhabitation of a life-place, Pezzoli et al. (2014) clearly show how a bioregionalist planning approach can address social and economic inequality, by merging place-based health planning and ecological restoration along the USA-Mexico border. This example illustrates how "the concept of bioregionalism is evolving through a process of place- and context-driven adaptation" (Aberley 1999, p. 25). Ways to propose more just and participatory ecological restoration approaches, to build integrative planning, acknowledging the potential positive moral and political values of cities for social justice, are some of the challenges currently debated in the bioregional community.

Acknowledgments The author received financial support for the research behind this chapter from the French National Research Agency under the program JASMINN Anr-14-CE18-0001.

References

Aberley, D. (1993). *Boundaries of home: Mapping for local empowerment*. Gabriola Island/Philadelphia: New Society Publishers.

Aberley, D. (1999). Interpreting bioregionalism: A story from many voices. In M. V. McGinnis (Ed.), *Bioregionalism* (pp. 13–42). New York: Routledge.

Agyeman, J. (2013). *Introducing just sustainabilities*. Zed Books. http://www.press.uchicago.edu/ucp/books/book/distributed/I/bo20842679.html.

Agyeman, J., & Evans, B. (2004). 'Just sustainability': The emerging discourse of environmental justice in Britain? *The Geographical Journal, 170*(2), 155–164. http://www.jstor.org/stable/3451592.

Alexander, D. (1990). Bioregionalism: Science or sensibility? *Environmental Ethics, 12*(2), 161–173.

Anguelovski, I., Shi, L., Chu, E., Gallagher, D., Goh, K., Lamb, Z., Reeve, K., & Teicher, H. (2016). Equity impacts of urban land use planning for climate adaptation: Critical perspectives from the global north and south. *Journal of Planning Education and Research, 36*(3), 333–348. https://doi.org/10.1177/0739456X16645166.

Barnett, C. (2011). Geography and ethics: Justice unbound. *Progress in Human Geography, 35*(2), 246–255. http://oro.open.ac.uk/28485/.

Blanchon, D., Moreau, S., & Veyret, Y. (2009). Comprendre et construire la justice environnementale. *Annales de géographie, 665–666*(1), 35–60. https://doi.org/10.3917/ag.665.0035.

Booth, P., Breuillard, M., Fraser, C., & Paris, D. (2007). *Spatial planning systems of Britain and France: A comparative analysis*. London: Royaume-Uni de Grande-Bretagne et d'Irlande du Nord.

Born, B., & Purcell, M. (2006). Avoiding the local trap scale and food systems in planning research. *Journal of Planning Education and Research, 26*(2), 195–207. https://doi.org/10.1177/0739456X06291389.

Campbell, H., & Marshall, R. (2006). Towards justice in planning: A reappraisal. *European Planning Studies, 14*(2), 239–252. https://doi.org/10.1080/09654310500418192.

Carr, M. (2004). *Bioregionalism and civil society: Democratic challenges to corporate globalism*. Vancouver: UBC Press.

Church, S. P. (2014, March). Exploring urban bioregionalism: A synthesis of literature on urban nature and sustainable patterns of urban living. *S.A.P.I.EN.S. Surveys and Perspectives Integrating Environment and Society, 7*(1). https://sapiens.revues.org/1691.

Curtis, F. (2003). Eco-localism and sustainability. *Ecological Economics, 46*(1), 83–102. https://econpapers.repec.org/article/eeeecolec/v_3a46_3ay_3a2003_3ai_3a1_3ap_3a83-102.htm.

Evanoff, R. (2011). *Bioregionalism and global ethics: A transactional approach to achieving ecological sustainability, social justice, and human well-being*. New York: Routledge. http://myaccess.library.utoronto.ca/login?url=http://www.tandfebooks.com/isbn/9780203843086.

Fainstein, S. S. (2009). Spatial justice and planning. *Justice Spatiale/Spatial Justice, 1*, 1–12. http://www.jssj.org/article/justice-spatiale-et-amenagement-urbain/.

Fainstein, S. S. (2010). *The just city*. Ithaca: Cornell University Press.

Fanfani, D. (2018). The urban bioregion as form and project of the co-evolution between urban and rural domain. The case of the Florence Metropolitan Area. *International Journal of Engineering & Technology, 7*(1.4), 61–68. https://doi.org/10.14419/ijet.v7i1.4.9264.

Feagan, R. (2007). The place of food: Mapping out the 'local' in local food systems. *Progress in Human Geography, 31*(1), 23–42. https://doi.org/10.1177/0309132507073527.

Fincher, R., & Iveson, K. (2008). *Planning and diversity in the city: Redistribution, recognition and encounter*. Houndmills/Basingstoke/Hampshire: Royaume-Uni de Grande-Bretagne et d'Irlande du Nord.

Fincher, R., & Iveson, K. (2012). Justice and injustice in the city. *Geographical Research, 50*(3), 231–241. https://doi.org/10.1111/j.1745-5871.2011.00742.x.

Fraser, N. (1997). *Justice interrupts: Critical reflections on the "postsocialist" condition*. New York: Routledge.

Gervais-Lambony, P., & Dufaux, F. (2009). "Justice... spatiale !" *Annales de géographie, 665–666*(January), 3–15. http://www.cairn.info/resume.php?ID_ARTICLE=AG_665_0003.

Godschalk, D. R., & Rouse, D. C. (2012). *Sustaining places: Best practices for comprehensive plans* (PAS report 567). APA Planning Advisory Service.

Guthman, J. (2008). Neoliberalism and the making of food politics in California. *Geoforum, 39*(3), 1171–1183. https://doi.org/10.1016/j.geoforum.2006.09.002.

Harvey, D. (1973). *Social justice and the city*. Baltimore: Etats-Unis d'Amérique/Johns Hopkins University Press.

Kymlicka, W. (Ed.). (1992). *Justice in political philosophy* (2 vols). Aldershot: Royaume-Uni de Grande-Bretagne et d'Irlande du Nord/Etats-Unis d'Amérique.

Lefebvre, H. (1974). *La production de l'espace*. Paris: Éditions Anthropos.

Magnaghi, A. (2014). *La biorégion urbaine: Petit traité sur le territoire bien commun*. Paris: Eterotopia France.

Magnaghi, A., & Fanfani, D. (2010). *Patto Città-Campagna. Un Progetto Di Bioregione Urbana per La Toscana*. Luoghi. Alinea. https://www.ibs.it/patto-citta-campagna-progetto-di-libro-alberto-magnaghi-david-fanfani/e/9788860554758.

Marcuse, P., Connolly, J., Johannes, N., Olivo, I., Potter, C., & Steil, J. (2009). *Searching for the just city: Debates in urban theory and practice*. London: Royaume-Uni de Grande-Bretagne et d'Irlande du Nord, Etats-Unis d'Amérique.

Menser, M. (2013). The bioregion and social difference: Learning from Iris young's metropolitan regionalism. *Environmental Ethics, 35*(4), 439–459. http://connection.ebscohost.com/c/articles/94960459/bioregion-social-difference-learning-from-iris-youngs-metropolitan-regionalism.

Pezzoli, K. (2013). *Bioregional justice: a framework for ecological restoration* (Draft statement prepared for the good neighbour environmental board) (pp. 1–7). San Diego: Global Action Research Centre.

Pezzoli, K., & Leiter, R. A. (2016). Creating healthy and just bioregions. *Reviews on Environmental Health, 31*(1), 103–109. https://doi.org/10.1515/reveh-2015-0050.

Pezzoli, K., Kozo, J., Ferran, K., Wooten, W., Gomez, G. R., & Al-Delaimy, W. K. (2014). One bioregion/one health: An integrative narrative for transboundary planning along the US–Mexico Border. *Global Society: Journal of Interdisciplinary International Relations, 28*(4), 419–440. https://doi.org/10.1080/13600826.2014.951316.

Rawls, J. (1971). *A theory of justice*. Cambridge, MA: Etats-Unis d'Amérique: The Belknap Press of Harvard University Press.

Reynolds, K., & Cohen, N. (2016). *Beyond the kale: Urban agriculture and social justice activism in New York City*. Athens: Etats-Unis d'Amérique: The University of Georgia Press.

Sale, K. (1985). *Dwellers in the land: The bioregional vision*. San Francisco: Sierra Club Books.

Smith, D. M. (1994). *Geography and social justice*. In *Oxford*. Royaume-Uni de Grande-Bretagne et d'Irlande du Nord: Blackwell.

Soja, E. W. (2009). La Ville et La Justice Spatiale | Jssj.Org *Justice Spatiale/Spatial Justice*, 1. http://www.jssj.org/article/la-ville-et-la-justice-spatiale/.

Soja, E. W. (2010). *Seeking spatial justice*. Minneapolis: Etats-Unis d'Amérique: University of Minnesota Press.

Sonnino, R. (2010). Escaping the local trap: Insights on re-localization from school food reform. *Journal of Environmental Policy & Planning, 12*(1), 23–40. https://doi.org/10.1080/15239080903220120.

Thayer, R. L. (2003). *LifePlace: Bioregional thought and practice*. Berkeley: University of California press.

Visser, G. (2001). Social justice, integrated development planning and post-apartheid urban reconstruction. *Urban Studies, 38*(10), 1673–1699. https://doi.org/10.1080/00420980120084813.

Walzer, M. (1983). *Spheres of justice: A defense of pluralism and equality*. New York: Etats-Unis d'Amérique: Basic Books.
Winkler, T. (2012). Between economic efficacy and social justice: Exposing the Ethico-politics of planning. *Cities, 29*(3), 166–173. https://doi.org/10.1016/j.cities.2011.11.014.
Young, I. M. (1990). *Justice and the politics of difference*. Princeton: Etats-Unis d'Amérique, Royaume-Uni de Grande-Bretagne et d'Irlande du Nord.

Part II
Fields for (Re)framing Planning in Bioregional Sense

Bioregional Planning and Biophilic Urbanism

Peter Newman and Agata Cabanek

1 Introduction

Bioregionalism has been part of cities from the beginning. Cities grew out of the opportunities they created but could only do this if their bioregional services – food, fuel, materials, water, waste absorption and ecological services – were adequate and well managed (Mumford 1961). When cities forgot this link or deliberately denied it, they collapsed (Diamond 2009). Prophetic voices like George Perkins Marsh said this in the nineteenth century (Marsh 1864), but the same can be seen in ancient times. The biblical prophet Isaiah railed about Babylon (a real city but also representing any city that developed such arrogance about its environmental context); Isaiah predicted the collapse of Babylon due to its overcutting of its surrounding forests (14:8) 2700 years ago.

In more recent times, bioregionalism has been rediscovered in the environmental movement, the territorialist movement (in Italy), the natural resource management or landcare movement (in Australia) and a multiple of expressions through urban and regional sustainability (Magnaghi 2005; Cork et al. 2007; McHarg 1969; Fanfani, 2009, 2013; Thayer 1997, 2009; Beatley 1999, 2012).

The link between bioregionalism and cities is not always made. Some bioregional perspectives, like those based around McHarg's environmental mapping, give a sense that a bioregion would be better off without the city. Such an approach, often described as romanticism, has a long history of reaction to industrial

P. Newman (✉)
Distinguished Professor of Sustainability, Curtin University Sustainability Policy (CUSP) Institute, School of Design and the Built Environment, Curtin University, Perth, Australia
e-mail: P.Newman@curtin.edu.au

A. Cabanek
Curtin University Sustainability Policy (CUSP) Institute, School of Design and the Built Environment, Curtin University, Perth, Australia
e-mail: agata.cabanek@postgrad.curtin.edu.au

D. Fanfani, A. Matarán Ruiz (eds.), *Bioregional Planning and Design: Volume I*,
https://doi.org/10.1007/978-3-030-45870-6_7

modernism (Pepper 1996). But new movements are now appearing that are re-establishing the inherent integration of cities and their bioregion which are more positive about how the city can help recreate a better bioregion (Newman and Jennings 2008; Hes and Du Plessis 2015). One of these movements is biophilic urbanism. This chapter will show how bioregionalism and biophilic urbanism are related. It will attempt to show that cities can indeed begin their bioregional strategies from the biophilic design strategies. It will demonstrate this in some case studies, especially in Singapore.

2 Bioregionalism

A bioregion is defined by natural borders rather than by political borders, as in the Yellowstone to Yukon bioregion, which traverses state and national borders. Bioregional natural systems are critical for cities to function, but they are usually assumed to be separate from the built environment. These natural systems that surround the city include the water supply, local food and timber supplies; local materials for building; local waste-absorbing processes in air, water and soils; local biodiversity that provides the fundamental life forces of the regional ecosystem; and bioregional recreation spaces for the city. Such bioregional perspectives have been studied to minimise urban impacts for some time and are now part of a bioregional science (Thayer 1997, 2009; Fanfani 2009, 2013).

As cities consume or erode their natural environments, there has been growing concern that they must move from minimising their impact to rejuvenating their bioregional natural systems. If the natural systems are impacted too heavily, they can collapse, so the idea of regeneration is now being highlighted to not only minimise this but to repair the generations of damage that went before. The new ideas of resilient or regenerative design are now being applied (Lyle 1985, 1994; Thomson and Newman 2018). For example, many ideas for managing the increasing effects of climate change rely on green infrastructure which is multi-use infrastructure that uses natural systems to provide functions that traditionally were achieved by grey infrastructure systems, for example green space to absorb flooding, oyster beds to revive rivers and bioretention basins and swales (Matthews et al. 2016). Many of these projects go beyond resilience to actually regenerate the centuries of damage to their surrounding bioregion.

The more recent addition to bioregionalism is how cities can be even more regenerative through biophilic urbanism.

3 Biophilic Urbanism

Biophilic urbanism is based on the knowledge that humans have an innate connection with nature that should be expressed in their daily lives, especially in cities. Bringing nature onto and inside buildings has become the new focus and requires a new science and a new governance. This has not been a strong feature of architectural principles and practice (even though there has been a long tradition of landscape architecture) yet potentially offers great rewards if it is implemented in the structure of the built environment.

Biophilia was a term first brought to life in 1964 by the psychoanalyst Erich Fromm in his exploration of the *Essence of Man*. He saw that humans' awareness of their "mortality" separates them from nature, causing deep anxiety and conflict (Fromm 1964). Humans try to overcome this anxiety by either a regressive path of narcissism, incestuous symbiosis, violence and necrophilia or a progressive path of altruism, freedom and biophilia. "Biophilia" was defined as a love of life and living processes.

The concept of the biophilic human being was then examined and popularised in 1984 by a sociobiologist, E.O. Wilson, in his book *Biophilia.* Wilson defined biophilia as "the innate tendency to focus on life and lifelike processes". He utilised the term "biophilia" to describe his deep feelings of connection to nature during a period of exploration and immersion in the natural world. Wilson's special insight was that this biophilic propensity developed as part of evolutionary survival so it encompasses certain characteristics that remain with humans even in modern cities and thus must be built into its everyday architecture (Wilson 1984; Kellert and Wilson 1993).

Today biophilic urbanism has become a major social movement within city policy and practice. The movement from ecology to the built environment can be seen in the collected work edited by Stephen Kellert and others, *Biophilic Design: The Theory, Science, and Practice of Bringing Buildings to Life* (Kellert et al. 2008), largely focused on the building level, to Timothy Beatley's book, *Biophilic Cities: Integrating Nature into Urban Design and Planning* (2011). There is now a Biophilic Cities Network with membership across the globe; the network enables cities to share information on how to mainstream biophilic urbanism into the policies and practices of cities.

The special niche of biophilic urbanism has been its focus on how to apply greenery into and onto the buildings that make up our cities, predominantly through green roofs and vertical greenery that have changed buildings from being concrete and steel designed to separate urban life from nature to living walls and roofs that are now seen as habitat sites with a new kind of design aesthetic (Kellert et al. 2008; Kellert 2008). As a result, a wide range of designs and methods for integrating nature into the built environment have emerged and continue to evolve with the potential of linking into bioregional regenerative outcomes.

3.1 Green Roofs

Green roofs are being developed across the world based on a range of new materials and new technologies as well as new science of what species will thrive in different areas (Dunnett and Kingsbury 2008; Wood et al. 2014). They are also being built for different reasons. North America is discovering that they are a very effective and popular option for managing stormwater and reducing the urban heat island effect. Basel, in Switzerland, has been installing green roofs for the past 16 years with a focus on increasing biodiversity. Where there may be a sole initial driver for the green roof installation, the multiple benefits are discovered which then tends to lead to a ripple effect of further green roofs being installed in the surrounding area (Soderlund and Newman 2015).

Chicago first conducted a green roof trial on their City Hall, and its success led to incentives and regulations to encourage further green roofs in the City of Chicago. The driver for this was the need to cool the city and reduce the urban heat island effect. By 2010, Chicago had 359 green roofs totalling 51 hectares, and the Chicago City Hall green roof has become an icon for Chicago's sustainability movement.

Green roofs can be intensive or extensive like the California Academy of Sciences in San Francisco or Millennium Park in Chicago which is an extensive (10 hectare) green roof built over parking lots; this project has resulted in increasing tourism and further development bringing $3–5 billion economic benefit to the area (Soderlund 2016).

Green roofs can become part of a city's building policy with strong incentives such as extra density if provided or just the encouragement of a city policy. Germany began with incentives in 1983 followed by Basel, Switzerland, in 2000. Both countries currently have a high number of green roofs, and it is now an accepted form of practice. Washington initiated a green roof rebate program in 2005 and, as part of their Sustainable DC strategy, aims to have 20 million sq. ft. green roofs by 2020. Many global cities have initiated some form of incentives encouraging green roof construction in their cities. Austrian cities Vienna, Linz, Salzburg and Graz provide multiple grants and subsidies to support various green infrastructures being installed, including green roofs. Globally there is a growing tool kit of options for biophilic urbanism policy. This requires not just green roofs but green walls as well.

3.2 Green Walls

French botanist Patrick Blanc was the first to demonstrate extensive green walls; he created large, artistic and prominent green walls with plant species selected from waterfall rock-face plants. Blanc's walls are hydroponic panel systems which are quite thin, thus enabling them to be large and tall. Since these spectacular examples, green walls of all kinds have sprouted across the world (Blanc 2008).

Green walls are suitable for both indoor and outdoor locations. The resulting benefits will vary with the site, and, in some climates, indoor placement brings greater benefits. Toronto has discovered this with indoor biofilter green walls developed from NASA space technology research. These biofilter green walls significantly improve indoor air quality through a filtering system primarily involving the plant roots and soil microbes. Biofilter walls are also beginning to be recognised scientifically where a 2-year study of an installation in Sydney suggested impressive results of significant indoor particulate and carbon dioxide reductions (Burchett and Torpy 2011).

There is a growing body of evidence about such projects as the Toronto indoor biofilters, which have been a popular addition in developments, that they have multiple social, environmental and economic benefits.

3.3 Benefits of Biophilic Urbanism

Socio-psychological and environmental benefits are the most studied elements of biophilic urbanism (Newman et al. 2017). These are likely to combine and contribute to significant economic benefits such as better workplace productivity, improved health and healing, increased retail potential, decreased crime and violence, increased property values and employee attraction and increased liveability in dense areas. These are set out in Table 1 along with some estimates of economic benefit from each.

There are many obvious benefits of biophilic urbanism, but most of the literature and work by the biophilic urbanists are on how it can benefit cities as though they weren't part of a bioregion. So how does biophilic urbanism help with bioregional agendas and how can bioregionalism help the biophilic urbanism agendas?

4 Linking Bioregionalism and Biophilic Urbanism

In order for biophilic urbanism to assist with a broader bioregional agenda, it will need to focus on how the natural features that are being introduced onto and into built structures can improve bioregional outcomes. Like all landscape architecture, bioregional-oriented biophilic urbanism needs to see how the choice of plants and their ecological structures can assist in a range of outcomes being sought by bioregionalism. It can also start as a bioregional policy which is translated into a local biophilic urbanism policy and extends the potential outcomes. There are several ways that biophilic urbanism can help with the bioregionalism agenda; the three examined here to illustrate the links are ecosystem services, biodiversity and sense of place.

Table 1 Economic benefits of biophilic urbanism

Area of benefit	Estimated economic and environmental benefit
Better workplace productivity	\$2000 per employee per year from daylighting \$2990 per employee over 4 months when desks angled to view nature
Improved health and healing	\$93 million per year in reduced hospital cost of natural features provided in the US hospitals
Increased retail potential	Skylighting in a chain store would result in a 40% sale increase, ±7% 25% higher sales in vegetated street frontage
Decreased crime and violence	Public housing with greenery had 52% reduction in felonies Biophilic landscapes introduced across New York City would have \$1.7 billion through crime reduction
Increased property values	Biophilic buildings attract higher rental prices, 3% per square foot or 7% in effective rents, selling at prices 16% higher
Employee attraction	Biophilics attract and retain high-quality workers
Increased liveability in dense areas	Green features increase saleability of densely built apartments blocks
Carbon sequestration	In Singapore, aboveground vegetation sequesters 7.8% of the total emitted daily carbon dioxide
Reduced urban heat island effect and reduced energy consumption	Due to shading provided by urban trees, in Los Angeles, annual residential air-conditioning (A/C) bills can be reduced directly by about US\$100 million, additional savings of US\$70 million in indirect cooling, US\$360 million in smog-reduction benefits
Water management and quality	Up to 70% of stormwater retention capability depending of the local climate and other conditions
Air quality	Urban street canyons full of greenery can reduce particulate matter by up to 60% and nitrogen dioxide by up to 40%
Biodiversity conservation	A study of 115 wildly colonised green roofs in north of France found that 86% of species were native to the area

Source: Newman et al. (2017)

4.1 Ecosystem Services

The choice and type of biophilic services in a city can greatly assist bioregional watershed management, waste management and the provision of resources such as energy, materials, food and water. Cities covered in hard surfaces need to slow down stormwater flows, and there is much evidence of this now being mainstreamed, for example permeable and porous pavements infiltrate rain water which can be stored in underground tanks as in Vitoria-Gasteiz. Cities with substantial vegetation can clean the air and water; they can absorb grey water through bioswales and rain gardens to help grow biophilic landscaping, especially in areas where water is scarce at certain times of the year. Cities can provide particular types of food such as vegetables, herbs and spices because they are so labour-intensive, reducing food miles as many restaurants are now using to attract customers. Cities can provide water through their own urban catchments as well as drawing from their bioregional surrounds as in Singapore (outlined below). Cities can provide their own energy from local renewable sources thus reducing the impact on bioregions or working in partnership to share resources like biofuels as in Perth's White Gum Valley project (Newman et al. 2017).

The key, as to whether cities do this, will be whether cities plan for this or not. Modernist planning expectations certainly did not include such agendas, but new technologies for small-scale water, energy, waste and materials can combine with the expertise from biophilic scientists to enable such agendas to be mainstreamed (Newman 2005; Beatley 2011).

4.2 *Biodiversity*

With declining global biodiversity, increasing the availability of habitat in cities through increased urban vegetation is an obvious focus for progressive cities. The United Nations 2012 conference on biodiversity combined most of the world's nations in a pledge to increase commitment and spending on halting the rate of species loss; but it will be cities that mostly are able to do this. Green roofs and green walls have multiple benefits, but if carefully integrated into urban landscaping and bioregional ecosystems, they can also help with biodiversity.

Cities in Switzerland, particularly Basel, have been studying the progression of biodiversity associated with their green roofs with encouraging results, resulting in mandatory green roofs on new flat-roofed buildings similar to Toronto. Some bird species are beginning to colonise Swiss green roofs. In a study of 115 "wild-colonised" green roofs in northern French cities, 86% of the colonies were found to be native plants. This suggests that, once established, biophilic architectural features could act as important sites for biodiversity colonisation from the surrounding bioregion (Brenneisan 2006; Baumann 2006; Madre et al. 2014).

The key to enabling a biodiversity link is to see how plant species and habitat structures can be designed with a bioregional perspective, not just a local aesthetic perspective. This will take scientific monitoring and studies to ensure it is working.

4.3 *Sense of Place*

A bioregional approach to urban design helps to create a sense of place. Beatley and Newman (2013) make a case that biophilic cities are overlapping in their desire to be sustainable and resilient through a range of place-oriented strategies that are trying to make the built environment more sensitive to its local, regional and planetary environment. Newman and Jennings (2008, p 144–155) developed five strategies for cities to enable them to foster a sense of place. One of those is "to connect the urban form to the wider bioregion". To achieve that, local planning authorities must provide planning criteria and tools and fund necessary biophilic structures to connect the city to its bioregion. Cities located in a particular bioregion need to have the characteristics of their regional ecosystem at the heart of their biophilic systems.

In Europe, planning regional ecological networks to connect urban and rural natural systems has a long tradition. A flagship example of biophilic urbanism linking to regional ecosystems has been delivered in Vitoria-Gasteiz in Spain. The capital city of the Basque Country has had a policy for some time to join urban and rural natural systems creating a network that provides a number of eco-services as well enhancing humans' well-being (Beatley 1999, 2012). The sense of place that has been generated permeates from the bioregion through to its parks, boulevards, and buildings. The green infrastructure creates channels connecting the greenbelt and its parks to the greenery in the city. The green network provides favourable conditions for enhancing urban and rural biodiversity recreating lost habitats. One of the important biophilic projects was naturalisation of a stream, which once was channelled in a concrete pipe. The stream, boarded by native riparian vegetation and traditionally reinforced embankment, runs along Gasteiz Hiribidea Avenue. Together with an impressive green envelope at the Palace of Europe, the stream creates a biodiversity hotspot in the city centre providing habitat to more than 70 butterfly species, many insects, and small animals (Beatley 2012) (Fig. 1).

5 Singapore: Biophilic City

Few cities have gone as far as Singapore with their biophilic urbanism. The island state has revegetated much of its previously cleared areas increasing canopy cover by 40% between 1986 and 2007. The goal of the city is to move from being a "garden city" to a "city in a garden" or even a "city in a forest". Canopies have been built over most major roads and parks with different levels of habitat as well. Corridors of greenery have been built across the city called Park Connectors providing walking and cycling access only. Perhaps most impressive though has been the commitment to green roofs and green walls into hundreds of buildings based on a new science of how to apply it in Singapore's climate developed by the government and freely provided. The enthusiasm of government, private sector and community groups for their biophilic city is evident in a number of films about Singapore (Newman et al. 2012).

Biophilic urbanism is now being mainstreamed into the town planning system in Singapore. New buildings in Singapore are now required to have a Green Floor Plate Ratio which requires them to replace the floor plate of the development with at least the same and sometimes twice as much greenery as the floor plate area (Newman 2014; Ong 2003). WOHA, the architects of Singapore's award-winning Park Royal Hotel also known as the "jungle hotel", took great advantage of Singapore's green area ratio (GAR) to maximise green space and biodiversity, achieving a 5 to 1 ratio (Fig. 2).

Singapore's global leadership in biophilic urbanism has been recognised (Newman 2014), so other cities are now copying them. For example, Washington D.C. recently created a green area ratio (GAR), modelled after Singapore's, which requires developers to replace the green space they have built over into their

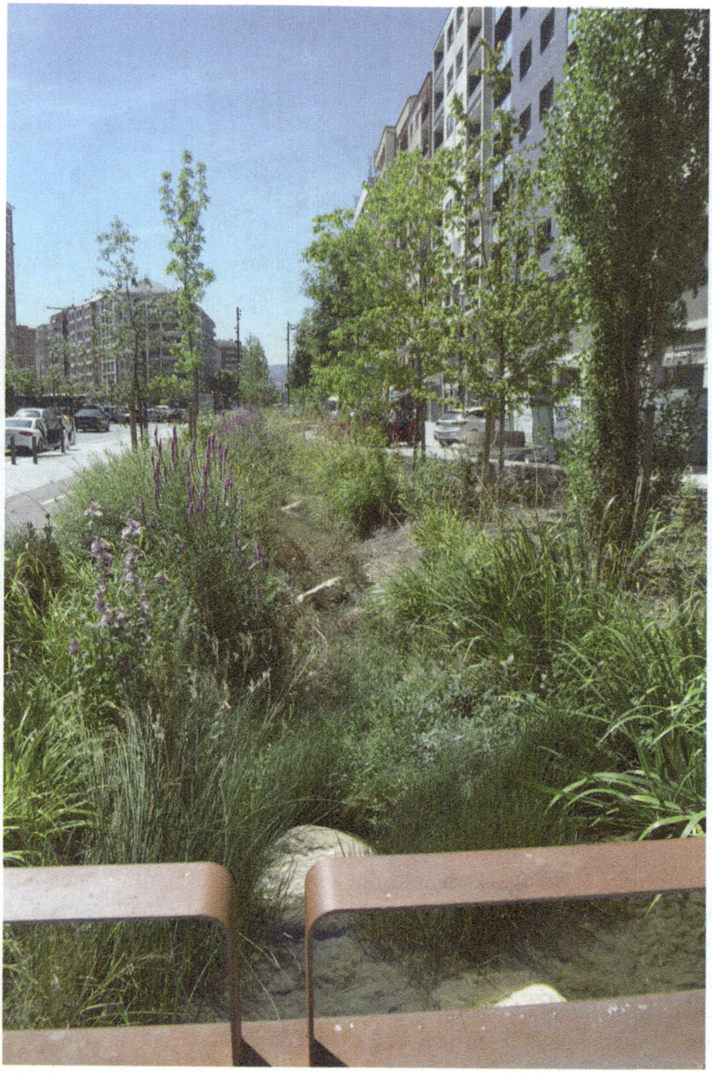

Fig. 1 Regenerated urban stream from stormwater pipe in Vitoria-Gasteiz, bringing bioregional biodiversity into the city. (Source Photo Agata Cabanek)

building's roof and facade. D.C.'s new stormwater runoff and GAR fees are expected to pay for many more biophilic projects (https://doee.dc.gov/GAR).

The goals of linking ecosystem service, biodiversity and sense of place are seen to overlap in all the new biophilic projects being built in Singapore such as the Gardens by the Bay which an educational area is showing the whole variety of biodiversity in its bioregion and creating multiple habitat sites to demonstrate them (Fig. 3).

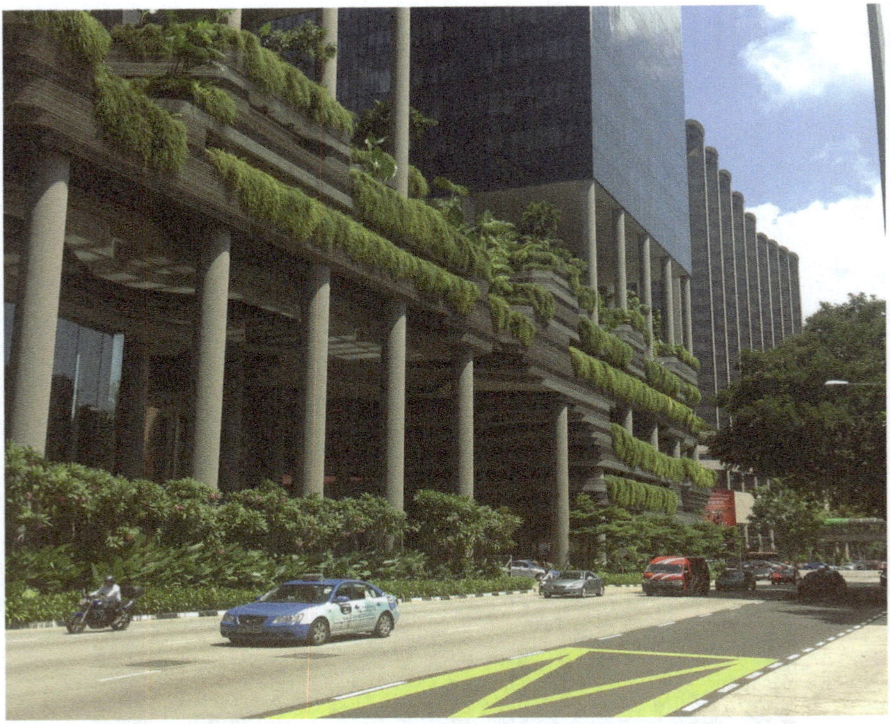

Fig. 2 Singapore's Park Royal Hotel which achieved a green floor ratio of 5:1. (Source Photo Peter Newman (Color figure online))

Singapore's KTP hospital incorporated greenery and biophilic design throughout the hospital in the hope that it would not only improve healing rates but that this initiative would encourage butterflies back. Both have happened. A goal of 100 butterfly species was set, and after 3 years, 102 species were sighted at the hospital (Newman and Matan 2012) (Fig. 4).

Three key conclusions about the value of biophilic urbanism and how it is relating to bioregionalism can be drawn from Singapore:

(a). *Singapore shows how the stigma can be removed from density as not being a feature of green cities.*

Singapore's biophilic urbanism has shown the world how a dense city can regenerate natural systems and create far more natural urban systems. It is doing this between buildings and all over buildings using their structures to create new urban ecosystems never considered possible before (Fig. 5) of a high-rise green facade. This is countering the problems of modernist buildings and their unattractive qualities to many people.

Singapore has demonstrated that density probably helps in two ways: (a) it enables concepts like Park Connectors and the Gardens by the Bay to be developed

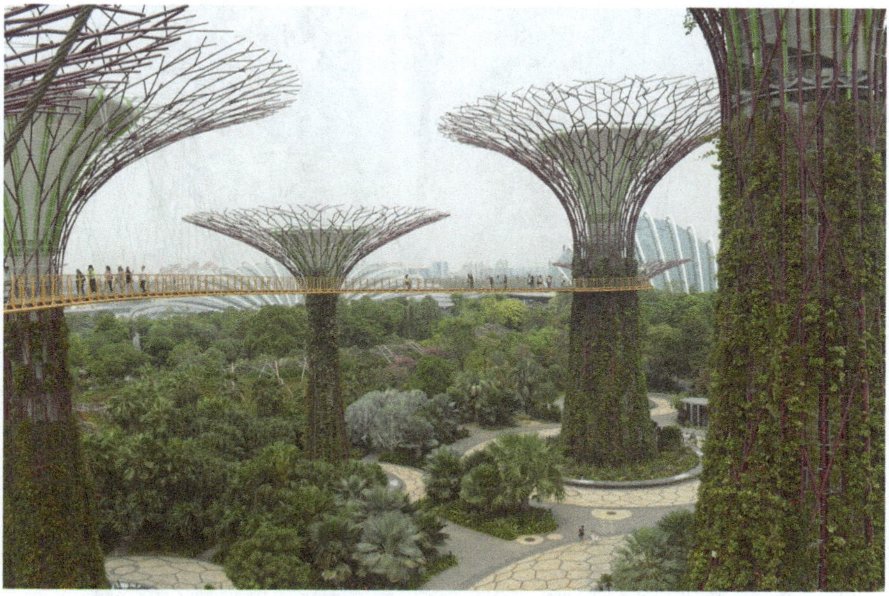

Fig. 3 Singapore's Gardens by the Bay replaced a reclaimed area with a range of technologically creative habitats and educational facilities for demonstrating bioregional biodiversity. (Source Photo Agata Cabanek)

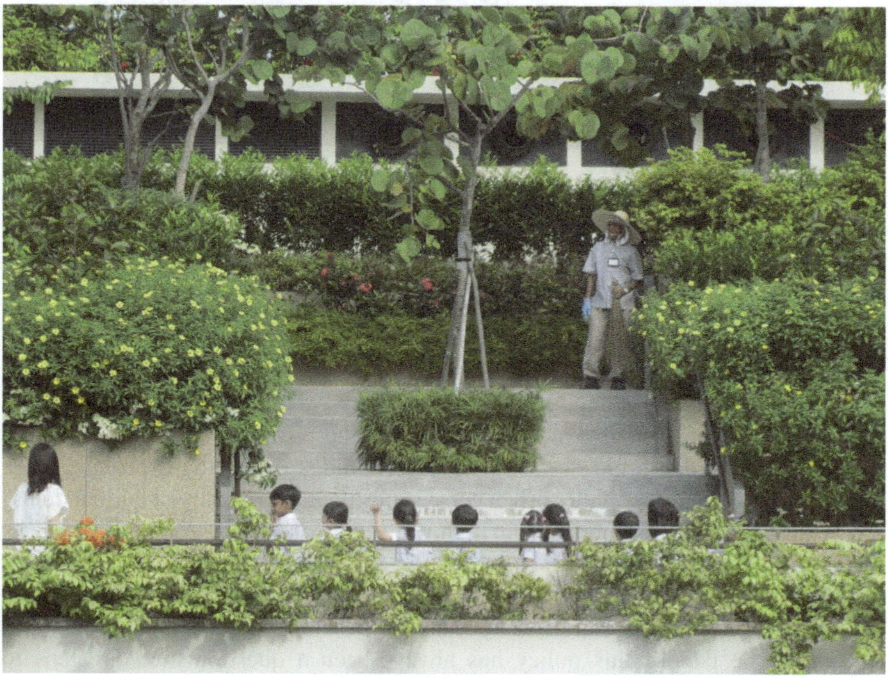

Fig. 4 KTP hospital in Singapore showing biophilic features that have made the hospital into a tourist attraction. (Source Photo Peter Newman)

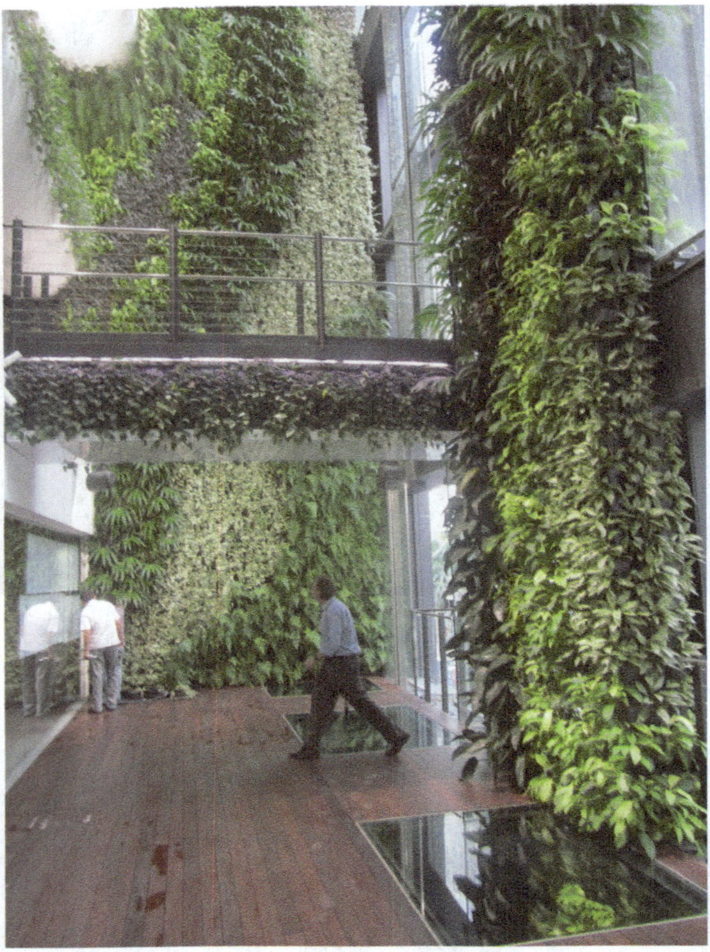

Fig. 5 High-rise green façade in Singapore high-rise office building. *Source* Photo Peter Newman (Color figure online)

as they need intense land uses where distances are short; and (b) it enables the height of buildings to be used to help create a third dimension in an urban ecosystem. This means that a structure for biological activity can be created around buildings similar to the structure of tall forest. Thus the positive element of biophilic urbanism is that dense cities with high-rise buildings can perhaps provide more opportunities to build biophilic urban ecosystems than low-density suburbia, due to their extra habitat opportunities from high walls and flat roofs. This is a big issue as the world is trying to find ways of preventing car-dependent urban sprawl with all its oil, climate, health and economic implications, and most cities point to a powerful need for increased densities (Newman 2006). However, the need for natural systems to be part of this policy has always been a question that threatens to undermine the value in more compact cities. Perhaps biophilic urbanism is a way to facilitate green and attractive cities that are also far more efficient in resources? To take away the stigma of density would be a significant bioregional planning contribution from biophilic urbanism now clearly demonstrated in Singapore.

(b). *Singapore has shown how a city can make a contribution to local and bioregional biodiversity.*

Singapore's NParks started measuring biodiversity when they began their biophilic experiments. They have pioneered the Singapore Biodiversity Index which has been adopted by many cities around the world. These data are now showing that new and rare species are being found in Singapore long after they were thought to have disappeared from the urban area. The many local examples set out in a series of beautiful publications from the city all show rapid increases in birdlife and other biodiversity as soon as habitat is provided, whether it is using local species or not. Indeed many of the tree species used to provide the structure of their urban ecosystems are not native, like the rain trees used to structure canopy cover over roads and parks (because their root systems fit into urban areas). KTP Hospital measures biodiversity in birds, fish and butterflies, and all are going up as their biophilic features mature.

Biophilic urbanism like that demonstrated in Singapore is unlikely to recreate the pre-urban ecosystem nor is that ever claimed. But it can do far more to recreate the structure of the ecosystem in any area as it can use the diversity of a city's built forms and microclimates to create urban ecosystems far more biodiverse and complete in their structures than in the unidimensional urban parks and gardens we are used to. In this, it is more like the regenerative design paradigm mentioned earlier.

(c). *Singapore has shown how new kinds of bioregionally oriented urban ecosystems can be imagined developing if biophilic urbanism is taken seriously.*

As the biophilic urbanism in Singapore spreads and matures into a more complete coverage of the urban environment, it can be expected that not only will local biodiversity rise but a better understanding of how urban ecosystems can help bioregions regenerate. It is not the same as the pre-city rain forest, but it will have many features of a rain forest except it will also contain a city full of people.

6 The Next Stage in Singapore's Biophilic Urbanism

There are two new projects that take Singapore's biophilic urbanism into new territory and can help show bioregional outcomes. The projects are new urban areas being built on sites that are highly degraded – one is a degraded industrial area and the other is a section of coastline that has been reclaimed using earth fill and recycled rubbish. Their biophilic design strategies as part of their strategic planning are providing a new opportunity for bioregionalism.

The two new projects are redeveloping areas for extra housing and in the process are regenerating the natural features of the area using bioregional principles and then bringing these back into the biophilic urbanism being used in and on buildings. One is taking a former river delta area that had been drained and channelised into concrete drains and will recreate some of the former river mouth ecosystem. It will then take some of the features of this ecosystem back into how the landscape is created around and on the buildings for the new housing area. It is thus joining the natural features of the area into the built form and regenerating the former ecosystem. The other project is on the coast and will be using coastal ecosystem features to regenerate the area from a reclaimed concrete wall into a thriving natural area; it will then bring these features into the green roofs and green walls of the new housing area (Ming et al. 2010; Yabuka 2018).

Biophilic urbanism has emerged in the USA but is not just an American phenomenon. Singapore has shown, perhaps more than any other city, how a dense Asian city can bring nature into the city in new and exciting ways. Perhaps the most important outcome of Singapore's biophilic urbanism is that it has proved not only that density does not preclude a city from bringing nature more intensely into the daily life of a city but in fact density may assist this.

The rapidity with which Singapore has made this transition from being a modernist city, where nature was kept at a distance from urban development to embracing it at every point of the city's development and buildings, suggests that any city wanting to make a contribution to biodiversity and to creating a healthier and more complete urban ecosystem can now do it. The technology of green walls and green roofs is now available and needs to be trialled in many different urban environments. The results can be a city where a new kind of urban nature develops that fulfils the functions of the original ecosystem replaced by the city and which contributes to bioregional outcomes.

7 Conclusions

Bioregional planning and biophilic urbanism are natural allies in many aspects of environmental planning. There is a need for bioregionalism to bring its insights and science right into the city and down to the detailed landscaping in and on buildings, and there is a need for biophilic urbanism to extend their science and insights out into the corridors and surroundings of the bioregion that supports every city. Such linkages will need to be demonstrated more and more such as the two new redevelopment case studies in Singapore. It is possible that a new kind of biophilic urbanism will be created that is more related to the local ecology and bioregional restoration, gaining its design motivation not from a collection of plants from around the world but from the restored local ecology. At the same time, the case studies could be rejuvenating bioregionalism because it grows out of the city and its development rather than being just what happens outside and around the city. Such potential integration of bioregionalism and biophilic urbanism is needed in all cities.

References

Beatley, T. (1999). *Green urbanism: Learning from cities in Europe*. Washington, DC: Island Press.

Beatley, T. (2011). *Biophilic cities: Integrating nature into Urban Design and planning*. Washington, DC: Island Press.

Beatley, T. (Ed.). (2012). *Green cities of Europe: Global lesson on green urbanism*. Washington, DC: Island Press.

Beatley, T., & Newman, P. (2013). Biophilic cities are sustainable resilient cities. *Sustainability, 5*, 3328–3345. https://doi.org/10.3390/su5083328.

Blanc, P. (2008). The vertical garden: From nature to the city. New York: W.W. Norton & Company,

Brenneisan, S. (2006). Space for urban wildlife: Designing green roofs as habitats in Switzerland. *Urban Habitat, 4*, 27–36.

Baumann, N. (2006). Ground-nesting birds on green roofs in Switzerland: Preliminary observations. *Urban Habitat, 4*, 37–50.

Burchett, M. D., & Torpy, F. (2011). *How humble houseplants can improve your health, lecture recording, UTS Science in Focus, UTS, Sydney*. Available: https://www.uts.edu.au/about/faculty-science/partners-and-community/uts-science-focus/medical-and-biomedical-sciences/how-humble-houseplants-can-improve-your-health. Accessed 18 May 2020.

Cork, S., Stoneham, G., & Lowe, K. (2007). *Ecosystem services and Australian natural resource management (NRM) futures*. Canberra: NRMSC, Commonwealth of Australia.

Diamond, J. (2009). *Collapse: How societies choose to fail or succeed*. New York: Viking Books.

Dunnett, N., & Kingsbury, N. (2008). *Planting green roofs and living walls* (2nd ed.). London: Timber Press.

Fanfani, D. (2009). Multifunctional planning of the Periurban territory and limiting land consumption. The strategic scenario for the "Polycentric City of Central-Western Tuscany". In B. Badiani & M. Tira (Eds.), *Urban containment: The Italian approach in the European perspective* (pp. 55–70). Sant'Arcangelo di Romagna: Maggioli. isbn: 9788838743634

Fanfani, D. (2013). Local development and Agri urban domain: Agricultural Park as promotion of an 'Active Ruralship'. *Planum: The Journal of Urbanism, 27*(2), 38–47.

Fromm, E. (1964). *The heart of man*. New York: Harper and Row.

Hes, D., & Du Plessis, C. (2015). *Designing for Hope: Pathways to regenerative sustainability*. Abingdon: Routledge.

Kellert, S. R., & Wilson, E. O. (1993). *The biophilia hypothesis*. Washington, DC: Island Press.

Kellert, S. R., Heerwagen, J., & Mador, M. (2008). *Biophilic design: The theory, science, and practice of bringing buildings to life*. Hoboken, NJ: Wiley.

Kellert, S. R. (2008). Dimensions, elements, and attributes of biophilic design. In S. R. Kellert, J. Heerwagen, & M. L. Mador (Eds.), *Biophilic design* (pp. 3–19). New Jersey: Wiley.

Lyle, J. T. (1985). *Design for human ecosystems: Landscape, land use, and natural resources*. New York: Van Nostrand Reinhold.

Lyle, J. T. (1994). *Regenerative Design for Sustainable Development*. New York: Wiley.

Magnaghi, A. (2005). *The Urban Village: A charter for democracy and local self-sustainable development*. London/New York: Zed Books.

Madre, F., Vergnes, A., Machon, N., et al. (2014). Green roofs as habitats for wild plant species in urban landscapes: First insights from a large-scale sampling. *Landscape Urban Plan, 122*, 100–107.

Marsh, G. P. (1864). *Man and nature, or physical geography as modified by human action*. London: Samson Low Son and Marston.

Matthews, T., Ambrey, C., Baker, D., & Byrne, J. (2016). How green infrastructure can easily be added to the planning toolkit. *The Conversation*, April 26. Retrieved from: https://theconversation.com/heres-how-green-infrastructure-can-easily-be-added-to-the-urban-planning-toolkit-57277.

McHarg, I. L. (1969). *Design with nature*. New York: Natural History Press.

Ming, L. J., Suan, T. P., & Toh, W. (2010). HDB's next generation of eco-districts at Punggol and eco-modernisation of existing towns. *The IES Journal Part A: Civil & Structural Engineering, 3*(3), 203–209. https://doi.org/10.1080/19373260.2010.491259.
Mumford, L. (1961). *The city in history*. London: Penguin Press.
Newman, P. (2005). The city and the bush-partnerships to reverse the population decline in Australia's Wheatbelt. *Australian Journal of Agricultural Research, 56*, 527–535.
Newman, P. (2006). The environmental impact of cities. *Environment and Urbanization, 18*(2), 275–295.
Newman, P. (2014). Biophilic urbanism: A case study of Singapore. *Australian Planner, 1*, 47–65.
Newman, P., Beatley, T. & Blagg, L. (2012). *Singapore 'biophilic city'* [Online]. You Tube. Available: https://www.youtube.com/watch?v=XMWOu9xIM_k [Accessed 23/04/2014].
Newman, P., & Jennings, I. (2008). *Cities as sustainable ecosystems*. Washington, DC: Island Press.
Newman, P., & Matan, A. (2012). *Green Urbanism in Asia*. Singapore: World Scientific Publishing Company.
Newman, P., Beatley. T., & Boyer, H. (2017). *Resilient Cities. Overcoming Fossil Fuel Dependence* (2nd Edn.). Washington, DC: Island Press.
Ong, B. L. (2003). Green plot ratio: an ecological measure for architecture and urban planning. *Landscape and Urban Planning, 63*(4), 197–211.
Pepper, D. (1996). *Modern environmentalism: An introduction*. Abingdon: Routledge.
Soderlund, J., & Newman, P. (2015). Biophilic architecture: A review of the rationale and outcomes. *AIMS Environmental Science, 2*(4), 950–969. https://doi.org/10.3934/environsci.2015.4.950.
Soderlund, J. (2016). *Biophilic urbanism an emerging social movement,* PhD Curtin University, Perth, Australia.
Thayer, R. L. (1997). *Gray world, green heart: Technology, nature, and the sustainable landscape*. New York: Wiley.
Thayer, R. L. (2009). *LifePlace: Bioregional thought and practice*. California, CA: University of California Press.
Thomson, G., & Newman, P. (2018). Urban fabrics and urban metabolism - from sustainable to regenerative cities. *Resources, Conservation and Recycling, 132*, 218–229.
Wilson, E. O. (1984). *Biophilia*. Cambridge, MA: Harvard University Press.
Wood, A., Bahrami, P., & Safarik, D. (2014). *Green walls in high-rise buildings: An output of the CTBUH sustainability working group. Council of Tall Buildings and Urban Habitat*. Mulgrave, VIC: The Images Publishing Group Pry Ltd..
Yabuka, N. (2018). HDB begins applying Biophilic design framework to new towns, *Indesignlive.sg*, 10 August. Retrieved from: https://www.indesignlive.sg/insight/hdb-biophilic-design-framework-new-town

Co-evolutionary Recovery of the Urban/ Rural Interface: Policies, Planning, and Design Issues for the Urban Bioregion

David Fanfani

1 Background Framework of the Urbanization Process

The current waves of urbanization and the overall process of the so-called planetary urbanization if assumed in their more quantitative and diffusive forms – sometimes emphasized in manifold reports and scholars' reflections (Brugmann 2010; Glaeser 2011; Angel et al. 2011; UN 2018) – seem to entail a definitive dismission of the category of the "rural" or its oblivion under an overwhelming veil of "urban triumphalism" (Brenner and Schmid 2015, p. 156). Moreover, apparently opposite spatial forms of heavy density agglomeration – low density dispersion – in the context of different socio-geographical contexts mirror some dynamics operating at a subterranean level, in accordance with the global neo-capitalist accumulation forms (Sassen 2014), no matter of which parts of the globe or category of cities we are dealing with (Robinson 2006). Such different urbanization patterns, despite their spatial/morphological diversity, share a general effect and have a strong impact on rural territory resources depletion. This not only under the environmental point of view – land grabbing, desertification, land sealing, ecosystems disruption, etc. – but also by affecting socioeconomic values and community legacy, people displacement, agri-food production local system abandonment, and cultural and social heritage loss (Sassen 2014).

However notwithstanding this framework and reversing the matter in a "positive form," just for the pervasiveness of the urbanization process, the rural category seemed lately to gain momentum – at least in the western urbanized areas – because of the growing awareness of the problems and opportunities that stems from the increased and strong proximity between urban domains and practices and sometimes residual, rural areas and activities. Paradoxically the strong interference of urban places, facilities, and infrastructures on environmental systems and the

D. Fanfani (✉)
Architecture Department-Dida, Florence University, Florence, Italy
e-mail: david.fanfani@unifi.it

D. Fanfani, A. Matarán Ruiz (eds.), *Bioregional Planning and Design: Volume I*,
https://doi.org/10.1007/978-3-030-45870-6_8

disruption of patterns of rural productive systems contribute to shed light on the strategic values of maintaining and protecting rural embedded endowments, this mainly in the frame to provide conditions for settlements resilience, socioeconomic fairness, and sustainability. For this reason, all the mentioned impacts, despite their differences and specificities, call for a general awareness recovery of the relevance of the endowments and "commons" encompassed under the "rural" territorial category and systems and for a deepened knowledge of the undergoing phenomena in order to set viable policies and planning tools to best hamper and manage these harmful trends.

Moreover, the putatively called "new regionalism" strand of reflection – especially in the economic geography field – despite its multifaceted and also contradictory expressions and forms (Hettne and Söderbaum 1998, 2000; Lovering 1999; Söderbaum and Shaw 2003; Morgan 2004) contributed to shed light on the "thickness" and perspective of the regional scale as background frame to appraise, at least partially, spatial patterns reconfiguration and flows related to a wider process of mainly neoliberal economic forces. It shows, in particular, how settlements functionalities and patterns are affected at regional level mainly by a twofold dynamic of reterritorialization of economic regulatory schemes and productive systems on the one side and of globalization of capital flows and strategic decision nodes on the other side also (Jonas 2012; Wheeler 2002), according to a "glocal" hybrid paradigm (Swyngedow 2004). Moreover "new regionalism" triggered some intellectual reactions and strategic attentions toward the regional dimension that relates also to critical reflections about the blindly assumed neoliberal paradigm while proposing forms and concepts for the recovery of a "progressive" and fair regionalism (Kipfer and Wirsig 2004; Sites 2004).

In this sense it is worth to note how the scale and scope of the shortly accounted processes do not allow to set up limited, local, tactical, and short-sighted solutions. Indeed, urbanization processes and patterns have unfolded by now mainly at the scale of the city region (Brenner 2002; Rodriguez-Pose 2008; Neumann and Hull 2009) or, at least, at the supra-municipal scale, triggering thus also general opposite models to look at local development and resources exploitation, depending on if an heuristic "globalist" framework or critically "endogenous" is assumed.

City region concept-related contributions and debates fed indeed pivotal reflections focusing not only on the institutional and governance reframing needed to cope with processes, flows, and functionalities overcoming the institutional, sectoral, and scale borders inherited from the past but jointly with these on the new planning and design demands entailed by the process of metropolitan regions (re) structuring. This especially considering the impact of city region developments on environmental systems and related sustainability issues (Wheeler 2009) triggering a strong demand for designing sustainable settlement patterns and policies (Kelbaugh 1997; Ravetz 2000; Calthorpe and Fulton 2001).

For this reason, it comes in the foreground the importance to adopt a multi-scale approach to the analysis of urban/rural interactions, viable to appraise, and representing both local interactions at the level of urban/rural interface, as well as the wider regional settlement patterns and complementary ecosystem structure.

2 Reframing Spatial Planning and Policies Approach to Enhance and Preserve Urban/Rural Interface

2.1 The Changing and Strategic Nature of the "Rural" and the "Urban/Rural" Interface

As shown above, focusing the planning and governance issues at the city, region, or metropolitan scale, being aware of the mentioned spatial, functional, and symbolic pervasiveness of the urbanization process and of its consequences, more generally means to take dismissal from the idea that it would be possible to deal with spatial form and environmental issues concerning settlements planning and design, in simple way by repurposing urban-centered and dualistic, single city/countryside models. Patterns of urbanization, considering the scale and functional complexity, ask instead to tackle with the very drivers of the settlement transformation at the scale and level where they originate and unfold their forces and potentialities and then with the multi-scale effects of urban sprawl, especially considering the scope of the impacts on ecosystems.

Indeed rural or more natural featured territories surrounding the urban can no longer be represented as a still well-defined – environmental and social – world (the rural) facing the city domain (the urban) but rather as a sum of more complex natural/anthropogenic patterns, or envelope of structures, ranging from regional to local scale. Then, in this prospect, urban/rural interface assumes a strategic meaning in reframing and re-conceptualizing policies, planning analysis methods, and design tools.

This does not mean to give up completely with the inherited spatial planning tools and methods, but it entails firstly the necessity to re-conceptualize some categories and objects of territorial sciences as well as to innovate and better integrate the methods and tools themselves.

In fact, this does not necessarily entail the withering away of the category of the rural as such and the rise of a "post-rural" condition mainly framed according to a re-asserted and totally pervasive urban-centered prospect. It means rather that, contrary to the past, the category of "rural" cannot be taken for granted anymore, whereas, nevertheless, it can still matter, especially in some regional contexts (Carlow et al. 2016), under conditions that "...require careful contextually specific and theoretically reflexive investigation that may be seriously impeded through the unreflexive use of generic labels that predetermine their patterns and pathways of development and their form and degree of connection to other places" (Brenner and Schmid 2015, cit. p. 174).

Some years ago, referring to "global south countries" – erstwhile the so-called development countries – Adriana Allen pointed out on the opportunity to reconsider the urban/rural interface nature under the complex bundle of flows and relationships setting the interactions between these two putatively well analytically and operationally distinguished domains, especially while considering the twofold and hybrid nature of the urban/rural interface (Allen 2003, 2010). Partly anticipating the debates on urbanization forms in western – or global north – countries, especially related to low density settlement, or sprawl, expansion (EEA 2006), Allen statements best account for "…the artificial distinction between 'urban' and 'rural', a distinction that (mis)informs not only the setting up of institutional arrangements but , also, and more broadly, the deployment of planning approach and tools" (Allen 2003, cit., p. 135).

Acknowledging the paradigmatic shift in the planning approach entailed by the introduction of environment and ecologic matters, Allen went on upholding the importance of framing settlement spatial planning tool according a multi-scale and strategic approach aimed to overcome the "urban-rural dichotomy ingrained in planning systems" (Allen 2003, cit. p. 135) and reasserting how the "ecological, economic and social functions performed by and in the peri-urban interface affect either city and the countryside" (Allen 2003, cit. p. 135). It especially refers to the necessity of addressing and designing – according to a multi-scale prospect – a theoretical framework and operational approach suitable to gather rural, regional, and urban planning as three distinctive fields of action that overlap at the urban/rural interface. An approach that seems to be best suited to consider the increasing demand for settlements sustainability, resilience, and fairness especially underpinned by a new search for environmental and resource access justice (Fainstein 2011; Pezzoli 2013; Pezzoli and Leiter 2016).

2.2 *A Regional-Scale Model for Urban/Rural Joint Strategic Planning: The Co-evolutionary Prospective of the Urban Bioregion*

Drawing on Allen contribution, the regional scale turns out to be the best suited spatial level to set out policies and planning tools to frame either rural development planning or urban-focused planning as joint levels of regulation that could affect urban/rural interaction. Considering this, and especially the environment and ecosystemic requirements that underpin the pursue and establishment of resilient, self-relied, and sustainable settlement patterns, the bioregional prospect turns out to be of interest as possible conceptual operating paradigm and reference (Scott Cato 2013; James and Scott Cato 2014). This mainly drawing on its capacity to allow for jointly treat urban and rural/ecosystem issues considering urban settlements as a whole; a theoretical element that found lately a further deepening under the category of "urban bioregion."

Adopting a comprehensive reporting and a methodologically correct approach to bioregionalism allows to seize how the category of urban bioregion strongly draws on bioregional traditions and cultural legacy.[1] In this respect it is also argued

---

[1] The theoretical legitimacy to fully acknowledge and refer urban bioregion concept as a strand or more recent evolution of bioregional legacy deserves at least some short caveats aimed to recall how:

that – according to a vision of "urban bioregionalism" – "...utilizing bioregional ideals in urban areas can contribute to an epistemological shift in the human relationship to the environment and natural resources from the current condition" (Church 2015, p. 2). As introduced by Atkinsons (1992), this model expresses a peculiar interpretation of the bioregional legacy that, without overlooking its eco-centric facets and origins, develops a vision of mutual supportive relationship between settlements patterns and form and ecosystems structure and functions. Atkinsons fully assumes the eco-centric bioregional starting point as a call not for a shift toward a utopic, bounded uncontaminated place where to rest, but as – according to Sale (1991) – a pragmatic and operational perspective to achieve places where to inhabit well, now and for the future. According to Atkinsons, sustainability hinges on a renewed urban regional symbiosis aimed to gain self-reliance in coping with the economic bias and unbalances stemming not as much from a destiny of backwardness, but especially from multinational corporate-driven global markets. In this direction the urban bioregion model is upheld as an alternative one, best suited to counter economic extractive and exhaustive forces, by recovering proximity economic relationship also recurring to "selective regional closure" enabling and fostering internal markets affordability and viability (Sthör and Tödtling 1977).

By the way it is worth to note that the mentioned underlying "extractive" streams lately concerned not only the so-called, erstwhile, "third world" regions but also – although with different forms and effects – the "global north" regions as they further developed and unfolded under a global trend lately fueled also by the hyper-financial and de-territorialized turn of global capitalism (Sassen 2014, cit.).

Furthermore, the paradigm of urban bioregion meets important analogies – and well fits to – with outstanding legacies in the field of regional planning and rural development. Among others we can refer to socio-spatial patterns that were yet envisioned with the *Agropolitan* model devised by Friedmann and Douglass that represents an interesting insight in this direction (Friedmann and Douglass 1978;

- Bioregionalism is not to conceive as a formally and definitively stated or static body of thought, rather a "tradition of many voices" (Aberley 1999), encompassing arts, habits expression, community relationships, and, also, spatial and environmental planning fields of action, often in advocacy and bottom-up form.
- Bioregionalism origins as a call for re-inhabiting practices according to places of nature and endowments (Berg and Dasmann 1977), and then it cannot be overlooked the intrinsic relationship between nature and culture that every inhabiting action entails and, for that, how, nevertheless in co-evolution with the ecosystem recovery and reproduction, settlement-related issues still matter.
- As well shown in credited and well-sounded contribution (Thayer 2003, pp. 155–156), bioregional spatial planning approach also strongly hinges on the "culturalist" and "organicist" roots of American regionalist movement where the outstanding contribution of RPAA members and, among others, of Lewis Mumford and Benton MacKaye addressed and tried for a – we could now say optimistic – "neo-technic" synthesis between nature, culture, and technology suited to harness, starting from the natural structure as "indigenous" "counter-mold" (MacKaye 1928), the metropolitan "deluge" and built up an inhabited region as a "collective artwork" (Mumford 1938).

Friedmann 1981). Indeed, despite its main and original focus on Asian developing countries, and for the previous considerations, this model deserves attention also in our reflection about western countries urbanized contexts. Such a model allows indeed it tries to cope with issues of integrated rural development related to the necessity to achieve and recover sustainable and balanced urban-rural relationships according to a bottom-up, self-relied development model and envision an ecologically tailored polycentric settlement pattern. In this prospect, a pro-active and socio-economic empowered role on behalf of the rural domain is assumed as opposed to the hierarchical urban-rural trickle-down based development mechanism.

3 Spatial Planning and Policies: A New Agenda for the Urban/Rural Interface in the Urban Bioregion

As underlined the special focus of this chapter is finally aimed to frame a set of issues and related tools aimed to best point out, manage, and master the complex interlocked wholeness of flows, relationships, and endowments entailed by conceiving a co-evolutionary view of the urban/rural domain development under the urban bioregion paradigm.

Such a paradigm allows to consider the urban/rural interface as a "membrane" suitable to best distinguish two well-defined, albeit communicating (energy, matter, information), domains that can cooperate for a healthy and fair settlement system (see also the Saragosa and Chiti chapter in this volume, 'Bioregion and Spatial Configurations. The Co-evolutionary Nature of the Urban Ecosystem). In this regard, Allen mentioned a contribution well focused on a methodological/operational reframing of policies especially based on an integrated, multi-scale strategic planning/policies approach. Although drawing on this contribution, a further deepening seems necessary – assuming the urban bioregion as a co-evolutionary model – to best cope with the western/European contexts and also considering the time lag that separates us from then and the related new issues entered in the debate.

In doing so it is worth to proceed by pointing out, on the one side, more directly some spatial planning general issues and, then, referring such issues to the current institutional framework of policies and planning methods and, on the other, addressing especially the necessity and conditions to overhaul them in order to achieve a better urban/rural integrated model of planning and governance.

3.1 New Matters and Themes for Spatial Planning at the Urban/Rural Interface

According to Friedmann and Weaver (1979*cit.*), adopting an urban bioregionalist approach calls for the overcoming of a mainly functionalist model of regional planning. It means, especially in the European contexts, to appraise the "local thickness" of historical, cultural, ecological endowments that triggered and sustained regional and local development as well as a thriving urban civilization.

In this prospect, spatial planning, conceived as an activity aimed to coordinate many disciplines and to enliven and feed a cross-disciplinary exchange, is asked to consider especially some, relatively, new interconnected fields of activity or issues, among which it seems worth to mention:

- The recovery of a new settlement's metabolism

Urban/rural interface turns out to be of increased relevance in allowing and supporting the recovery of the missed metabolism that historically – at least until the dawn of the industrial revolution – featured the relationship between urban environment and surrounding agro-ecosystems (Bellamy Foster 1999; Gallent et al. 2006; Andersson et al. 2016, pp. 275–331). Flows of energy and matter (e.g., power supply, food and drinking water provisioning, raw materials, sewage treatment and waste management, GhG emissions, etc.) are all currently mainly structured according to a linear strongly entropic and wide-ranging networks model. Re-localizing urban settlements according to a bioregional approach (Thayer 2013) entails a strong reduction of these networks' range and a general redirection toward circular flow schemes and a cut of harnessing of fossil fuel in providing commodities and facilities. As previously pointed out, urban/rural interface could be envisioned as the "membrane" through which many of these flows transit and that could allow to provide service to deliver resources (e.g., ecosystem services; see AA.VV 2005) in such a way to avoid the recourse to highly expensive and complex technological equipment and devices.

Moreover, this kind of ecosystemic turns in urban services and related management and delivering technologies, among other goals, will also allow for a general improvement of the quality of urban and periurban environment along with its amenities and attractiveness. This kind of shift entails, in terms of spatial planning and design tools and policies, to pay peculiar attention to the ecosystem dimension in accordance with a multifunctional and integrated mode of landscape ecological design (Jonhston and Lovell 2000) especially at the urban/rural "edge" (Tjallingii 2000). That either in analytical terms and in setting the various sectoral policies following an integrated and coordinated policy approach.

- Pursuing resilient and biophilic settlements and urban environment

The previous point firstly affects the spatial planning and territory design, whose action translates in a more complex and integrated approach to the urban/regional project. This especially concerns the approach to built environment structures recovery and retrofitting (Beatley and Newman 2013; Church 2015, cit.) and particularly the adoption and recovery of some nature-based techniques in reclaiming basic environmental functionalities of ecological systems. It is worth noting how in this prospect, turns out to be of relevance the "retro-innovation" concept, as – according to Stuiver (2006) – conceived as smart recovery of old affordable and context fitting methods and operating principles in a completely new socio-technic regime but assuming low-entropy models and techniques of intervention.

Multifunctional and integrated "eco-design" of ecosystemic services and "structures" allows to best cope with the challenging issue stemming from the dramatic effects of climatic change and global warming (Wilson and Piper 2010) but, at the same time, to operate with the prospect of a "transitional model" where ecological challenges play as a stimulus to enhance a livable, healthier, and vibrant built environment. It is not difficult to mention how in this new endeavor field we can gather many recent issues at the top of the list of public policies and design debate. Among these, it is worth to recall the wide-ranging theme of "green and blue infrastructure" mainly aimed to point out the necessity to cope with a regenerative management and design model concerning either the residual green spaces – be they biodiversity reserve, active farmland area, or also wastelands – or the complex and often disrupted hydraulic and riverine structures at both the watershed and local scale. This issue was fed, at the European level, by manifold research and program activities also aimed to point out policies and design criteria to support experiences and project of rivers and streams "daylighting." This as much to enhance landscape and ecological quality of the built environment as resilience in the face of climate change effects (run-off water catchment, urban microclimate improvement). Also, the growing attention paid to the design and management – sometimes according to bottom-up initiatives – of urban farming and urban agriculture practices can be considered as a step forward in the direction of urban resilience achieving based on the recovery of some urban/rural metabolism functionings. In a wider sense, that encompasses also social, educational, and cultural meanings. This field of policies, design, and action can also be referred to the new conception of the urban and settlement entailed by the "biophilic city" concept as contended especially by some scholars (Beatley and Newman 2013) and also by Newman and Zingoni De Baro themselves in Vol. II of this book.

- Morphological/spatial issues: devising integrated design methods for polynuclear settlement and urban systems

The approach to urban/rural interface not as a result of a footloose and unchecked urbanization process – and then as a space, at the best, to mitigate as much as possible urban impact – but as a "counter-mold" which underpins new balanced settlement forms at the various scales, entails some main design and policy design implications. First of all, to operate in the direction to "fix" the inherited metabolic rift of the modern city and metropolis and of steady resilience gains facing climate change and global warming effects – based on a retrieved green-blue wide-ranging infrastructure – means to explore the necessity to "split" the modern hierarchical city region form and pursue a well-balanced and cooperative polycentrism. In this direction it is not possible quoting in few lines the wide-ranging literature that concerns this aspect in terms of spatial analysis and settlements models, addressing sustainability matters related to urban form conceived either as in its various patterns at the regional scale or as a complex mix of spatial and functional land use patterns at the urban and local one (Alexander et al. 1977, pp. 3–40; Kohr 1976; Batty 2001; Banister 2005; Magnaghi 2010, pp. 208–241; Lambregts and Zonnenveld 2003; Cook and Lara 2013; Ravetz et al. 2013). Moreover it is also worth to note how this issue also affects governing power matters mainly related to the opportunity of devolution of political and administrative power at the local level (Wills 2016), in order to reframe development and resource uses and decisional processes, underlying especially the re-rapprochement of ecological economy and political ecology (M'Goonigle 1999). In general terms it seems worth to recall the relevance of a methodological stance aimed to explore the possibilities in the direction of the adoption of polycentric settlement patterns and models. In this direction, drawing on bioregional paradigm, some contributions get a step further beyond a functional/spatial approach, trying to deepen "how" to analyze and represent spatial patterns aimed to achieve sustainable design goals and environment and settlement recovery at the regional scale (Gotlieb 1996) based also on long-lasting built and natural environment heritage.

In this framework, Thayer, starting from Alexander's seminal concept of pattern language (Alexander et al. 1977, *cit.*), goes on in defining a more integrative idea of "bio-generative" spatial patterns that "...represent the best long-term fit of human intervention with geomorphic, climatic, biotic, and cultural influences" (Thayer 2003, p. 166). This concept of pattern is bio-generative since it is aimed to spatially represent – as a signature – a (life)place-specific co-evolutionary interaction between ecological and human (cultural) domain framed in the context of resource limits and their regenerative possibilities.

It is worth referring how, despite a bio-generative pattern, sequence moves on through some multi-scale operating levels – pattern model design method is also strongly underpinned on a fine-grained scale and bottom-up approach. This often calls for with an advocacy or facilitating commitment on behalf of planners in fostering and empowering participatory processes for local communities and for bringing in the foreground ordinary knowledge and skills enhancement. Concerning the aims of this chapter, bio-generative pattern concept is clearly at odds – how also Thayer points out – with market-driven model of settlement where suitable and co-evolutionary interaction between urban and rural domain fades out, replaced by low density housing patterns mirroring metropolization and hierarchical processes at the regional scale.

Drawing especially on Thayer's contribution, and landscape studies legacy, Silbernagel envisions patterns as a result of an eco-cultural integrative approach to landscape analysis and representation (Silbernagel 2005). In this framework, place-based patterns are the result of the complex composition of natural and material (mainly quantitative) elements and qualitative ones, related to socio-cultural features represented through manifold sources (e.g., oral, drawn, arts, etc.), also employing GIS tool in innovative way. These patterns set the ground to compose spatial "horizontal" narratives – conceived as opposed to the traditional "vertical" landscape ecology overlay mapping method – which result as syntactic articulation of ecological and cultural facts. Moreover, according to Silbernagel, this model of bio-cultural spatial pattern tailoring and application hinges on an historical and cross-disciplinary prospective, and it is aimed to unfold and feed a planning and design process that allows to foster sense of place belongings and stewardship concern.

Place-based and cross-disciplinary description of regional historical thickness, aimed to point out some long-lasting regional patterns, also represents the basic elements of the approach in the regional analysis and design of the Italian territorialist school. Starting from the previously described urban bioregion model, territorialist approach (see Magnaghi 2010*cit.*, pp. 208–241) sets the issue of the urban/rural – in either analytical or design terms – by reversing the prevailing hierarchical core-periphery and urban-centered relationship which features the current development of metropolitan region settlement pattern, by opposing and envisioning a multi-centered pattern of "city of cities" or "city of villages" based on (Figs. 1, 2, 3, and 4):

- Acknowledgment and representation of the long-lasting and "living" heritage ("Territorial Patrimony") issued by the co-evolutionary relationship between natural endowments and anthropogenic and cultural action.
- Definition of the main living patterns of the built environment ("structural invariants") and/or of the "long-lasting" territorial structure that can support – at various scales – a sustainable design approach and goals (strategic scenario and "territory design") and a renewed settlement polycentric structure.
- Bottom-up and advocacy planning action aimed to enhance, support, and empower local society grassroots and socially produced initiatives and goals, in setting planning targets and local development projects (Img. 1 and 2). This also with the aim to feed and foster as much as possible self-government practices and a federalist approach vs. hierarchical and exogenously driven settings, strongly embodied in the current deliberative and decisional processes.
- Definition of a shared strategic scenario design and of a territory project aimed to jointly recover the agro-ecosystem structure and a multi-centered settlement pattern.

The roughly rendered cognitive, spatially framed, and political sequence is aimed either to feed a new vision for spatial arrangements and settlement design at the various scales or to interact, also in critical and dialectical terms, with the inherited, market-driven, institutional bodies and practices.

Referring to urban/rural interface issues, the described approach turns out to be suitable to completely reframe business as usual approach to settlement design, appreciating especially long-lasting living patterns in supporting and weaving a new polycentric city form and settlement structure. What once was classified as periphery becomes the center of a completely reframed "identity-based" settlements structure. In this vision, heritage and local endowments at the urban/rural interface allow to devise "…new city walls (that) go newly to define and bounding the urban landscape as 'common': green belts and biotic corridors that enmesh as a system urban, periurban and regional parks, (agricultural, fluvial, naturals) thrusting down as 'green hands' in the city open spaces by regenerating public spaces and connecting them with surrounding agricultural spaces; water systems – be they natural or artificial-, managed as city and territory metabolic systems that redesign the urban and agrarian landscape threads; (…) the densification of the built environment and the

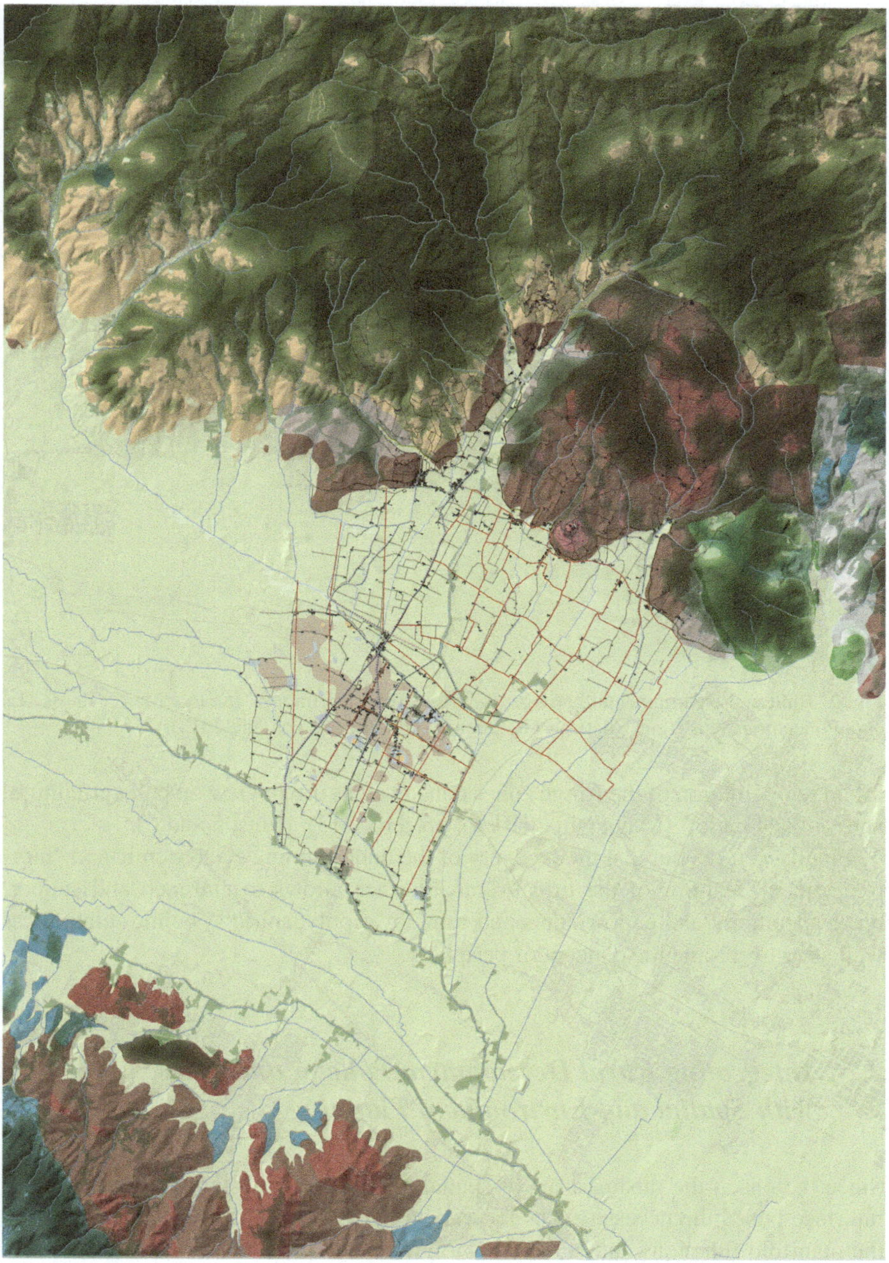

Fig. 1 Long-lasting settlement structure. (*Source* Master thesis "La città Policentrica dell'Agna", dott.ssa F. Giallorenzo, Dir. Prof. D. Fanfani, 2017)

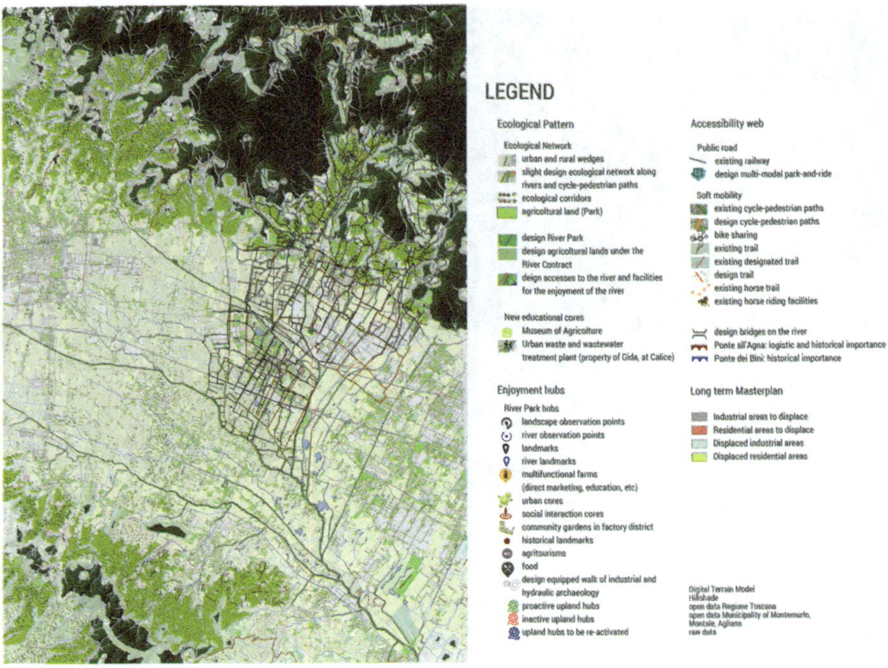

Fig. 2 Built and environmental heritage: the "Territorial Patrimony." (*Source* Master thesis "La città Policentrica dell'Agna", dott.ssa Giallorenzo, Dir. Prof. D. Fanfani, 2017)

urban rehabilitation of the fringe zones conceived as urban view on belt agricultural and wooded parks" (Magnaghi 2010*cit.*, pp. 212–213)[2] (Figs. 5 and 6).

Finally, it turns out that the recovery of the underpinning ecosystemic and "morphogenetic" features of the urban/rural interface allows to entrench and support place specificity and endowments and to recover polycentric systemic relations as well as to overcome the concept of periphery.

3.2 Integrating Rural Development Policies and Tools with Spatial and Environment Planning

Since the onset, the raising issue of spatial planning and design at the urban/rural interface posed the necessity – as far as dealing with a domain where run through the manifold functions and activities – to go beyond or, at least, to integrate traditional land use-based planning tools (Andersson et al. 2016) or master planning approach (Allen 2003, cit) for the recovery of a strategic relational approach (Abeele and Leinfelder 2007). Later – mainly in relation with the emergence of a multidimensional call for settlement resilience, especially entailed by climate and social

[2]Author's translation

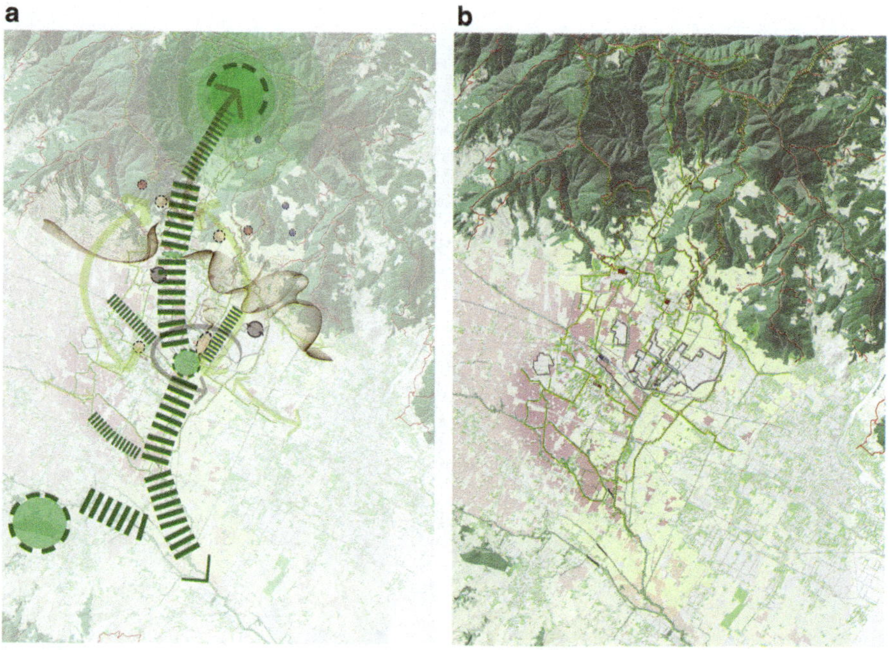

Fig. 3 Strategic scenario for a bioregional settlement recovery in the Prato-Pistoia area. (*Source:* Master thesis "La città Policentrica dell'Agna", dott.ssa F. Giallorenzo, Dir. Prof. D. Fanfani, 2017). (**a**) The Strategic Scenario: concept. (**b**) The Strategic Scenario Spatial Project

changes – this shared awareness between planners, practitioners, activists, and policy agents slightly shifted to address issues mainly related to some "metabolic or ecosystem services" (AA.VV. 2005, cit.) that the surrounding rural areas can deliver for the urban environment. In this framework urban/rural interface becomes the strategic domain and pivotal resource where it is possible to develop and re-embed, among others, local food systems (Morgan and Sonnino 2010) and the regional renewable energy system (Van den Dobbelsteen 2008) and, generally, to try and find out the room for the recovery of regenerating circular resources employment schemes. Beyond these issues of local development, treated in the following paragraph, this kind of shift poses the twofold question of the strategic role performed by agriculture and farmland in – possibly – delivering such a service and, moreover, of a general reframing of such an activity in multifunctional, rentable, and sustainable terms, not only for the sake of urban resident but also for the farmers' health and farming economic viability.

Pursuing joint goals of agriculture qualification and profitability, ecological and urban/rural landscape enhancement, calls to focus about the way how to best match traditional rural development tools – referring mainly to Agriculture European policy (CAP)for farm activity support and related to agri-environment measures – with spatial planning procedures at the various scales. Farming on the urban surrounding areas gains in this framework an active role of co-production – jointly with the urban domain – of "commons" and of a more sustainable built environment that can

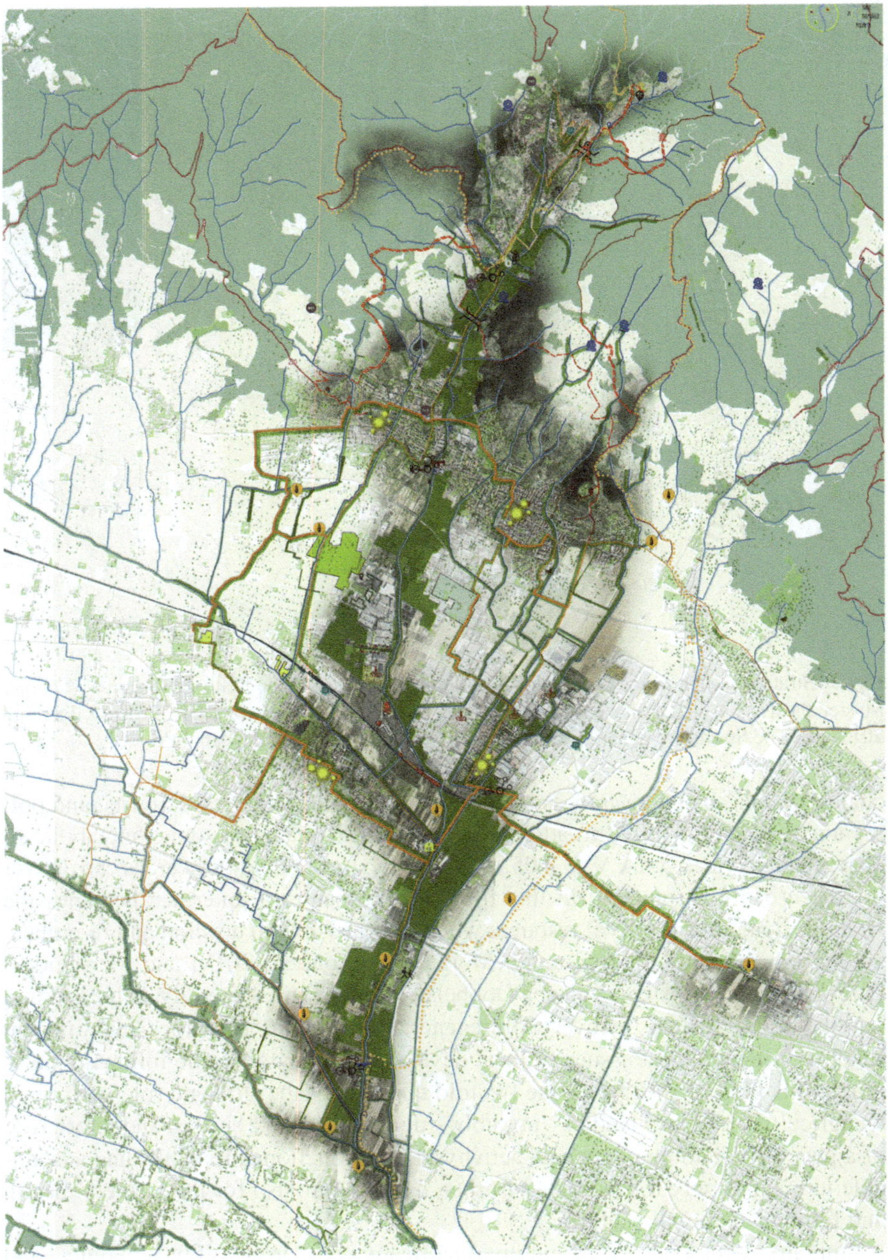

Fig. 4 Master plan of the polycentric urban system. (Source: Master thesis "La città Policentrica dell'Agna", dott.ssa F. Giallorenzo, Dir. D. Fanfani, 2017)

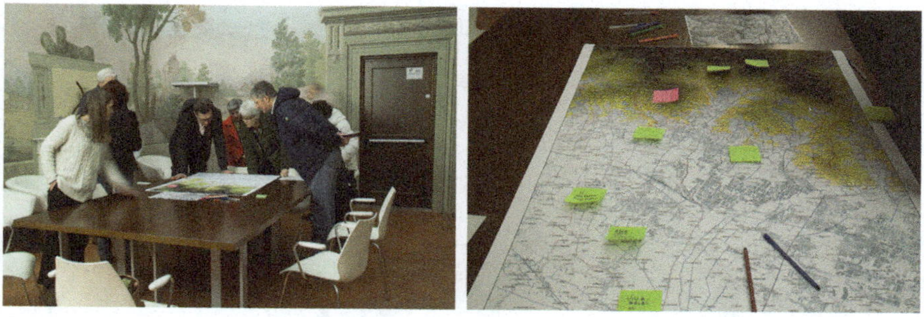

Img. 1 and 2 Participative design sessions activities. (*Source* Photo F. Giallorenzo courtesy)

be best pursued by adopting a strategic approach to planning also by reinforcing partnership and bottom-up and multi-level governance (Andersson et al. 2016, cit, pp. 181–200; Lazzarini 2019). Some main points that address the mentioned recovery of planning/rural development matching refer especially to:

- Adopting the regional landscape planning level as a multi-scale framework which allows to enforce the adoption and implementation of the rural development strategies by supporting especially – also with ranking rewards mechanism – place-specific measures, addressing ecosystems regeneration and local rural market jointly with agri-food systems enhancing
- Conceiving the sub-regional landscape planning goals as strategic elements and guidelines to match with strategic choices, land use directives, and rules adopted at the municipal level
- Promoting local actors and stakeholder's involvement in setting projects and actions at the local or also intermunicipal level
- Establishing and promoting specifically tailored periurban management tools (e.g., agricultural parks, rural districts, agri-urban contracts) supported by formal public-private partnerships and agency also adopting CLLD governance model
- Strongly reinforcing inter-sectorial and cross-scale collaboration between public bodies and offices as ordinary government practice for policies and project setting and delivering

Finally, this set of issues features the call to achieve a new policy and planning agenda without which it seems hardly possible to grasp with the goal of a renewed "pact" and metabolism between city and countryside.

3.3 Urban/Rural Place-Based Development Policies as Expression of Self-Relied Re-embedded Economies

Regarding urban/rural interface, drawing on urban bioregion approach, it clearly comes out that the point is not so much how to best accommodate urban housing developments or "services and equipment" for urban life in a pleasant and,

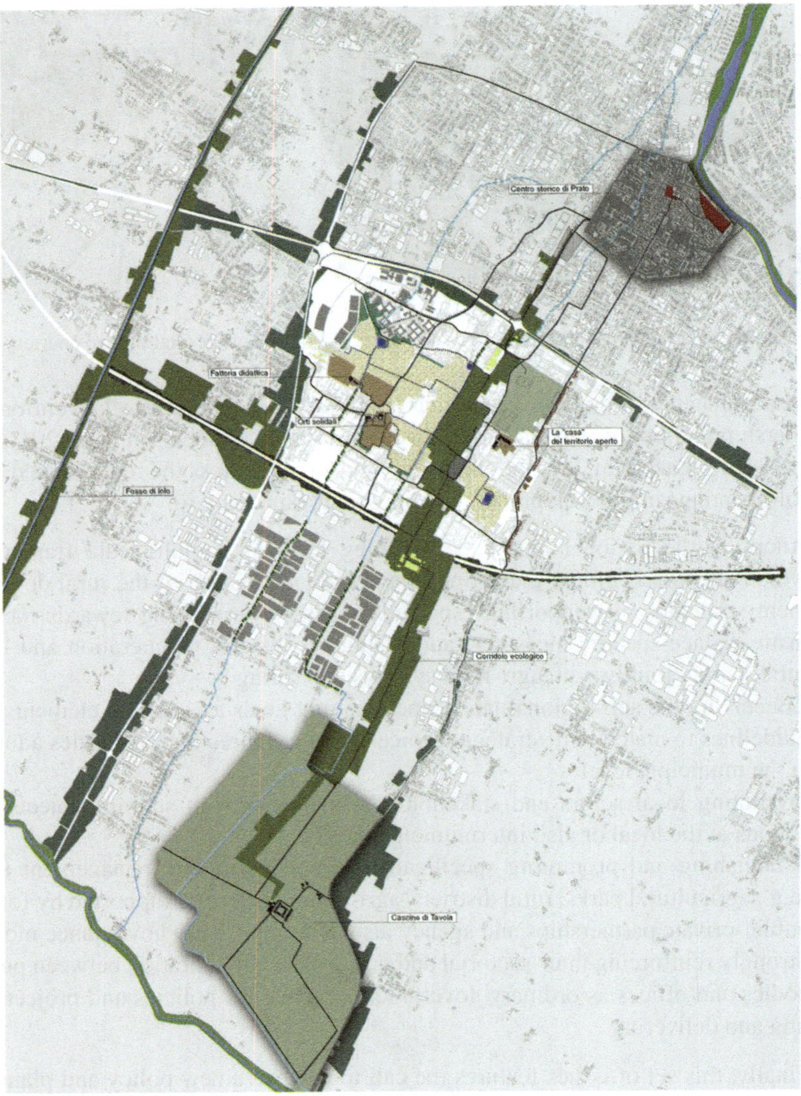

Fig. 5 Commune of Prato (Tuscany), green agri-urban inner fringe, and recovery of territorial connections. (Source Bachelor Degree Thesis, R. Rosa, C. Margaritelli, Dir. Prof. D. Poli, Co.dir. Prof. D. Fanfani)

putatively, sustainable way but to conceive urban/rural interface as an "active" domain suitable to feed new place-based economies aimed especially to regional and local market and to feed urban/rural metabolism. That means to explore and design this domain not as what is "neither urban and no more rural" to support as much as possible urban "external dis-economies," but as underpinning endowment of new proximity, self-relied, and resilient economies for "proto-bioregions" (James

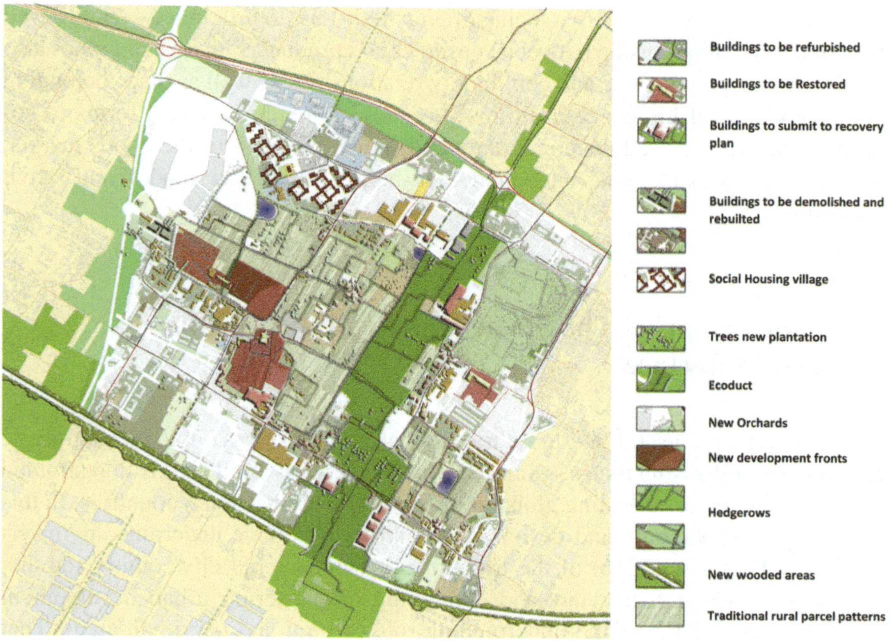

Fig. 6 Commune of Prato (Tuscany), Master Plan Project of the green agri-urban inner fringe. (Source Bachelor Degree Thesis, R. Rosa, C. Margaritelli, Dir. Prof. D. Poli, Co.dir.Prof. D. Fanfani)

and Scott Cato 2014) based on regional amenities and places endogenous values (Power 1996). In this prospect, some of the goods and services that this domain can deliver are encompassed by the previous mentioned category of ecosystem services (MEA 2005, cit.) as basic functions for the re-inhabiting and re-embedding process, strongly related to the "transitional age" also echoed in the title of this book, and envisioning a completely reframed energy regime (Hopkins 2008; Thayer 2013 cit.). According to MEA, these services are aimed to different goals – sustaining, regulation, and delivering – which correspond to a different way of economic appraisal and expression. Indeed, not all of them are valuable according to the market price system even though they do embody some real "use" or "existence" economic values. Some others, instead, allow to trigger and feed some new re-localized exchange economies and value chains with strong multiplier effects for the local economic system, especially based on retrieved and regenerated amenities and regional heritages (Power, cit. pp. 7–13). In this latter category, we can surely mention and ascribe, as the most meaningful but no single example, the creation of agri-food local systems (Morgan and Sonnino 2010, cit.), the re-embedding of smart and "vernacular" (Dobbelsteen 2008) regional energy system suitable to exploit the potentialities of place renewable energy sources or touristic system based on "slow" practices and fruition of local heritage and amenities (Paquot 2014). Anyway, despite the market values that can be assigned to this latter kind of economic chains, it should not be overlooked that, being often based – due to proximity – on retrieved trust and direct relationship between consumer and producers, these economies also allow to recreate new civic and community relationships as well as place belonging sense and stewardship concern. In this way they are really based on forms of co-production that can feed the community and social thickness of the goods market, toward a responsible and integrated well-being production model and "civil economy."

4 Final Remarks: The Strategic Role of the Urban/Rural Interface

Reflection on urban/rural interface "transitional" domain turns out to be of strategic relevance in addressing issues stemming from the pervasive and mainly unrestrained urbanization process affecting global north as well as global south countries. In this framework the planning and design of urban/rural interface underpins an "inversion" (De Lestrange 2016) of the traditional urban-centered city/countryside discourse, by reversing the view and countering or mastering urban development starting from a vision of the underpinning role of rural and periurban areas. That entails to think about urban/rural interaction no more in oppositional terms but in co-evolutionary ones. This means that the matter is no longer how to best master and design urban developments according to real estates, housing markets, or land rent values providing smaller damage to natural values, but how to co-produce and recover a co-evolutionary relationship and sustainable and livable settlement patterns starting from the "counter-mold" constituted by ecosystem/metabolic functioning and farmland economic, cultural, and landscape values. The chapter shows how the urban bioregion model – as also better described by Magnaghi in the contribution to this volume – allows to best frame the urban/rural topic conceiving human settlements and built environment according to, although sometimes weakened and withered, their specific regional wholeness and long-lasting and regenerative features, where natural ecosystems, as well as cultural and natural structures and meanings, act and develop as mutually reproductive. This underpinning and fostering thriving (re)inhabited places as well as regionally based and self-relied economies. For planning policies and tools as well as for design approaches that shift toward a co-evolutionary prospective, this entails some consequences. Indeed, agro-ecologic patterns recovery, enhancement, and design ask planners and the institutional planning system to adopt and strongly try to develop integrated approach, tools, and practices, also fostering bottom-up and inclusive methods. The latter point especially aims to sustain "co-production" and mutuality between urban and rural "agents" or citizens, creating a sense and awareness of belonging to a common place to be looked after together and, finally, periurban farming and farmer empowerment for an "active ruralship" (Fanfani 2012). On the planning and policies system side, the previous considerations entail a not easy endeavor, especially to overcome "path-dependent" behaviors. Indeed, the need to retrieve the relationship between agro-ecosystem issues and settlements regeneration goals – especially in addressing resilience and self-reliance aims – asks for a deepened approach to multi-level and inter-sectorial policies. This is a suitable approach to overcome an urban/rural divide which, despite its endurance and helpfulness in codifying spatial rules and allowing the appraise of functional equipments disposal, seems to be no more fruitful and effective in the heuristic, operational, and conceptual terms. An approach to be pursued is especially by adopting relational analysis and design frameworks to reveal and acknowledge new spatial practices and by supporting effective planning and design tools and policies for more balanced, self-relied, and regional-based settlement patterns.

References

AA.VV. (2005) *Millennium Ecosystem Assessment, 2005. Ecosystems and human well-being: Synthesis.* Washington DC: Island Press. file:///C:/Users/Acer/Downloads/document.356.aspx(1).pdf. Accessed March 19, 2019.

Abeele, P. V., & Leinfelder, H. (2007). *Strategic zoning plan for open spaces.* Paper presented at the 20th Congress of the International Housing and Planning Federation.

Aberley, D. (1999). Interpreting bioregionalism: A story from many voices. In M. V. Mc Ginnis (Ed.), *Bioregionalism* (pp. 13–42). London/New York: Routledge.

Alexander, C., Ishikawa, S., & Silverstein, M. (1977). *A pattern language. Towns, buildings, construction.* New York: Oxford University Press.

Allen, A. (2003). Environmental planning and management of the periurban interface: perspectives on an emerging field. *Environment and Urbanization, 15*, 135–147, http://eau.sagepub.com/content/15/1/135, Accessed 9 Feb 2019.

Allen, A. (2010). Neither rural nor urban: Service delivery options that work for the periurban poor's. In M. Khurian & P. McCartney (Eds.), *Periurban water sanitation services: Policy, planning and method* (pp. 27–61). Dordrecht: Springer.

Andersson, K., Sjöblom, B., Granberg, L., Ehrström, P., & Marsden, T. (Eds.). (2016). *Metropolitan ruralities, in research in rural sociology, 23.* Bingley: Emerald.

Angel, S., Parent, J., Civco, D. L., & Blei, A. M. (2011). *Making room for a planet of cities* (Policy focus reports). Lincoln Institute of Land Policy.

Atkinsons, A. (1992). The urban bioregion as sustainable development paradigm. *Third World Planning Review, 4*(14), 327–354.

Banister, D. (2005). *Unsustainable transport: City transport in the new century.* Abingdon: Routledge.

Batty, M. (2001). Polynucleated urban landscapes. *Urban Studies, 38*(4), 635–655.

Beatley, T., & Newman, P. (2013). Biophilic cities are sustainable, resilient cities. *Sustainability,5*, 3328–3345. https://www.researchgate.net/publication/277377188_Biophilic_Cities_Are_Sustainable_Resilient_Cities. Accessed 19 Feb 2019.

Bellamy Foster, J. (1999). Marx's theory of metabolic rift: Classical foundations for environmental sociology. *American Journal of Sociology, 105*(2), 366–405.

Berg, P., & Dasmann, R. (1977). Reinhabiting California. *The Ecologist, 7*(10), 399–401.

Brenner, N. (2002). Decoding the newest metropolitan regionalism in the USA. A critical overview. *City, 19*(1), 3–21.

Brenner, N., & Schmid, C. (2015). Toward a new epistemology of the urban? *City, 19*(2–3), 151–182.

Brugmann, J. (2010). *Welcome to the urban revolution*. New York: Bloomsbury.
Calthorpe, P., & Fulton. (2001). *The regional city. Planning for the end of sprawl*. Washington: Island Press.
Carlow, V. M., Kvorning, J., Steinführer, A., & Oltmann, C. (2016). *Ruralism. The future of villages and small towns in an urbanizing world*. Berlin: Jovis.
Church, S. P. (2015). Exploring Urban Bioregionalism: a synthesis of literature on urban nature and sustainable patterns of urban living. *S.A.P.I.E.N.S Surveys and Perspectives Integrating Environment and Society, 7*(1), 1–11.
Cook, E. A., & Lara, J. J. (Eds.). (2013). *Remaking Metropolis: Global Challenges of the Urban Landscape*. Abingdon: Routledge.
De Lestrange, R. (2016). *Le paysage comme matrice del la fabrique du territoire. Buenos Aires Genève Bruxelles Transposition(s)*. PhD thesis UCL-Université Catolique de Louvain. Presses Universitaires de Louvain. https://pul.uclouvain.be/book/?GCOI=29303100497970. Accessed 17 Mar 2019.
European Environment Agency. (2006). *Urban Sprawl, the ignored challenge, (EEA report 10/2006)*, Luxemburg. file:///C:/Users/Acer/Downloads/eea_report_10_2006.pdf. Accessed 16 Mar 2019.
Fainstein, S. (2011). *The just city*. London/Ithaca: Cornell University Press.
Fanfani, D. (2012). Local development and "agri-urban" domain: agricultural park as promotion of an "active ruralship". In Perrone, C. (Ed.), *Living landscape /landscapes for living*. Policies, practices, images, conference proceedings. University of Florence, February – June 2012, pp 39-47. http://issuu.com/planumnet/docs/living_landscapes_conference___full_4a0b8848 3b3e0f?e=3882228/5389668. Accessed 17 Mar 2019.
Friedmann, J. (1981). The active community: Toward a political-territorial framework for rural development in Asia. *Economic Development and Cultural Change*, *29* (2), 235–261. https://www.jstor.org/stable/1153287?origin=JSTOR-pdf&seq=1#page_scan_tab_contents. Accessed 16 Mar 2019.
Friedmann, J., & Douglass, M. (1978). Agropolitan development: Towards a new strategy for regional planning in Asia. In P. C. Lo & K. Salih (Eds.), *Growth pole strategy and regional development policy: Asian experience and alternative approaches* (pp. 163–192). Oxford: Pergamon Press.
Friedmann, J., & Weaver, C. (1979). *Territory and function. The evolution of regional planning*. Chicago: Edward Arnold.
Gallent, N., Andersson, J., & Bianconi, M. (2006). *Planning on the edge. The context for planning at the rural-urban fringe*. London: Routledge.
Glaeser, E. (2011). *Triumph of the city*. New York: Tantor.
Gotlieb, Y. (1996). *Development, environment and global dysfunctions*. Belray Beach: St. Lucie Press.
Hettne, B., & Söderbaum, F. (1998). The new regionalism approach. *Politeia, 17*(3), 6–21.
Hettne, B., & Söderbaum, F. (2000). Theorising the Rise of Regionness. *New Political Economy*, 5(3), pp. 457–473. Available at SSRN: https://ssrn.com/abstract=2398942
Hopkins, R. (2008). *The transition Handbook. From oil dependency to local resilience*. Vermont: Chelsea Green Publishing.
James, R. F., & Scott Cato, M. (2014). *From resilient regions to bioregions: An exploration of green post-Keynesianism* (PKES working paper 1407). http://www.postkeynesian.net/working-papers/1407/. Accessed 17 Mar 2019.
Jonas, A. E. G. (2012). City-regionalism: Question of distribution and politics. *Progress in Human Geography, 36*(6), 822–829.
Jonhnston, D. M., & Lovell, S. T. (2000). Creating multifunctional landscapes: How can the field of ecology inform the design of the landscape? *Frontier of Ecology and Landscape, 7*(4), 212–220.
Kelbaugh, D. (1997). *Common place: Toward neighborhood and regional design*. Seattle: University of Washington Press.

Kohr, L. (1976). *The city of man: The Duke of Buen Consejo*. Puerto Rico: Editorial de La Universidad de Puerto Rico.

Kipfer, S., & Wirsig, K. (2004). From contradiction to coherence? A review symposium on the US American "new regionalism". *Antipode, 36*(4), 728–732.

Lambregts, B., & Zonnenveld, W. (2003). *Polynuclear Urban Regions and the transnational dimension of Spatial Planning*. Eurbanet report 3, Delft, Delft University Press. file:///C:/Users/Acer/Downloads/OTB2003%20HUPS026%20web(2).pdf. Accessed 17 Mar 2019.

Lazzarini, L. (2019) *Urban/rural co-productions Planning and governance approaches for improving the relationships among city and countryside in Italy and England*. PhD thesis dissertation doctoral program in Urban & Regional Development Turin Polytechnic School, Supervisors: Prof. G.Cinà, DiST/Politecnico di Torino, IT, Dr. Matthew Reed, CCRI/University of Gloucestershire, UK, Co-Supervisor.

Lovering, J. (1999). Theory led by policy: The inadequacies of the "New Regionalism" (Illustrated from the case of Wales). *International Journal of Urban and Regional Research, 23*(2), 379–395.

M'Goonigle, R. M. (1999). Ecological economics and political ecology: Towards a necessary synthesis. *Ecological Economics, 28*, 11–26.

MacKaye, B. (1928). *The new exploration. A Philosophy of regional planning*. Urbana/Champaign: University of Illinois Press.

Magnaghi, A. (2010). *Il Progetto Locale* (IIth edition reviewed). Torino: Bollati Boringhieri. English translation of first edition: (2005) *The urban villages: A charter for democracy and local self-sustainable*. London: Zed Books.

Millennium Ecosystem Assessment. (2005). *Ecosystems and Human Well Being: Synthesis*. Washington: Island Press.

Morgan, K. (2004). Sustainable regions: Governance, innovation and scale. *European Planning Studies, 12*(6), 871–889.

Morgan, K., & Sonnino, R. (2010). The urban foodscape. World cities and the new food equation. *Cambridge Journal of Regions, Economy and Society, 3*(2), 209–224.

Mumford, L. (1938). *The culture of the cities*. Orlando: Harcourt Brace, Jovanovich Publisher.

Neumann, N., & Hull, A. D. (Eds.). (2009). The futures of the city region. *Regional Studies (Special Issue), 43*(6), 777–787.

Paquot, T. (2014). *Le Voyage contre le tourisme*. Paris: Coll. "Rhizome"-Etérotopia.

Pezzoli, K. (2013). *Bioregional justice: A framework for ecological restoration* (Draft statement prepared for the good neighbor environmental board). San Diego: Global Action Research Centre, pp. 1–7.

Pezzoli, K., & Leiter, R. A. (2016). Creating healthy and just bioregions. *Reviews on Environmental Health, 31*(1), 103–109.

Power, T. (1996). *Lost landscapes and failed economies, The search for a value of places*. Washington, DC: Island Press.

Ravetz, J. (2000). City-region 2020: Integrated planning for a sustainable environment. *International Journal of Sustainability in Higher Education, 1*(3), 305–308. https://doi.org/10.1108/ijshe.2000.1.3.305.3. Accessed 10 Apr 2019.

Ravetz, J., Fertner, C., & Sick Nielsen, t. (2013). The dynamics of peri-urbanisation. In K. Nilsson, S. Pauleit, S. Bell, C. Aalbers, A. Thomas, & T. Sick Nielsen (Eds.), *Peri-urban futures: Scenarios and models for land use change in Europe* (pp. 13–44). Dordrecht: Springer.

Robinson, J. (2006). *Ordinary cities: Between modernity and development*. London: Routledge.

Rodrìguez-Pose, A. (2008). The rise of the 'City Region' concept and its development policy implications. *European Planning Studies, 16*(8), 1025–1046.

Sale, K. (1991). *Dwellers in the land. The bioregional vision*. Santa Cruz: New Society Publisher.

Sassen, S. (2014). *Expulsion. Brutality and complexity in the global economy*. Cambridge, MA: The Belknap Press of Harvard University Press.

Scott Cato, M. (2013). *The bioregional economy, Land, liberty and the pursuit of happiness*. London: Routledge.

Silbernagel, J. (2005). Bio-regional patterns and spatial narratives for integrated landscape research and design. In B. Tress, G. Tress, G. Fry, & P. Opdam (Eds.), *From landscape research to landscape planning: Aspects of integration, education, and application* (Wageningen UR frontis series) (12th ed., pp. 107–118). Dordrecht: Springer.
Sites, W. (2004). Progressive regionalism: A "deliberative" movement? *Antipode, 36*(6), 766–778.
Söderbaum, F., & Shaw, M. T. (Eds.). (2003). *Theories of new regionalism*. London: Palgrave.
Stöhr, W. B., & Tödtling, F. (1977). Spatial equity-some anti-theses to current regional development doctrine. *Regional Sciences, 38*(2), 33–53.
Stuiver, M. (2006). Highlighting the retro side of innovation and its potential for regime change in agriculture, Between the local and the global: Confronting complexity in the contemporary agri-food sector research. *Rural Sociology and Development, 12*, 147–173.
Swyngedouw, E. (2004). Globalisation or 'glocalisation'? Networks, territories and rescaling. *Cambridge Review of International Affairs, 17*(1), 25–48.
Thayer, R. L. (2003). *LifePlace, bioregional thought and practice*. Berkley: California University Press.
Thayer, R. L. (2013). The world shrinks the world expands: information, energy and relocalization. In E. Cook & J. J. Lara (Eds.), *Remaking metropolis* (pp. 39–59). Abingdon: Routledge.
Tjallingii, S. (2000). Ecology on the edge: Landscape and ecology between town and country. *Landscape and Urban Planning, 48*, 103–119.
United Nation–Desa/Population Division. (2018). *World urbanization prospects 2018*. https://population.un.org/wup/. Accessed 10 Mar 2019.
Van den Dobbelsteen, A. (2008). *Smart vernacular planning: sustainable regional design based on local potentials and optimal deployment of the energy chain*. In Proceedings of the world conference SB08, Melbourne CSIRO- Commonwealth Scientific and Industrial Research Organisation, Australia, pp 967–974 http://www.irbnet.de/daten/iconda/CIB15946.pdf. Accessed 17 Mar 2019.
Wheeler, S. (2002). The new regionalism: Key characteristics of an emerging movement. *Journal of the American Planning Association, 68*(3), 267–278.
Wheeler, S. (2009). Region, megaregion and sustainability. In M. Neuman & A. Hull (Eds.), *The futures of the city region. Regional Studies* (special issue), *43* (6): 863–876.
Wilson, E., & Piper, J. (2010). *Spatial planning and climate change*. Milton Park, Abingdon, Oxon: Routledge.
Wills, J. (2016). *Locating localism. Statecraft, citizenship and democracy*. Bristol: Policy Press University of Bristol.

Agriurban Commons. Which Resistance and Adaptation Processes to Metropolization?

Pierre Donadieu

1 Introduction

Metropolitan regions are currently vulnerable, much more than yesterday and less than tomorrow. Due to a growing concentration of populations in often very dense urban areas, citizens are exposed to environmental, health and alimentary risks that question the security of property and people. In the face of these real (or sometimes imagined) dangers and of these changes in current climatic and energy transitions, the possibilities of resilience[1] of the inhabitants are very variable. They depend above all on the political and economic capabilities of public authorities to organize these adaptations in an effective and equitable way. When these capacities are reduced or insufficient, an alternative (among others) exists: the pooling of projects, values, goods and services which favours the initiatives of the inhabitants to self-organize and take charge of their own resilience, with or without the assistance of the state and the public authorities of territorial collectivities.

In France as in other countries, the renewed idea of commons has emerged in the last few years as an opportunity offered to the democratic exercise on a territorial scale, for land planners and inhabitants alike. This text sheds light on this emergence in France, by privileging a category of commons whose purpose focuses on the agricultural and food issue in and around the cities: the *agriurban commons.*[2] It will

[1] Capacity for the inhabitants, after a disruption or a crisis of some kind, to restore their initial state, either physical or psychological or either to adapt to an evolution of this state

[2] Many definitions of agriurban agriculture have been given for the past 20 years. We will define it as any activity of vegetal and animal production located in or nearby urban areas, on native or artificial soils. In addition to food and non-food goods, it produces environmental ecosystemic, social, and cultural services that make these practices become "a social movement of re-appropri-

P. Donadieu (✉)
École Nationale Supérieure du Paysage de Versailles, Marseille, France
e-mail: p.donadieu@ecole-paysage.fr

D. Fanfani, A. Matarán Ruiz (eds.), *Bioregional Planning and Design: Volume I*,
https://doi.org/10.1007/978-3-030-45870-6_9

first define agriurban commons, then the way agriurban commons projects are built. Finally, it will sketch out some ideas to think about the future of urban agriculture.

2 Agriurban Commons

In France, the idea of preserving or creating agricultural activities in the urban communities, instead of eliminating them, has become a political project during the past 15 years (Donadieu 1998, 2013). These initiatives may involve social oppositions to the urbanization of agricultural areas or the development of new or former food supply proximity activities (short sales channels, so-called organic agricultural products). They all share the idea of pooling common interests between producers and consumer inhabitants.

2.1 *The* Common

Commons includes what is built and pooled, (Dardot et Laval 2014): goods (common), services, human relationships, projects, moral values, relationships with space and nature …. this simple definition, although tautological, given by a philosopher and a sociologist, should not make us forget the long history of the notion of common: in Roman law, then in the reflexions of the Fathers of the Church (i.e. Thomas d'Aquin), in the sociological and economical works of Pierre-Joseph Proudhon and Karl Marx in the nineteenth century, in those of socio-economist and economy Nobel Prize Elinor Ostrom (1990, 2010) and in many others that followed, in France in particular (Orsi 2013; Coriat 2015; Calame and Ziaka 2015).

It should be remembered that the idea of common is under the control of moral, political, legal and economic sciences and that its essence is based on the necessary pooling of interests between *commoners*, English term that can be translated as "appropriateurs" in French (Ostrom 2010). Let us remember that the notion of common is not given but co-constructed by societies in a specific historical and cultural context. It implies communities, institutions and rules for the reproduction and transmission of what is shared by goods' users: water, pastures and wood ... just as much as the moral and spiritual values of societies that rely to this good (Donadieu 2014a, b; Donadieu 2016a). There are no commons without interest or destiny communities.[3]

ation of the urban area" (Duchemin 2015). The expression "agriurban" is a contraction of urban agriculture.

[3]The destiny community assumes the solidarity and responsibility of those who are involved in an unclear process (the future of Europe for instance), while the community of interest mainly ensures the defence of the identity and values common to its members (professional community, trade union).

The co-constructed common converges with the legal idea of "a resource [for which] are established a repartition system of rights (access, extraction, addition, disposal…) and a governance structure ensuring that the rights and obligations of each of the participants in the common are respected" (Coriat, *Le retour des communs,* p. 47). In this respect, this co-construction involves both private and public logics, going thus beyond them or integrating them. It generally involves chosen modalities of common governance of the goods and services concerned.

2.2 *Territorial Common*

Let us use again the definition of a French geographer: "Territory is at the same time an economic, ideological and political (therefore, social) appropriation of the area by some groups that give a particular *representation* of themselves and of their history" (Di Méo 2000).

In a more general way, territories are interaction areas between physical and human areas. They are appropriate, governed and claimed by human groups of all kinds. They are mainly jurisdiction areas. They can be hierarchized, and their perimeter is variable in time and space. Their administration, thanks to the regulations elaborated by their governance, is at the heart of social organization which is seeking compromise between two very different goals: on one hand, to meet the demand and interests of local scale stakeholders, structured by the family, social, professional and institutional networks, and, on the other hand, to manage in a sustainable way the availability and the fair allocation of resources and the use of natural resources (soil, water, biodiversity, etc.) on a local and global scale. Built through historical, social and political processes, the relationship to soil and space in a territory concerns the supranational scale, the nation, the region, a group of municipalities, or a single municipality, as well as an urban or rural neighbourhood. "Territory is of course a space with variable geography, but it still remains a space organized to act together" (Vial et Dhérissard 2015).

The idea of territorial common is thus referred to the social and political construction of goods, of services and of places pooled together as commons on these different scales with the contradictions, tensions and conflicts generated by interests often divergent. It is the reduction of these divergences that is at work in the emerging experiences of current agriurban projects.[4] Their meaning can be appropriated by a collective "we" in the perimeter of the concerned territory. In opposition to what is defined as "their" or "his/her" good, the possessive pronoun creates a shared sense of solidarity, responsibility and real or symbolic appropriation by a plurality of individuals. For instance, in the jurisdiction area of an agriurban municipality, "our" market gardeners and "our" gardens" may be designated spontaneously by

[4] The idea of agriurban project was born in the early 2000s from a policy of the French Ministry of Agriculture, implemented on an experimental basis in the Ile-de-France region (12 projects).

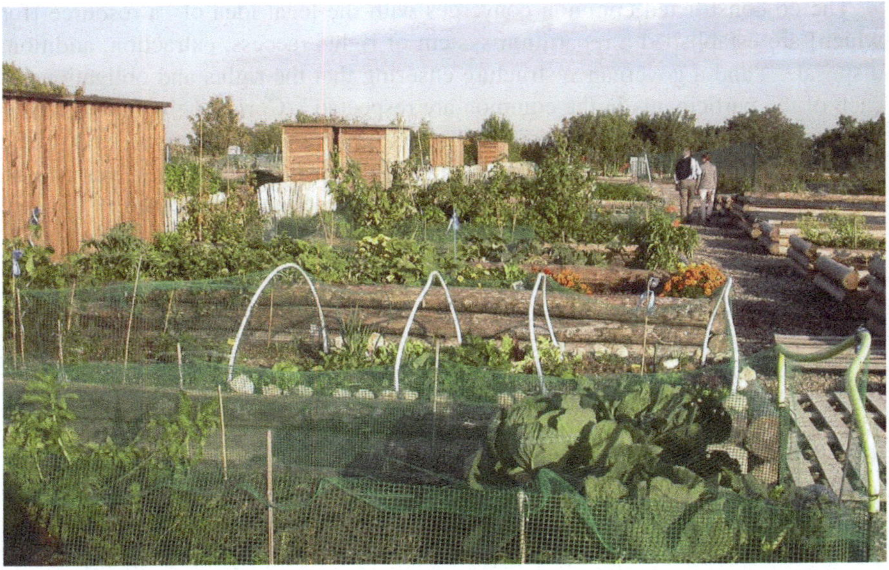

Fig. 1 Vegetable gardens to rent, Gally's farms, Versailles' plains (west of Paris), 2016. *Source* Photo Pierre Donadieu

some inhabitants, while others may indicate "their fields and their greenhouses" if the usages and perceptions of space by groups different from one another separate places with distinct or even opposed representations. There would therefore be as many territorial commons, of shared or unshared spatiality, as there are many different ways to make use of physical space in several[5] (Fig. 1).

2.3 Resist Together: A Form of Common

In France, there are many forms of social and economic self-organization which translate these urban collective resistances. Some of them mobilize agricultural or gardening practices, for instance, in Paris, the Urban Orchards association (*Vergers Urbains*) created in 2012 and the hundred or so shared gardens that have flourished in the capital, often with the support of municipalities.[6] They follow the wake of the *Green Guerrillas* (*or Guerilla Gardening*) initiated in New York by the artist Liz

[5] This anthropo-geographical position can be reconciled to the eco-culturalist theory of bio-regionalism (Berg and Dasman 1977) which seeks to integrate, as Alberto Magnaghi (2014) does, locally, the notions of territory and environmental ecology.

[6] In the Île-de-France region, the Francilian observatory of urban and biodiversity agriculture, established in 2015, estimates at about 750 the number of family and community gardens. Only 1% has a market economy.

Christy in the 1970s. Movement which triggered birth to the *community gardens* worldwide (Paquot 2016, pp. 99–103; Lagneau, in *Urban Agriculture op. cit.*, p. 71).

In France, the *Pedagogic Millar's Farm* (*la ferme pédagogique des Meuniers*) in the Val-de-Marne area, next to Orly Airport, is close to this urban culture of self-organization. Since 1995, it has become a social local centre of youth insertion and listening, organized around work in collective workshops. A social and solidarity economy self-managed company, supported by the VINCI Foundation, which has 800 members and 8 employees, educators and teachers and contractual relationships with municipalities, appears as a place built by and for the inhabitants. In its reference chart, it writes in the preamble: "The farm project was developed on the basis of the observation that the social bond has been deteriorating, that is to say on the capability of people to live together with respect for differences (age, colour, belief, social status) in a framework of social and solidarity cohesion". In Stains, in Seine-Saint-Denis, north to Paris, the same process of resistance and self-organization can be observed in the *Farm of Possible* (*la ferme des Possibles*). This place of agricultural production, in an urban environment, has a vocation for social integration of people in need (unemployed, in particular). It is an agroforestry farm engaged in an organic farming approach that produces vegetables and fruits. It highlights the importance of cultivated biodiversity and the ancestral figure of peasantry.

Some people claim the agroecological and spiritual principles of the *Colibris* movement founded by Pierre Rabhi, French theoretician of the "declining" of "happy sobriety" and of the "insurrection of consciences"; others illustrate explicitly a social agriculture implied in social inclusion practices with a very variable financial assistance of public services.

In all these new forms of resistance (or rather resilience), supported or not by public administrations, common goods and values which have been privatized or badly managed by neo-liberal practices are claimed: relationship to the land, social solidarity and human dignity as much as water and soil qualities, for instance. Private property is also questioned, and collective forms of social and spiritual life are revived. Alternative methods of agricultural production are preferred within communities and, more generally, a hope in the idealized virtues of life together with vegetable and animal, wild and cultivated nature.

The idea of territorial common expressed by these resistance practices sometimes corresponds to a withdrawal into oneself, to a critical posture of today's world functioning and to a survival surge of the disappointed and the excluded of the city and of life. In other cases, it is about real utopias (as food autonomy of urban areas), considered as chimerical by some people (by the scientists for metropoles in particular) or realistic by international movements as *Incredible Edible*. In any case, it is about hopes in better worlds initiated by producing food goods but, above all, facilities paid by public services (social inclusion, sharing, pedagogy, biodiversity). So many initiatives and innovations, alternative or not, that we will describe as agri-urban matters, and that can be better understood through the notion of landscape.

2.4 Towards Territorial Landscape Governance

Perceiving a territory as a landscape, as an accessible fragment to the senses, immediately brings the critical sense, aesthetic or not, which is given to it by the user. For the same scenery, this sense is different according to the practices of the users who remember different or similar characters. What "makes landscape" for some "does not make it" for the others.[7] Some resort to the *genius of the place*: "emotions that we feel in front of some places, with the conviction that they are inhabited, animated by a sort of aesthetic and mystical genius that would belong to them in their own right" (Roger, *Mouvance II*, 2006, p. 52). Some others to a *shared subjectivity* implying "for the landscape architect to accompany the passage of the individual feeling towards collective acknowledgement of the sensitive characters of a place or of a landscape" (Aubry, *Mouvance II,* op. cit., p. 95). But, most of the time, this collective feeling derives from a socio-political construction that brings the users of a space to a common comprehension of the meanings of places.

Let's take an example. In Fig. 2's landscape image (a fragment of the Angevines Low Valleys, floodable, in the perimeter of Angers Metropole), the farmer breeder holds of it essentially the meadows which allow him to patrol his herd and harvest his hay; the poplar grower values the poplars of which he appraises the economic profitability and expands it as much that he can; the ornithologist, the moor and the bushes where corncrakes nest (*Crex crex*), locally protected bird species; and the

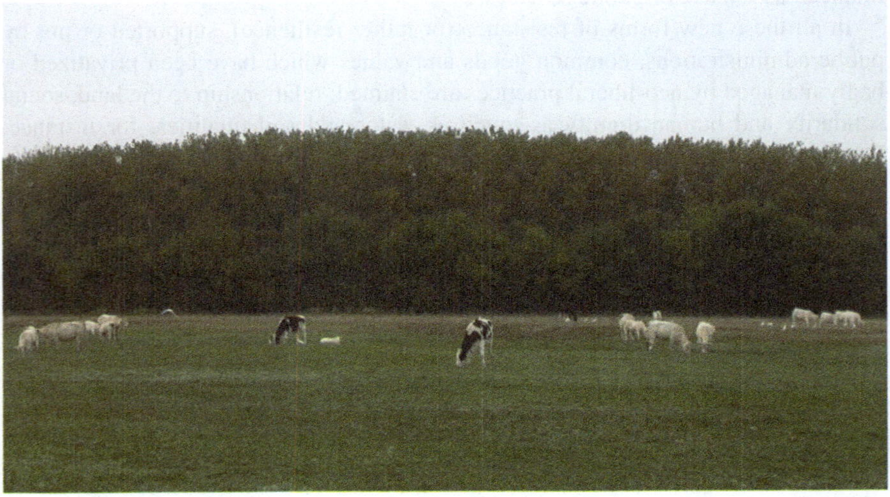

Fig. 2 Angevines Low Valleys (Metropole of Angers, France): a co-produced agriurban common. *Source* Photo Pierre Donadieu

[7] It is the same for the expression "Make territory" (*Faire territoire*), i.e. resolve together recognized issues as common on a pertinent area" (Vial et Dhérissard, *op. cit.*, p. 201).

wanderer living in Angers indicates the place where he regularly comes for a change of scenery in the middle of the flowery meadows during summer time.

Not only does this territory have as much meaning as there are landscape interpretations, but for the same places, distinct commons of landscapes are thus formed: those of the poplar growers who support poplar monoculture; the breeders who wish to expand their sources of hay threatened by the poplars' extension; those of the naturalists, botanists and ornithologists who are seeking to keep the meadows abandoned by the breeders thanks to public subsidies; and those of the strollers who want to keep this vast space accessible, model of friendly nature for most of Angers inhabitants. Tension is often latent between the users of these areas, and sometimes conflict may break out if the uses become rivals.[8] But it is the awareness of a responsibility to share that engages the emergence of the common between the stakeholders of the future of the landscapes of the place.

For this reason, since the 1990s, it has been possible to build the rules for the pooling of commons specific to these users, after several years of discussions between the elected representatives of Angers Metropole, the farmers, the land owners and the technicians of breeding, nature protection, landscape and poplar farming. This is in order to share the territory to the best of the interests that are pooled by all the stakeholders. *This landscape governance of a common territory* includes the contradictory and convergent interests of the users in an agreement that goes beyond them and of which each of them is the protector but takes part to its evolution. The community evolves: some leave and others stay and count new users.

If the common character to all the private soils of this valley is to be floodable and not constructible, the sharing of their uses is part of the construction of a *landscape and territorial common* that does not leave itself be imposed by exclusive poplars at the expense of any other economic use (cattle breeding), social (leisure activities), environmental (biodiversity, natural risks) or landscaped (individual and collective well-being). The common transcends individual interests in a given context but, not being sacralised, remains fragile when interests or local context change.

3 The Construction of Agriurbanity

The key issue of mixed landscaped and territory approaches is to reconcile the reasons for producing locally all or a part of the so-called eco-system-based services planned by the *Millennium Ecosystems Assessment* (2005): provisioning, environmental regulation, social and cultural services. The landscape and territorial scopes

[8]What geographer Hervé Davodeau says by analysing the conflicts linked to the landscape in Anjou: "We interpret the conflicts produced by landscape management as the revealers of the territorialisation of a landscape project that, by changing dimension, must change content". *Des conflits révélateurs de la territorialisation du projet de paysage.* Exemples from the Loire Valley. In Territoires de conflits, analyses des mutations de l'occupation de l'espace. L'Harmattan, pp.49–61/322, 2008. <Hal-00788157>

are of the same nature: to create shared relationships with the qualified places that make the territories liveable according to the inhabitants and stakeholders' tastes and preferences and not only as per public administrations.

The landscaped approach (or rather landscape-based) favours perceived topographic forms, multi-sensoriality, perceptible singular characteristics, local memories, nature facts and *in fine* the multiple senses – and not only functional – of what is perceived.

When it is designed by professional space planners, the project subscribes in time and space in a multiscale way. There lies its desired coherence, if it is implemented and respected (Donadieu 2014b, op. cit.).

Since the European Landscape Convention of 2000 (ELC) was signed, and sometimes before (in France, particularly), the landscape territorial project rather pursues purposes of aesthetic, societal and environmental satisfaction for the inhabitants, than those of strict aesthetic pleasures.

As a result, it managed to improve the urban and territory project without merging with him. The theoretical notion of landscape used by researchers is then referred to that of social, political and cultural construction of landscapes or of societal project of landscape (Donadieu 2016b). The challenge of choice of soil uses then clearly appears, as the space landowners and users become the main needed actors of the process of territorial landscape project. It is the notion of local individual and collective responsibility that should then rule public decisions (Fig. 3).

The way in which land use is democratically decided therefore depends on how territory and landscape projects are built and gathered together. These practices, which generally call on the notion of landscape only in patrimonial or naturalist perspectives, are very different according to the countries, from the most authoritarian to the most democratic.

One of the major obstacles relates to the soil property right, even if it is not absolute (with the usufruct in particular). Yet, as a result of the works of the American E. Ostrom, it has become possible to consider the rational dissociation of the different usage rights of a fund, from strict usage, contractual or not, until the right to alienate (Orsi, on 2013).

3.1 Dissociate Land Use Rights

When Garrett Hardin writes its famous article of 1968: *The Tragedy of Commons*, he is faced, as many researchers of that time, with the necessity to explain the degradation of tropical soils. He takes over his own account the long-standing criticism, by the agronomists and doctors, of common property, and he perpetuates, successfully, the idea that this land regime only brings misery to the societies that use it due to the depletion of the fragile resources concerned.

The only alternative to this status, as in the case of the collective pasture in North Africa, becomes private property that replaces the collectives, most of the time through a sharing and a cultivation which consecrates this change in land status.

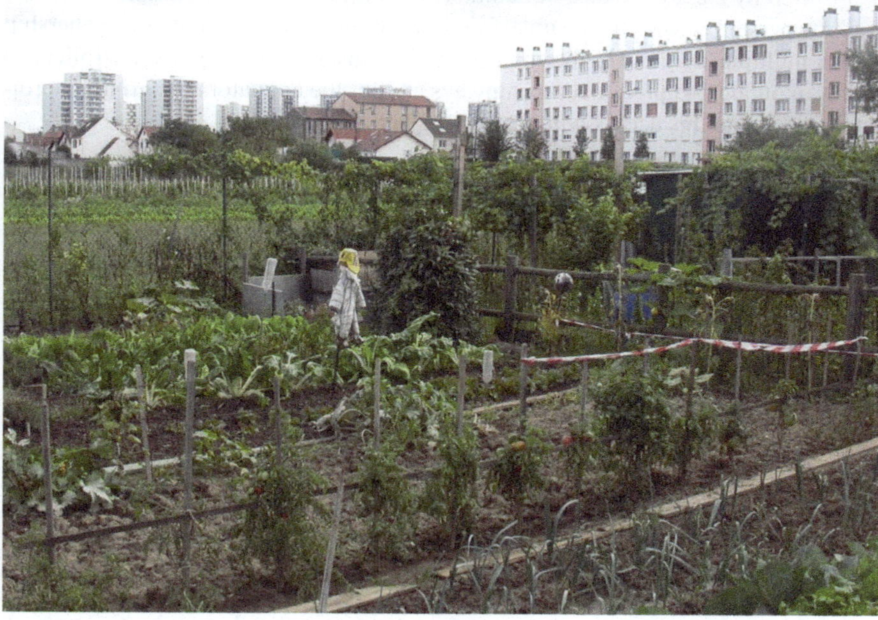

Fig. 3 Seine-Saint-Denis, Pierrefitte/Seine, north of Paris, agricultural soils, left by the market gardener, will they be built for housing or converted into family gardens as requested by the inhabitants? (see Fig. 6). *Source* Photo Pierre Donadieu

Once they have become owners of their lands, the former collectives' members are in this way supposed to integrate into their private heritage the risks of destruction of the good by uncontrollable users (the "stowaways" of Hardin), by producing more and fertilizing the soils. Yet, as Fabienne Orsi points out (2013, p. 20), in England as in France, the regime of land property community in the former regimes "not only implied the lack of freedom to dispose of the thing (*l'abusus*) but authorized the superposition (or juxtaposition) of various rights of property or usage of a same thing".

By decomposing property right into four types of right, Elinor Ostrom distinguished several types of users of a fund (Orsi 2013, 77 and ff.):

- *The authorised users* who only hold access and collection rights, for instance, a shepherd and its herd on a collective pasture or strollers in an agricultural area open to the public
- *The usage and regulation right holders* who add to the previous rights the authorization to manage the good, for example, the delegate of the grazing collective or the *landscape manager* (the animator) of an agriurban park
- *The owners of the good without the right to alienate (proprietors)* who have all the previous rights, for example, the fund tenants

– *The absolute owners*, public or private, who have all the rights including to sell

Inspired by the governance of natural resources, this plural definition of "at several" ownership allows to imagine forms of common agricultural soil ownership whose multiple usages are the main issue, for instance, the right for strollers to access to public and private rural pathways and for the animators of agriurban projects to negotiate this access with the owners and the farmers.[9]

3.2 Some Cases of Agriurbanity in the Greater Paris Metropolitan Area and Elsewhere

In a loop of the Seine, at the extremity of the axis of the Défense area to the west of Paris, the market plain of Montesson gathers on 400 hectares 17 market gardeners who produce half of the salads consumed in the region of Paris. This plain was long promised to urbanization, but social resistance has been organized there with the help of legal tools of protection of agricultural soils. The Region Ile-de-France (Land Agency of the Green Areas, *Agence foncière des Espaces verts*) and the department of Yvelines (Sensitive Natural Areas, *Espaces Naturels Sensibles*) bought more than 60 hectares of lands in order to re-rent them to the farmers. But a project of detour road threatens! The stakeholders (elected representatives, farmers, owners, associations) then created the *Plain of Future* organization in 2012. The *Territorial Coherence Scheme* (SCOT, inter-communal urban plan) has approved its agriurban project. Indeed, a pluri-territorial agriurban governance (from the municipality to the state), whose origin dates to the early 2000s, was installed (Fig. 4). For one year, a collective ZAD *Patate* is planting potatoes along the roadways to support the defence of the plain and protect religious mantises that live there (Lagneau and al., op. cit., pp. 91–93).

The same processes of landscape and territorial governance have been developed with success on the Saclay plateau since the end of the 1990s (2400 hectares, 12 farmers, the multi-actors organization "*Terre et Cité*" in the south of Versailles; in the west of Versailles, with the patrimonial association of the *Versailles plain and the Alluets plateau* (25 municipalities, 10,000 hectares), since 2003, which set up an inter-community landscape charter.

Outside Paris region, many opportunities are thus seized by the socio-political collectives to stabilize agricultural activities and, in some cases, to establish young farmers. It is the case in Lille (Wavrin project, 47 hectares, 10 farmers not accommodated on site), on the former military base of Brétigny (50 hectares of project market gardening in organic agriculture) in the south of Paris, in Mouans-Sartoux (Maritime-Alps), to create a municipal farm dedicated to school catering or in order to favour, with municipalities, the set-up of community gardens and of (micro)urban

[9] These practices are easier to install in countries of jurisprudential law (e.g. the common law in the United Kingdom) than in the countries of codified law (France).

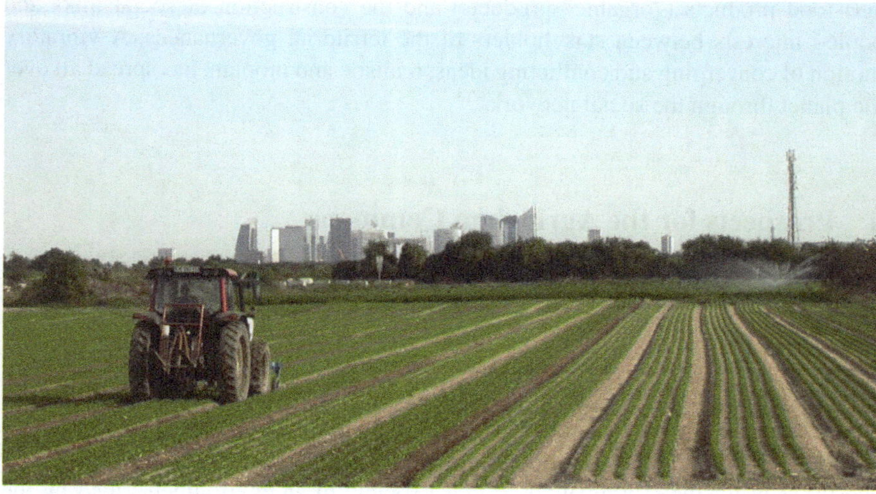

Fig. 4 *Plaine d'Avenir*: the Montesson plain (West Paris, France). *Source* Photo Pierre Donadieu

farm experimentations. It is also the case of the *Ville comestible* initiatives,[10] *Ville résiliente*, *Ville fertile*, *Ville végétale*, *Ville nature*, *Incroyables Comestibles* (Incredible Edible)[11]... : municipalities or collective militants of urban agriculture in Nantes, Arcueil, Bordeaux, Paris, Albi, Rennes, Montesson etc.

In all these cases, social, economic, ethical and spiritual values are shared separately. According to the concerned collectives, identifiable on social networks, their mobilization contributes to mitigate the perceived negative effects of globalization, metropolization and of the unregulated or poorly regulated urbanization. These values concern economic profitability, land stability of urban agriculture farms, producer and consumer proximity and the *high- or low-tech* techniques of innovating start-*ups*.[12] In addition to this, especially in the world of militancy and resistance, solidarity with the most deprived can be added to the list, as well as the responsibility of individual commitment, self-care, sanitary and gustatory quality of the

[10]They often highlight the systematic principles of permotherapy and permaculture: "which enables to see the city as a global eco-system, in which the overall elements interact with each other, are self-regulated and productive". Permaculture was theorized in 1970 by the Australians Bill Morisson and David Holmgrem critiques of industrial agriculture. https://villepermaculturelle.wordpress.com/objet/.

[11]Since the founding initiative of the English city of Todmorden in 2008, this international movement of urban agriculture, based on permotherapy, makes available for free all the vegetables cultivated in the public area. It is looking for towns and villages' food autonomy and encourages consumers to look for food supply in the vicinity of urban areas. 80 towns and villages (including Rennes and Albi) have joined this movement in France.

[12]We will admit the distinction between cultures outside *low-tech* ground (the vegetable and orchard garden of the Pullman Hotel in Paris by the Topager company) and *high-tech* (hydro, aqua and aeroponic) medium to high financial investment.

agri-food products ("organic" products) and the construction of social links and pooled interests between stakeholders of the territorial governances. A vibratory motion of converging and conflicting ideas, realistic and utopian, has spread all over the planet through the social networks.[13]

4 Prospects for the Agriurban Commons

4.1 The Three Commons

The previous overview of agriurban practices shows that there are three main ways to make common, to combine pooling interests. The first one registers in the merchant exchange between an agricultural producer and a food goods consumer aiming for economic models of profitability. The second regards the agriurban factory and the way for the city dwellers to make society in an environment ruled by the urban politics. And the last one, consequence of the first two, tries to resist or adapt to the dysfunctions that they generate by inventing new self-produced life environments.

4.1.1 Commons of Economic Interest

To talk about economic commons is like talking about markets, about the exchange area where the interest of the parties, the seller and the buyer, is to agree on a fair price. Most agricultural companies located in urban areas are part of a market, where the stakeholders (producers, {re-} sellers, consumers) are either relatively close to one another (vegetable and fruit sales on urban markets or in short circuits), distant (European markets) or very distant (globalized meat, wine, cereals and proteaginous markets).

Some companies achieve their whole turnover in close urban proximity, but for most of them, customers are both close and (very) distant from the places of production. Merchant communities, which are economic interest communities, export in the regulatory national or supranational framework (international commercial agreements).

The *Luffa Farm*, created in 2010 in Montreal, falls into this category – 2880 sq. on top of the roof of a commercial building in hydroponic market gardening – and is distributed in short circuits. This is also the case of most of the fields, market and floral greenhouses of agriculture companies, which have been long established in

[13] See three recent works: Collectif, *Agriculture urbaine: aménager et nourrir la ville,* Vertigo, Montréal, 2013, 388 p.; Guiomar X. (edit...) *Dossier agricultures urbaines,* Revue POUR, 2015, 415 p.; and *Agriculture urbaine, vers une réconciliation ville nature,* Natureparif, le Passager Clandestin edition, 2015.

the urban network of most of the cities of the planet and supply closer and distant markets.

Except for technical and economic prowess, as the Luffa Farm in France or as the urban farms' pioneers of Gally and Viltain in the west of Paris, this economic world occupies a modest position in the recent publications on urban agriculture, a weakness that can be explained by the alternative agriurban solutions that are proposed. In fact, many of them are part of the declining economic model born in the 1970s, following Denis Meadows' report (*The Limits of growth,* 1972). This very critical sensitivity of capitalism and productivism, agricultural in particular, has been embodied in many national and international publications which inspire most of "urbifarmers".

However, entrepreneurial commons that are visible through agricultural professional organizations, land agencies and technical institutes are very different from societal commons of allotment, shared and community gardens. The first ones are essentially motivated by market conquests, the protection of agricultural professions and biotechnological innovation that provides competitive benefits, which is not the case of the second ones that mainly provide social, educational, patrimonial and spiritual services and create urban communities in form of alternative and militant social networks. In practice, in the ethical framework of social and solidarity economy, they produce a part of the urban positive externalities of the economy that intensive specialized production, the merchandizing of world and the modernist conception of the city have made disappear without enough compensation.

4.1.2 Commons of Urbanistic Interest

Urban agriculture social trend, attached to food crops and to the land, finds an attentive echo in the alternative urban thought that the philosopher "of the urban" T. Paquot (*Les faiseurs de ville*, 2010) has made known to the francophone public. We can include, for example, some historical figures as botanist, pedagogue and theoretician of the city, English Patrick Geddes (1854–1932), who makes reference for the bio-regionalists (Magnaghi 2012, 2014). Nowadays, the current rules of the urban factory generally do not favour the welcoming and persistence of agriculture. The French code of urbanism appears to be too rigid to easily welcome the multiple agriurban initiatives, market and non-market. Indeed, by giving the choice to the elected representatives to classify agricultural lands in A (agricultural and productive), N (natural) or U (urban, real or potential), it makes way for regrettable ambiguities in local urban plans often too restrictive. The N zoning supposes so much naturalistic qualities (heritage) as landscape ones (cultural, aesthetical and functional for eco-systemic services), and zoning U is sometimes given to shared garden areas and educational farms. In all three, agricultural or social entrepreneurship activities are not facilitated in the long run as municipal objectives of accommodation, transport or nature preservation can put them into question (Chalot 2015), while agriurban projects could combine all these objectives if individual or collective mentalities and interests did not separate them.

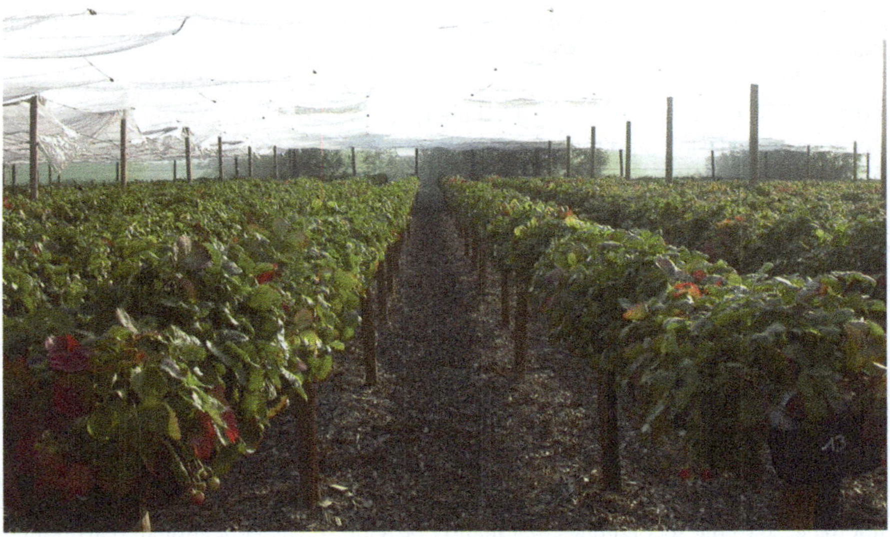

Fig. 5 Raspberry cultivation for pick on your own, *indoor*, Gally farms, Versailles. Economic and urbanistic commons. *Source* Photo Pierre Donadieu

But sometimes urban communities, owners of the land, invest in a real (sub) urban agriculture open to the city dwellers. In 2010, the municipality of Toulouse chose to preserve 240 hectares and to drive them in majority and under direct control in organic agriculture (cereals, soya, lentils, apiaries, viticulture) by giving access to the public for leisure activities. It is the same in Montpellier (Mas-Nouguier wine agriparc). In most cases where progress is being observed, urban agricultural commons require the meeting of all stakeholders: elected representatives, inhabitants, associations, future farmers, ecologists, town planners, landscape designers, etc. That is how the 100-hectare Noisiel park, in the conurbation of Val-Maubuée in the east of Paris, is now managed, thanks to a cattle farm providing economic value to public areas. In 2014, the "*le Vivant et la Ville*" cluster, the *Institut national de la recherche agronomique* (National Institute for Agronomic Research) and the *AgroParistech* enable to set up an experiment, near Versailles, with the Gally farms specialized in the production of vegetables aboveground under shelter, in circular economy (Fig. 5).

In almost all these cases, the commercial purpose of these projects is achieved through alliances between public institutions and private project owners and then in trade commons of public and private roots. Indeed, it contributes to build agriurban areas. They can take very different shapes: urban stockbreeding in large housing complexes (the Clinamen company in Courneuve, north of Paris), permaculture production tubs (*Incroyables Comestibles*), protection perimeters of former suburban rural areas opened to the public (agricultural parks in practice) or *low-* or *high-tech* experiments in and close urban conurbations.

This type of agriurbanism can limit to supply the neighbourhood. It can also give city dwellers a pedestrian or cycling access to the suburban rural landscapes and to the farms. These practices can be observed elsewhere, in Italy, for instance, in the large agricultural park in the south of Milan. So that de facto sketches of agri-neighbourhoods are born – future ephemeral communities or stable ones of a new kind – whose population density remains very variable along a gradient from the centre to urban periphery.

Still, another trend, very distant from the pooling process, regards green urbanism, whose decorative, environmental and sometimes food-related purposes are showed in many Parisian architects' projects. The responses to *The Call for Urban Innovative Projects* of the city of Paris (Pavillon de l'Arsenal publishing editions), in 2016, are the testimony of it.

In practice, this green and/or horticultural urbanism draws the attention of many urban elected representatives. It can create, to the advantage of the city, communities of public and private interest, thanks to a territorial governance. But the latter is not yet codified, if the agriculture/city hybridization forms are not stabilized. Urban gardenings have a symbolic economic place there, due to the relative weakness of their trade agricultural activity.

They have been generated over the past 20 years by a context of recurring urban and societal crisis, whose most significant effects are unemployment, environmental and food risks and the questioning of the societal consequences of neo-liberalism and metropolization.

4.1.3 Commons of Social Interest

In the perimeter of an urban region, the numerous areas of private and public gardening are a part of the urban factory, as well as the gardener/"urbifarmer" communities.[14] The conditions of their emergence (historical tradition and questioning of the trade world and of regulatory urban planning) sometimes turn them into counter powers of the city production dominant modes.

Here too a categorization is useful. On one hand, you can find *private gardens,* around the pavilions, in the gardens of buildings, on balconies and terraces, which belong to a family or co-proprietary common. On the other hand, you can find *labourer and allotment gardens*, which have flourished in central and western Europe for more than a hundred and fifty years: more than 60,000 in Berlin and approximately 240,000 in the Netherlands today. And more recently, *the community gardens* (collective or of social integration) appeared in North America at the end of the last century. They extended to the whole world where people in precarious situation (unemployed, refugees, sick and convalescent, isolated and homeless people, migrants, etc.) could meet help and solidarity.

[14] The urbifarmer is a neologism used by the *Guide of Urbifarmers* (*Guide des urbiculteurs, Natureparif*, May 2016).

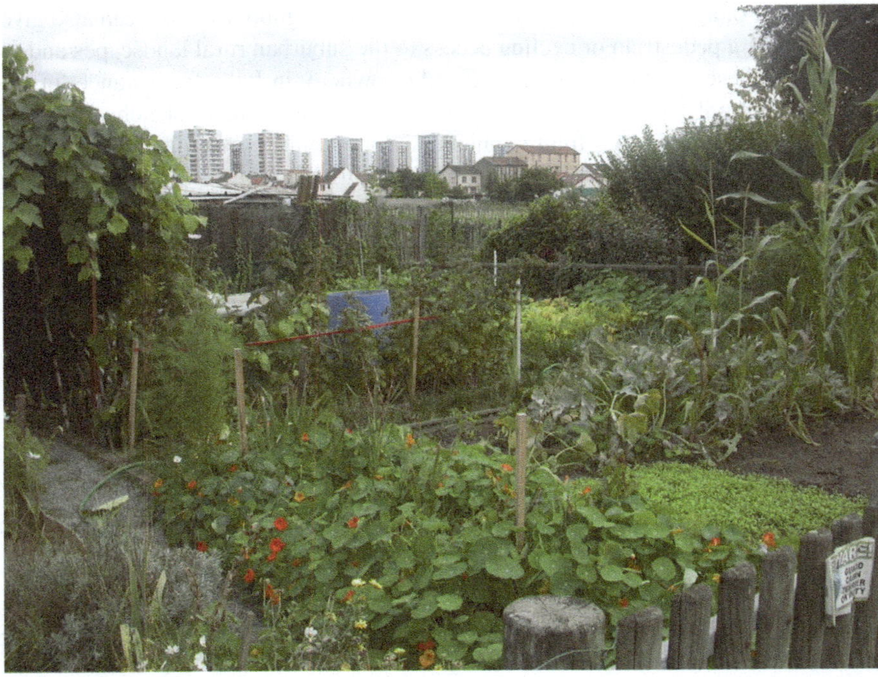

Fig. 6 Allotments gardens, Saint Denis, north of Paris. Social and urbanistic commons. *Source* Photo Pierre Donadieu

In France, the Cocagne gardens (organic vegetable farming with baskets) are a well-known example. Can be added to the list *the food crisis gardens,* national or local as in Cuba, the *shared gardens (jardins partagés)* by those who, as in Paris with the *Green Hand (Main verte)* charter, or through the regional collective *Graine de Jardins (Garden seed)*, wish to gather together in order to cultivate abandoned places of all types, public and private. There they can find conviviality and the sharing of a citizen consciousness (Lagneau, *op. cit.*, pp. 45–51) (Fig. 6).

The construction of commons around a cultivated place (or of breeding) and the sharing of alternative ideas (decreasing or of solidarity in particular) is clear in the community gardens that have taken place in urban wastelands. However, the limit with the shared gardens is not always clear, depending on the people who make use of it (neighbourhood inhabitants or homeless people!). The pooling of a place, which can "make territory", often hides social exclusions.

Finally, urban public parks and gardens, inherited from history, or recent, represent public authorities' responses for the provision to urban dwellers of what are now called ecosystemic services (environmental regulation, leisure and sport services, pedagogy, spiritual, aesthetic and aesthesic). Yet, they are not sufficient for the social categories that create commons of social interest. So, it is not uncommon that public parks welcome associative vegetable gardens. As in the case of the three categories of commons: economic, urban, and social, which are aimed, for example, to hybridize in Montreuil's site of "Murs-à-pêches" in the east of Paris.

4.2 Which Philosophical Support?

If we think that neither utilitarian or Kantian approaches nor libertarian principles provide enough lighting on the choices to be made, can we rely on pragmatic philosophy?

Is there a fourth way that would allow agriculture and urban gardening stakeholders not to care about the merits caused by their decisions and actions? And that would draw attention to the practical consequences of their actions only and lean on democratic debate to decide what is desirable to do or not?

Following psychologist William James, the American philosopher and pedagogue John Dewey (1859–1952) imagined a method (the survey and the mobilization of the "public") to facilitate the human adaptations to the evolution of societies and of their economic and political context. Dewey's pragmatic approach wanted thus to promote, in *The Public and its problems* (1927), self-realization through the participation of the individual to collective action.[15]

If we mobilize this moral and political philosophy, little known in Europe, to shed light on the problems raised by the presence or the project of agricultural activities in the city, the field of territorial agriurban governance practices already mentioned opens. It means that each agriurban case has its own problems and solutions related to the stakeholders involved. Entrepreneurial farmers and militant urbifarmers, the State and local authorities or associations hold a part of the problem and the solution. It is within the framework of goods and services thus jointly constructed that the stakeholders find their freedom of action and thought. These commons continue afterwards to adapt to new situations within the framework of a deliberative or participative democracy.

However, pragmatism is not the panacea, otherwise as a method of resolution of territorialized issues, since it is at the origin of social-liberalism (American and English mainly) as part of the market economy. So, applied to this field, it does not guarantee fair wealth redistribution. Let us rather retain from pragmatism the methods and not the ideologies derived from it. This method can be experimented in every territory, with success, by the way, as we have shown, but without mentioning its philosophical origins, which is not incompatible with the shared choice of moral cardinal values like justice, freedom, dignity and responsibility (Nussbaum, on 2011).

[15] The use of pragmatism from J. Dewey is developed in P. Donadieu, *Paysages en commun, pour une éthique des mondes vécus*, Presses universitaires de Valenciennes, 2014.

5 Conclusion

Commons are pooled socio-political constructions of goods and services. The notion of *agriurban common* allows to highlight and to account for very different forms of resistance and adaptation of urban societies to the loss or inadequacy of agricultural activities in metropolitan areas.

It favours the idea of the building of territories and agriurban landscapes thanks to the territorial and landscape governance tool. Its purpose is not only to preserve the farmland and farmers but also to focus on the democratic expression of the *collective choices* of the stakeholders, and of the public, associative and private parts. Processes result in social and sometimes political organizations of the communities of three types: (1) autonomous, alternative and often libertarians; (2) associated to political, economic and institutional local authorities, national or international, and (3) hybrid between these two poles.

The idea *of agriurban common* expresses the societal consequences of the multifunctionality which is assigned to agriculture (by the Agricultural Orientation Law of 1999 in France in particular). When (intra)urban agriculture initiatives do not lean on robust economic models, the services that they provide to city dwellers (social insertion, pedagogy, biodiversity, etc.) can be remunerated by public services and by the concerned cities in particular. Thus, communities of interest emerge which can become communities of destiny.

This idea allows above all to understand how a collective government of natural resources (soil and water mostly) and of their food usage is possible when urban political representation seeks alternatives to real estate market pressures; when legal, agronomic, urbanistic or landscape skills struggle to associate because they have been split up by the professional trainings and practices; and when local social forces, especially agricultural, become aware of their political power, not by confining thought and action within the limits of the local but by relying critically on the imaginary inspired by the landscapes created within the framework of the globalization of exchanges and networks, not by claiming additional rights from the State but by building, beyond public and private property, the local rules that will manage in a responsible way the goods and services common to the users of a territory (Calame and Ziaka, on 2015).

Producing the rules of *agriurbanism*[16] and of its many forms of territorial adaptation still remains an embryonic project. However, it is enriched every day by the common experience of the elected representatives, town planners, urban farmers, militants and agriurban project managers. These agriurban commons testify that one part of the citizens has the ability and wish to live with the agricultural world (and not just anyone), and they can therefore only be ruled through the pooling of interests acknowledged by the audiences of the urban factory. This practice, which

[16] Which may be defined as the art, science and technique of the urban factory with the farmers and gardeners, for and with the proximity inhabitants. See Robin Chalot's article, *Inventer un nouvel urbanisme en cultivant la ville,* in Agriculture urbaine, *op. cit.*, 2015, pp. 103–137.

is now inscribed in the duration, will experience successes and failures. It will request a long time to stabilize, characteristic inherent to territorial governance processes and to the evolution of mentalities and urban cultures.

References

Aubry, P. (2006). *Mouvance II, 70 mots pour le paysage* (A. Berque édit.). Paris: Éditions de la Villette.

Berg, P., & Dasmann, R. (1977, décembre). Reinhabiting California. *The Ecologist*, *7*(10).

Calame, P., & Ziaka, Y. (2015). Les biens communs et l'éthique de la responsabilité. *Ethique publique*, *17*(2), put-on line on May 6th 2016, http://ethiquepublique.revues.org/2306.

Chalot, F. (2015). Écologie et urbanisme : comment les experts du vivant peuvent-ils contribuer à la conception du cadre urbain ? *in VertigO - la revue électronique en sciences de l'environnement [Online], Débats et Perspectives*. Accessed 5 May 2020. http://journals.openedition.org/vertigo/16561, https://doi.org/10.4000/vertigo.16561

Coriat, B., (Éd.). (2015). *Le retour des communs, la crise de l'idéologie propriétaire*. Paris: Les Liens qui Libèrent.

Dardot, P., & Laval, C. (2014). *Communs, essai sur la révolution au XXIe siècle*. Paris: La Découverte.

Di Méo, G. (dir.) (2000). *Les territoires du quotidien*. Paris: L'Harmattan.

Donadieu, P. (2013). *Campagne urbane, Una nuova proposta di paesaggio della città*, introduzione di M. V. Mininni (1998), Donzelli, 2nd edition.

Donadieu, P. (2014a). *Paysages en commun, pour une éthique des mondes vécus*. Presses universitaires de Valenciennes.

Donadieu, P. (2014b). *Scienze del paesaggio, tra teorie e pratiche* (translation from Andrea Inzerillo). Pisa: édizioni ETS.

Donadieu, P. (2016a). Building urban agricultural commons: A Utopia or a reality? *Challenges in Sustainability*. http://www.librelloph.com/challengesinsustainability/article/view/cis-4.1.3.

Donadieu, P. (2016b). Contribution à une science de la conception des projets de paysage. In C. Chomarat-Ruiz (Éd.), *Paysage en projets*. Presses Universitaires de Valenciennes.

Duchemin, E. (2015). L'agriculture urbaine d'hier à aujourd'hui, en Île-de-France, en France et dans le monde. In A. Lagneau, M. Barra, & G. Lecuir (Eds.), *Agriculture urbaine, vers une reconciliation ville-nature* (p. 14). Naturparif, Neuvy-en-Champagne, Le passager clandestin.

Hardin, G. (1968). The tragedy of the commons. *Revue Science, 162*(3859), 1243–1248.

Magnaghi, A. (2012, mai-juin). Entretien avec Thierry Paquot. *Urbanisme, 384*.

Magnaghi, A. (2014). *La biorégion urbaine, petit traité sur le territoire bien commun*. Paris: Eterotopia France/Rhizome.

Millenium Ecosystem Assessment. (2005). *Rapport de synthèse de l'Évaluation des Écosystèmes pour le Millénaire*. http://www.millenniumassessment.org/documents/document.447.aspx.pdf.

Nussbaum, M.(2011). *Les émotions démocratiques : comment former le citoyen du XXIe siècle ?* Flammarion Climat.

Orsi, F. Elinor Ostrom et les faisceaux de droits : l'ouverture d'un nouvel espace pour penser la propriété commune. *Revue de la régulation* [En ligne], 14 | 2e semestre/Autumn 2013, put-on line on February 14th 2014, consulted on April 25th 2016. URL: http://regulation.revues.org/10471.

Ostrom, E., *Gouvernance des biens communs, pour une nouvelle approche des ressources naturelles* (1990), révision scientifique de Laurent Baechler. Bruxelles: De Boeck, 2010.

Paquot, T. (2016). *Le paysage*. Paris: La Découverte.

Roger A. (2006). *Mouvance II, 70 mots pour le paysage* (A. Berque édit.). Paris: Éditions de la Villette.

Vial, A.-C. et Dhérissard, G. (2015). Faire territoire aujourd'hui, enjeux et défis. In *Des territoires à penser* (p. 199). Éditions de l'Aube et Passions Céréales.

Urban–Rural Relations as Assemblages: A Conceptual Framework for Urban Food Policies

Gianluca Brunori and Paolo Prosperi

1 Introduction

In the twentieth century, the vision of rural development has been influenced by a modernization approach, which has seen the past in the countryside and in the city the future. The countryside, with this approach, has been perceived as territory waiting for urbanization, and rural development has been conceived of as application of urban models to rural areas.

This model has been strongly contested at the end of the 1970s, when endogenous development approaches have started to consolidate. They have focused their attention on the need for rural actors and communities to gain autonomy – first of all cultural – and to look for development models and trajectories based on distinctive characteristics of the rural territory.

The endogenous development approach has inspired the initial LEADER programs in Europe, and in many cases, it has been turned into strategies of relative 'distantiation' of rural areas and their economic activities from urban markets and technologies (Van der Ploeg 1994). Examples of endogenous rural developments have been found in the revitalization of remote rural areas based on back-to-land movements looking for alternative lifestyles. Soon, however, it has been recognized that strategies based on isolation could bring to 'green traps', situations where available resources would not be sufficient to achieve a minimum of social welfare (Cumming et al. 2014). Rural areas, in fact, don't escape from the logic of the 'space of flows' and its tendency to destructure the homogeneity and the identity of places (Castells 2011); the reconstruction of local identities embedded in space, the new 'spaces of places', is now to be understood as the outcome of relational strategies aimed at locally regulating the speed, and the patterns, of global flows.

G. Brunori (✉) · P. Prosperi
Department of Agrarian, Food and Agro-environmental Sciences, University of Pisa, Pisa, Italy
e-mail: gianluca.brunori@unipi.it; paolo.prosperi@unipi.it

D. Fanfani, A. Matarán Ruiz (eds.), *Bioregional Planning and Design: Volume I*,
https://doi.org/10.1007/978-3-030-45870-6_10

Endogenous approaches have thus evolved into neo-endogenous approaches (Lowe et al. 1995; Ray 1999) that focus on the capacity of rural areas to better position themselves in the globalized networks through the mobilization of local resources and local identities. In the strategies based on neo-endogenous approaches, local identities are shaped by the interplay with global trends, and their construction is moved by the need to build differences that embody into products and services demanded by global consumers (Ray 1999).

After the 2007–2008 crisis, things have changed. On one hand, the recession and the retrenchment of the public sector have put into evidence the dependency of rural areas from public spending and from incomes earned from outside the rural areas. Processes of abandonment, especially in the most remote areas, have thus intensified (Verburg et al. 2010). On the other hand, the crisis has hit strongly the trust in urban models. Mass unemployment has created a disillusion on the capacity of urban models to respond to social expectations and stimulated a new 'back to land' movement (Kasimis and Zografakis 2014). Facing new sustainability issues such as climate change, mass migration and resource scarcity, the question is to what extent will cities be able to cope and to anticipate future catastrophes.

It is now clear that the way out of the economic and social crisis cannot be found without a careful study of urban–rural links. An improved understanding of those interconnections would also contribute to build the pathway towards sustainability. Urban administrations are increasingly aware that life of cities depends strongly on the countryside as well as life of rural areas depends on cities. This new awareness implies a deep revision of the paradigms that so far have guided city administrations. Strategies to build resilient cities will have to envisage a transition to new and more sustainable lifestyles, production models, regulatory patterns and governance arrangements, considering explicitly rural areas as components of the urban life. The present paper develops a reflection on the governance principles, regulating the urban–rural links, that are necessary to address new sustainability challenges.

2 Transition as a Cognitive Process

The transition towards sustainability requires a deep change in the way people know and live the city. This change, in open and free societies, will require the construction of new visions and, even more important, new representations of the city. Shared visions and representations are necessary to coordination of independent actors (Gharajedaghi 2011). Making top-down visions accepted implies a vertical distribution of power and a hierarchical structure of cities, which rarely occur. In open, multipolar, complex societies, the only way to generate shared visions and representations is participation.

Shared visions (images of how a socio-technical system should be) and representations (images of how a socio-technical system is) can be considered as 'operating systems' of socio-technical systems, cognitive meta-rules that enable and constrain daily practices (Gharajedaghi 2011). Shared representations are stabilizers of a

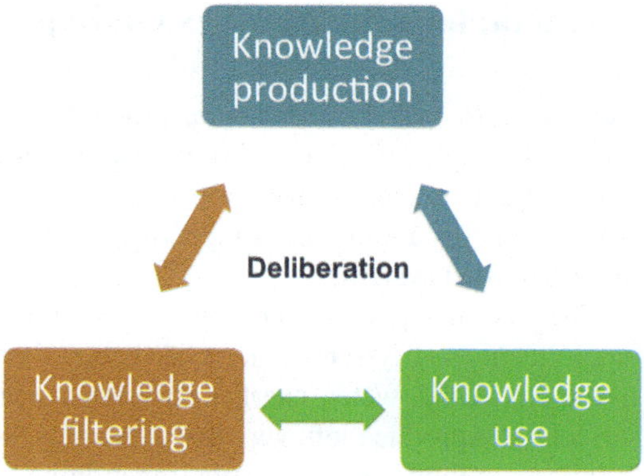

Fig. 1 Processes of deliberation and role of knowledge (Source: Adapted from Revi et al. (2014, p. 576)

society, but at the same time, they may be factors of resistance to change. Changing practices entails changing shared images. This is not an easy task, as a change of shared representations needs challenging strong assumptions embodied into cognitive and normative dimensions.

In a complex society, there are competing visions and representations, and each of them generates sets of practices. But if people don't live in separate realities, then visions and representations overlap to a certain extent. The challenge of transition to sustainability is to build upon these overlapping spaces. Deliberation, which is communication aimed at establishing common meanings in view of decisions, is the key to this process. In its 2014 climate change report (Revi et al. 2014), IPCC addresses this issue, highlighting how deliberation is affected by knowledge use, production and filtering.[1] In an information society, all are knowledge producers, users or filters, but some actors have more resources than others in performing them. Knowledge production is based on data collection and analysis. Knowledge use is related to decision-making and to communication. Knowledge filtering is about emphasis, priorities and translation. All actors are at the same time knowledge filters, producers and users, and shared images emerge when their knowledge is shared, questioned and improved through deliberation. Figure 1 illustrates the context wherein deliberation occurs. A new shared image (knowledge production) may be inspired by problems emerging in real life (knowledge use) by individuals or groups, communicated through the media (knowledge filters), embodied by other individuals and groups into their own images (knowledge production).

Knowledge use is at the basis of practices, as these are composed of meanings, skills and things (Shove et al. 2012). New knowledge can bring to modification of practices, and likewise novelties emerging from daily practices can contribute to new knowledge creation. The challenge of deliberative democracy is to open spaces where deliberation on issues of public interest is encouraged and the range of issues subject of deliberation is enlarged.

[1] In the IPCC report, knowledge users are named knowledge actors.

3 Metaphors for New System Representations

According to the above scheme, production of knowledge can bring to shared visions through processes of deliberation supported by knowledge filtering and knowledge use. Our contribution here aims to propose three metaphors that may improve understanding the complexity of urban–rural relationships when considering urban food systems.

The first metaphor we propose is 'metabolism'. With this, we look at cities as (socio-technical) systems whose life is based on circulation of resources that enter in the city (food, water, energy, materials), which are transformed into goods and services and produce leftovers that get out of the city as waste (Swyngedouw et al. 2006). As in living organisms, malfunctioning circulation may alter the functioning of the system. Socio-technical systems regulate these flows, and regulation and its outcomes are affected by power distribution, conflicts and cooperation between actors. The metaphor of metabolism is particularly useful to raise awareness about the limits to growth and the vulnerability of cities, as it makes visible the dependency of cities from a regular flow of resources coming from the outside, namely, from rural areas, and a correspondent outflow of waste to the outside. The metabolism metaphor also highlights the relevance of speed. A regular flow of resources entails an appropriate timing, adding the time dimension to the coordination among system elements and processes. A slow decision-making may alter the metabolism and make a crisis emerge. Moreover, given the same rate of consumption of inputs per unit of output, the concept of metabolism implies that the faster the processes of transformation, the higher the pressure on resources, as in a given unit of time more cycles of the same process can be performed. Strategies for slowing down the urban metabolism could, therefore, reduce the pressure on resources.

The second metaphor is 'circular economy' (Stahel 2016). Circular economy – which is "restorative and regenerative" (Ellen MacArthur Foundation 2015) and aims to keep and re-create the highest value of products for as long as possible, eliminating waste (European Commission 2015) – is generally opposed to the 'linear economy'. In a linear economy, in fact, exchange values don't embody the social costs of production, for example, pollution and resource depletion (Andersen 2007). Costs of waste management are only partially embodied into prices of the commodities, as a relevant part of waste management – as well as its costs – burdens on the shoulders of public administrations and citizens. As producers pay only a fraction of waste management, there is no incentive to reusing or recycling leftovers, unless the price of leftovers is higher than the costs of waste management. As a consequence, in a linear economy, there is not much distinction between leftovers and waste.

In a circular economy, waste tends to zero (Ellen MacArthur Foundation 2014). As producers and consumers pay the full cost (including social cost) of commodities, production processes are designed and organized in space so to make leftovers become inputs for other processes. A circular economy needs a systemic, rather than an analytical, approach. Whereas the linear economy is represented of a sum of individual activities, the circular economy is based on interdependence between production processes and active search for matching between leftovers' demand and supply. Unlike the linear economy, matching between demand and supply is not only based on exchange value but mainly on use value discovered through exchange of information about the physical, chemical and biological nature of the leftovers and through active research to exploit potential use. The rule of cascading (Ellen MacArthur Foundation 2014), a pillar of the circular economy, implies a ranking of value of successive uses of materials from the highest to the lowest value, so that, for example, before turning matter into energy – which has the lowest value per unit – a series of other transformation should be performed. Moreover, a circular economy implies a design of spatial proximities between producers so to minimize the logistic costs of leftover management.

The third metaphor is 'assemblage'. As known, the concept was proposed in the 1970s by the French philosophers Deleuze and Guattari and successively used by social scientists to make sense of the diversity and complexity of processes occurring into a society (De Landa 2016). In a city, people meet, talk, do things in common, fight, make projects, break out relations and transform their physical environment. Buildings, open spaces, infrastructures and technologies affect the way people interact and the way they operate on the environment (Moragues-Faus and Sonnino 2018). Assemblages are thus socio-technical entities, involving both human and non-human actors. The parts of an assemblage contribute to perform functions they were not necessarily designed to perform: a screwdriver is designed to screw, but it can be used as a weapon or as component of an artistic piece (Gharajedaghi 2011). In assemblages, order emerges through adaptation and learning rather than by design. In a city, power is distributed, so that any change needs to be carried out by coalitions of actors each of them having different visions and representations. Assemblages provide a metaphor to represent emerging order from interaction between independent elements and the contingency of this order.

The assemblage metaphor is useful both as a heuristic tool and as a strategic tool. As a heuristic tool, it helps to understand the drivers of urban change, the evolution of urban processes, the structures of power and the barriers to change. As a strategic tool, the metaphor of assemblage helps to identify forces that can be enrolled in processes of change and to design governance patterns (McCann et al. 2013). For example, it addresses the issue of establishing links between different policy, social, economic and administrative networks in the design of policies for multidimensional problems. It also tells us something about the long and complex processes of building shared goals between components with different interests.

4 New Representations for New Urban–Rural Relations

The above-described metaphors are particularly fit to the understanding of urban–rural relations towards transition to sustainability. With the development of trade, cities have emancipated from the constraints posed by the neighbouring countryside, becoming attractors of flows of material and symbolic resources from distant places (Woods 2009). Contemporary cities, if we abstract from their administrative boundaries, may be seen as urban–rural assemblages, wherein specific activities of rural areas, independently where they are located, are functionally linked to parts of the urban metabolism. For example, the present levels of European meat and dairy consumption could not be possible without the flows of soybeans, coming from Brazil or Argentina, feeding intensive livestock farms, nor the fresh fruit consumption patterns of the Londoners could be conceived without Spanish or African supply. These commercial patterns have become so consolidated that it could hardly be thought that an unexpected disruption of one part would leave other parts unaffected. For instance, after the garbage crisis in the city of Naples (Italy) in the early 2000s, the city administration signed an agreement with garbage incinerators in the North Europe to reduce the pressure on local landfills. It would not be possible to understand the management of the city of Naples without considering the existence of these plants.

With the emancipation from their neighbouring countryside, cities have lost a feedback function, signalling scarcity and depletion of resources. In an increasingly volatile environment, resource scarcity and depletion add up to instability of conditions for regular trade, to climate change and to backfires of the weakening of neighbouring rural areas, to make cities deeply vulnerable and unsustainable. As Cumming et al. (2014) suggest, these pathways bring to 'red traps'.

Transition to sustainability, according with the bioregional paradigm, should be imagined as a local/regional multi-scale process of disassembling and reassembling people, processes, relations and spaces. In an increasing volatile environment, a stronger connection to local resources, that is, a partial relocalization, is key to a risk management strategy, trading short-term advantages for long-term security (Thayer 2003). This would imply a progressive reconfiguration – based on the principle of local preference and circular economy – of socio-technical systems built around food, waste, water and energy.

This process of relocalization, however, could be thought – at least partially – as a return to self-sufficient, isolated spaces. In fact, a degree of independence of both rural and urban areas will be unavoidable and even desirable, as each of them will continue to look for opportunities linked to global networks and to keep a sufficient level of freedom and autonomy. Relocalization, then, needs to be based on economic, aesthetic and ethical appeal and requires negotiation among a variety of actors.

Adopting the metaphors of assemblages, metabolism and circular economy implies an approach to governance much different from past experiences. It implies integrating market regulation with social and technical rules. It gives public administrations and civil society a much greater say on market mechanisms, involving a diversity of actors, visions and representations in a common appraisal effort based on deliberation.

5 Building Sustainable Urban-Bioregional Food Systems

Food is an important component of urban metabolism. Every day people need food for their basic survival; for all people to be fed, production, processing, distribution and waste disposal processes are needed. The way these activities are organized, the available infrastructures and the rules that regulate the activities that affect the food and nutrition security of different groups contribute to the general welfare and to environmental health. Likewise, the way people behave can affect the way activities are organized in space and in time. The challenge of the transition to sustainable food systems is thus developing shared representations of the food system that affects daily people's practices.

Linear approaches represent food systems as mono-functional, as they generated only a limited set of outcomes, for example, stressing on the goal of food availability may imply a focus on production and producers and, therefore, an understatement of the role of social inequalities. Linear approaches cannot address the multidimensionality of food (Allen and Prosperi 2016) and the multiplicity of food system outcomes, such as health, environment and social outcomes. A system approach, on the contrary, postulates that actors and activities can generate a multiplicity of outcomes, not seldom implying trade-offs, dilemmas and unintended consequences, and that each outcome can be performed by a multiplicity of actors and activities. Updating the representation of food systems is thus a priority for transition also at a bioregional level.

For local food systems to be sustainable, an updated approach to food policies would then endeavour to answer questions like: what are the outcomes expected from a food system? What trade-offs may occur? What are the unexpected consequences of food system activities? Which are relevant actors and activities in producing sustainability and food security outcomes? How to regulate actors and activities so to have better outcomes? How to improve practices? How to overcome barriers to the achievement of better outcomes? How to trigger and develop self-reliant, fair and safe local food systems? The following scheme (Fig. 2) frames the transition strategies to food system sustainability.

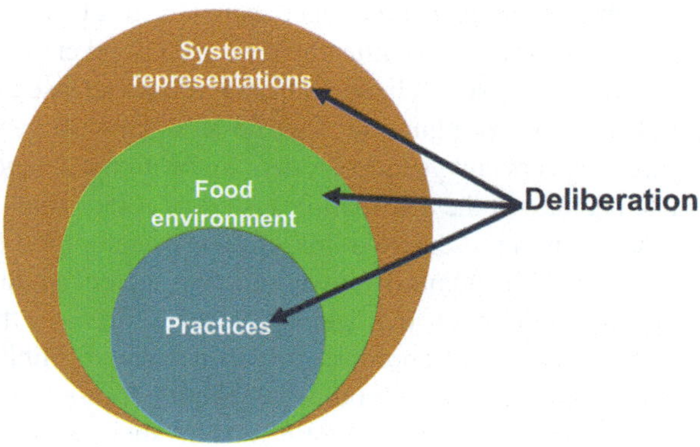

Fig. 2 Framework of deliberation-driven transition strategies towards food system sustainability. (Source: Authors' elaboration)

The scheme links the process of framing daily practices with governance of knowledge. Transition strategies should be able to change actors' practices through a democratic process centred upon deliberation. The challenge is to enlarge the area of issues being problematized through public deliberation and to guarantee deliberation mechanisms safe from manipulation. In the case of food, we assist to a growth in the number of issues that are discussed in the public sphere and submitted to ethical problematization, and problematization is a first step towards a change of frames and new rules for choice. For example, in Italy, the problematization of the origin of food has created a strong pressure to a relocalization of food consumption and production. As consumers increasingly ask to know the origin of the food they choose, producers reorganize the value chain in order to promote national or local products.

Food system representations – of the actors and their relations, their activities and their outcomes –frame the meanings people give to their food practices. New meanings for food, for example, in relation to environmental, health or social issues, encourage people to develop new skills and to embody new sets of things into their practices. The campaign on food waste, which started from grassroots initiatives and upscaled to national and international level, has helped people problematize their daily practices (Tucker and Farrelly 2016). However, it is to be recognized that top-down campaigns, aimed at imposing top-down representations, are not necessarily successful. System representations are filtered to consumers through their food environment, which determines the set of material, symbolic and relational conditions that affect consumers' choice. In a given food environment, people can have access to food through direct entitlements (self-production), indirect entitlements (income to buy food) and transfer entitlements (food provided through social networks or through state subsidies) (Brunori et al. 2013). People can have easy access to a larger or a narrower range of food items, depending on distance, mobility and income. The combination of these entitlements depends both on subjective conditions of people and to their food environment. Everybody has needs and preferences in relation to food, but needs and preferences are enabled, and constrained, by everyday life patterns (e.g. workplace, social life, house life) on one side and by systems of food provision on the other side. Blaming the consumers for wrong food practices may not be as successful as a thorough and shared understanding of the food environments that influence them (Evans 2011).

In the scheme above illustrated (Fig. 2), food choice embodied in food practices is a driver of system change. Decreased or increased demand can send signals to market actors to adjust the supply. New knowledge at consumers' level can be shared to peers and generate system innovation. Changes in shopping patterns stimulate changes in the distribution system, a component of the food environment.

A system representation linking food system, food environments and food practice gives public administrations and civil society an important room for manoeuvre that links, integrates and readjusts market forces in the creation of food environments conducive of appropriate food behaviour. Public administrations can affect people's entitlement to food by regulating access to urban gardens, by organizing public procurement, by promoting healthy dietary guidelines and by regulating food distribution. Circular economy patterns can be created through education, incentives and penalties and infrastructures (Suárez-Eiroa et al. 2019). As most of these matters are normally regulated by different bodies, appropriate governance patterns can foster communication between the relevant sectors.

The interplay between practices, food environments and system representation depends on the availability of deliberative spaces. Food policies coherent with a system approach would set forums to foster knowledge creation, develop data silos to monitor urban metabolism and its sustainability, establish cross-departmental strategic units and finance projects that address emerging problems with innovative approaches. Knowledge should reach all involved actors to raise awareness and provide feedback for individual and collective behaviour. In a logic of transition towards sustainability, a more secure, sustainable and healthier food environment – at local, urban and bioregional level – is the one that opens spaces of deliberation to all actors to reflect on food sustainability, healthiness and morality and to provide input for knowledge management and for policies.

6 Concluding Remarks

Emerging sustainability issues are increasingly challenging the capacity of cities to cope and anticipate future and uncertain adversities. An improved understanding of those drivers and related interactions, especially related to the urban–rural relations, can help urban administrators change paradigms of decision-making to build resilient cities through a transition to more sustainable practices and governance arrangements. The present work has disentangled a specific reflection on the governance principles, regulating the urban–rural links, that are necessary to address new sustainability challenges. The transition towards sustainability requires a deep change in the way people know and live the city. New knowledge brings to modification of practices, and novelties contribute to new knowledge creation. Within this framework, spaces of deliberation on large issues of public interest are needed to develop knowledge and share visions towards more sustainable practices regulating urban–rural interplays. To improve the understanding of the complexity of urban–rural relationships, when considering urban food systems, we have applied three metaphors: the metabolism concept, the circular economy and the assemblage metaphor. This triangulation of metaphors is particularly fit to the understanding of urban–rural relations towards transition to sustainability. It approaches governance much differently from past experiences, allowing for integrating market regulation with social and technical rules, giving public administrations and civil society a much greater say on market mechanisms, involving a diversity of actors, visions and representations in a common appraisal effort based on deliberation. Thus, according with the bioregional paradigm, transition to sustainability can be imagined as a progressive reconfiguration of socio-technical systems (composed of food, waste, water, energy) built on a local/regional multi-scale process of disassembling and reassembling people, processes, relations and spaces. With particular regard to urban and bioregional food system, local food policies can trigger tool applications to foster knowledge creation, retrieve data on urban metabolism and its sustainability, launch cross-cutting strategic groups and promote innovative projects. A regional – or local – foodshed based on knowledge sharing among all the actors can allow for transition to sustainability if spaces of deliberation are open, comprehensive and supported by appropriate policies oriented towards food sustainability, healthiness, morality and knowledge management.

References

Allen, T., & Prosperi, P. (2016). Modeling sustainable food systems. *Environmental Management, 57*(5), 956–975.

Andersen, M. S. (2007). An introductory note on the environmental economics of the circular economy. *Sustainability Science, 2*(1), 133–140.

Brunori, G. et al. (2013). *Creating resilient food systems for enhancing food and nutrition security*; TRANSMANGO: EU KBBE.2013.2.5-01 Grant Agreement No. 613532. Leuven, Belgium.

Castells, M. (2011). *The rise of the network society: The information age: Economy, society, and culture* (Vol. 1). The Atrium/Southern Gate/Chichester/West Sussex, UK: Wiley.

Cumming, G. S., Buerkert, A., Hoffmann, E. M., Schlecht, E., von Cramon-Taubadel, S., & Tscharntke, T. (2014). Implications of agricultural transitions and urbanization for ecosystem services. *Nature, 515*(7525), 50–57.

De Landa, M. (2016). *Assemblage theory*. Edinburgh: Edinburgh University Press.

Ellen MacArthur Foundation. (2014). *Towards the circular economy: Accelerating the scale-up across global supply chains*. Geneva: MacArthur Foundation.

Ellen MacArthur Foundation. (2015). *Delivering the circular economy: A toolkit for policymakers*. Geneva: MacArthur Foundation.

European Commission. (2015). *Closing the loop – An EU action plan for the circular economy*. Brussels: European Commission.

Evans, D. (2011). Blaming the consumer–once again: The social and material contexts of everyday food waste practices in some English households. *Critical Public Health, 21*(4), 429–440.

Gharajedaghi, J. (2011). *Systems thinking: Managing chaos and complexity: A platform for designing business architecture*. Amsterdam/Boston/Heidelberg/London/New York/Oxford/Paris/San Diego/San Francisco/Singapore/Sydney/Tokyo: Elsevier.

Kasimis, C., & Zografakis, S. (2014). *Economic crisis and return to agriculture*. Athens: Pedio Publishing.

Lowe, P., Murdoch, J., & Ward, N. (1995). Networks in rural development: Beyond exogenous and endogenous models. In J. D. van der Ploeg & G. van Dijk (Eds.), *Beyond modernization* (pp. 87–105). Assen: Van Gorcum.

McCann, E., Roy, A., Ward, e K. (2013). Urban pulse-assembling/worlding cities. *Urban Geography, 34*(5), 581–89. https://doi.org/10.1080/02723638.2013.793905.

Moragues-Faus, A., & Sonnino, R. (2018). Re-assembling sustainable food cities: An exploration of translocal governance and its multiple agencies. *Urban Studies*, 0042098018763038.

Ray, C. (1999). Endogenous development in the era of reflexive modernity. *Journal of Rural Studies, 15*(3), 257–267.

Revi, A., et al. (2014). Urban areas. In C. B. Field et al. (Eds.), *Climate change 2014: Impacts, adaptation, and vulnerability. Part A: Global and Sectoral aspects. Contribution of working group II to the fifth assessment report of the intergovernmental panel on climate change* (pp. 535–612). Cambridge: Cambridge University Press.

Shove, E., Pantzar, M., & Watson, M. (2012). *The dynamics of social practice: Everyday life and how it changes*. London/Thousand Oaks/New Delhi: Sage.
Stahel, W. R. (2016). Circular economy: A new relationship with our goods and materials would save resources and energy and create local jobs. *Nature, 531*(7595), 435–439.
Suárez-Eiroa, B., Fernández, E., Méndez-Martínez, G., & Soto-Oñate, D. (2019). Operational principles of circular economy for sustainable development: Linking theory and practice. *Journal of Cleaner Production, 214*, 952–961.
Swyngedouw, E., Kaika, M., & Heynen, N. C. (2006). *In the nature of cities: Urban political ecology and the politics of urban metabolism*. London/New York: Routledge.
Thayer, R. L. (2003). *LifePlace: Bioregional thought and practice*. Berkeley, CA: University of California Press.
Tucker, C. A., & Farrelly, T. (2016). Household food waste: The implications of consumer choice in food from purchase to disposal. *Local Environment, 21*(6), 682–706.
Van der Ploeg, J. D. (1994). *Born from within: Practice and perspectives of endogenous rural development*. Assen: Van Gorcum.
Verburg, P. H., van Berkel, D. B., van Doorn, A. M., van Eupen, M., & van den Heiligenberg, H. A. (2010). Trajectories of land use change in Europe: A model-based exploration of rural futures. *Landscape Ecology, 25*(2), 217–232.
Woods, M. (2009). Rural geography: Blurring boundaries and making connections. *Progress in Human Geography, 33*(6), 849–858.

Looking Forward: Some Opportunities and Challenges for Bioregional Planning in Current Policies and Planning Framework

David Fanfani

1 Regionalisms and Bioregionalism: Fostering Pro-activity and Subsidiarity

Regional scale, even if in accordance with different disciplinary "nuances" and heuristic aims, turned out to be in recent decades one of the more relevant issues in (re) framing the discourse about concepts such as places and regions, economic/local development issues, and government/governance models and institutions (Paasi 2002, 2009) and about related human settlement patterns and disposals. Despite the accent posed on the role of regional/local endowments – either in terms of embedded skills and knowledge and of natural resources and landscape qualities – new regionalism mainly conceived regional, geographical, and institutional spaces as helpful elements to better rearticulate the overwhelming global economic model either in terms of corporate competitiveness or of governance institutions, aimed more to pursue economic effectiveness than social cohesion and environmental fairness and sustainability (Morgan 2004). Obviously it is not this kind of regionalism, conceived as a latest – financial – stage of the capitalist accumulation process (Wheeler 2002), that can be assumed as a model to support the recovery of a bioregional discourse concerning planning and human development.

Moreover the same can be spoken out about some interpretive models that – related to the observed regional dimension assumed by the urbanization process – coined the framework of the "city region" (Rodrìguez-Pose 2008; Jonas 2012) as leading paradigm sometime adopted as "naturally" given, either in terms of analytical practices or as design reference model, and not submitted to any critical revision.

Notwithstanding, if these two approaches to regionalism and "city regionalism" – very roughly rendered in their possible mainstream interpretations – are not

D. Fanfani (✉)
Architecture Department-Dida, Florence University, Florence, Italy
e-mail: david.fanfani@unifi.it

D. Fanfani, A. Matarán Ruiz (eds.), *Bioregional Planning and Design: Volume I*,
https://doi.org/10.1007/978-3-030-45870-6_11

really close to the bioregional approach and to the regionalist legacy in which it entrenches, it is not to overlook the relevance that the proposed "shift" of the human geography discourse entails also for a bioregional reframing of regional planning and local development matters.

First of all it is worth noting how some remarkable strands of "progressive regionalism" (Mc Kinnon 2017) paired and enriched – addressing especially issues of economic and spatial fairness – the mentioned mainstream approach. Moreover, that combined with some renewed research on local productive systems – as exploiting long-lasting social capital and knowledge endowments – helped to best outline the underpinning and not negligible role of local/regional heritage in triggering "from below" local development processes. This, furthermore, also accounting for the very endogenous nature of development process itself and of self-relied import replacing economies.

This kind of vision finds room and echoes within the bioregional discourse, showing how current debate on human settlement and urban/metropolitan development could meet and cross some important issues of bioregionalism as well as be ignited and reframed by its integrated and holistic approach. In particular, that challenging crossed revision calls us to best focus at least on some issues that feature the bioregional discourse, which are not so explicitly considered in the general regionalist geography and territorial sciences.

1.1 Subsidiarity and Urban/Rural New Alliance for the City Bioregion

Co-evolution and Endogenous Approach

First of all for the bioregional approach – regardless of the various scales at which this paradigm is adopted (Sale 1991) – natural or ecosystem structures and functions constitute the measure to which refers either development goals and policies, as well as planning and design tools aimed to achieve a regenerative, biophilic, and fair settlement environment. That, according to a co-evolutionary approach (Norgaard 1994), points out innovation as a field of collaborative practices between nature and culture, aimed to integrated ecosystem recovery and "neo-ecosystems" creation (Magnaghi 2010). This according with le "genie naturel" (Clément 2012) through which mankind can cooperate in accordance with wider general "natural" laws and pursuing "co-development" endogenous processes (Jacobs 2001). This approach overcomes the passive, or at the best, adaptive role designed for ecosystem and long-lasting natural endowments in planning policies and assigns them a pro-active and underpinning role in defining spatial and development scenario (Becattini 2015). Moreover, it calls for the adoption and enhancement of a fitting scale and susbsidiarity principle according to which at each territorial level best pertain specific powers, committed functions and endeavors. This is according to joint sovereignty, responsibility, and solidarity principles in order to guide resources management and deliberative processes, especially in terms of self-relied development policies and fair "commons" exploitation (Ostrom 2013).

A Bioregional Place Identity: A New Urban/Rural Alliance and Bio-generative Patterns
Co-evolutionary approach and subsidiarity pose the consequent demand to reframe in terms of cohesion, solidarity, and integration of the urban/rural relationship. This with the aim to reframe this duality not in terms of mutual dissolution – as depicted in some "planetary urbanization visions" – but reaffirming the mutuality and complementarity between the two domains – even if not assured by taken for granted inherited categories – and contextually and reflexively re(de)fined in each case and regional/local context (Brenner and Schmid 2015). In particular, as it is well pointed out by Thayer in his chapter of this book, the bioregional discourse – as aimed to pursue balanced settlement patterns jointly with spatial and environmental justice and fairness – can't avoid to contour the key elements suitable to promote and support a new alliance between urban and rural domain and between the function of social actors and the forces that refer to them. These elements demand, indeed, for a "place specific" and more reflexive approach suitable and strong enough to render the innovative ways in which the urban and rural dimensions very often weave together and merge. All this exists in some spatial context where it is very difficult, sometimes – especially in Western and European countries – to envision the urban as a built inhabited core surrounded, at the supra-local scale, by wooded or farmland areas scarcely populated with small rural centers. Urban and rural now mutually define a dense thread of social, environmental, and cultural relations and flows that, otherwise, don't demand, in the bioregional vision, for a definitive dismissal of the rural as finally withering out in an overwhelming urban environment growth. On the contrary, it calls – as well highlighted by Thayer – to reverse the current unbalanced relationship between urban and rural that privileges the former. All that entails a strategic commitment aimed at the recovery of sustainable settlement patterns and to support a shared awareness about the values that rural and natural areas embody. This particularly concerning the ecosystem services those areas can deliver for the settlement's overall resilience, amenity, and for the inhabitant's well-being. In this context arises, among other matters, an important pressing challenge in the field of planning to come up with innovative and "bio-generative" design patterns (Thayer 2003) as heuristic and normative models. Those shifting patterns are the ones best suited either to take into account, appraise, and represent the complexity of the relationship between our anthropogenic world and our ecosystems, while at the same time providing us some new normative and also narrative models (EDORA-ESPON 2010), based on relational, integrated, and prestational elements.

2 Bioregional Communitarianism: Local Practices and Reframed Planning

As mentioned, subsidiarity, which casts the form of a new bioregional institutional project, needs to be fed and fostered by newly empowered bottom-up social activism and relationships. Ones that very often spontaneously rise up, whereas it has to find space and public hearings in open, participative, and often radical and strongly advocated planning practices and tools.

2.1 Local Bioregional Community by Practices

If the bioregion's design is properly contoured according to various scales (Sale 1991, p. 52–66), its progressive development will be primarily fueled and fostered by "community-oriented" actions at the human/local scale.

Nevertheless, this "movement" toward local empowerment needs to be fostered in its bottom-up origins and can't be conceived only according from a top-down devolution process, often rendered as the sole approach in administrative and bureaucratic terms. All that "movement" entails the necessity of reconnecting the institutional framework to a system of localized actions and socially shared needs with the fundamental aim to finally pursue joint goals of local development and ecosystem enhancement and protection (M'Goonigle 1999). That means pursuing a process of "democracy building from below," enabling and educating inhabitants to cope with issues of resource use and depletion at the appropriate scale. A process that results in the possibility to express on behalf of concerned people some deliberative powers and voices about those issues, then in bringing "back to the earth" dilemmas no longer treatable, in effective terms, at global level or according to the inherited dialectic between global and local (Latour 2017).

Manifold experiences and practices "on the field" reveal how the bioregion reconstruction process – be it conceived either to recover the relationship between urban and rural domain or to enhance the overall conditions of regional/local geo-ecosystems – is mainly triggered by localized and grassroots re-inhabiting and stewardship initiatives on behalf of population, activists, NGO associations, and similar groups. Practices that very often stem from conflicts related to public or private supported projects concerning local resource, values or "commons" exploitation (e.g. farmland consumption, water corporate management, landscape degradation, building waste treatment plants, infrastructure constructions, land grabbing, etc.).

In some other cases, such practices are aimed to reclaim, recover, and appropriate for community interest goals, abandoned and disrupted places, and/or the development of new "civic" bioregional fair economies based on mutual trust and self-help (e.g., agri-food communities and pacts, local renewable energy systems, local currencies, time banks, etc.).

It is from these spontaneous aggregations and practices – often very well organized – that sense of belonging originates and develops, which firstly paves the way to the reconstruction of stronger community-based relationships and trust starting from the places of stewardship and care.

Nevertheless, what is meant here it is not to recover and reintroduce a nostalgic and comforting idea of community – that in the age of global mobility of goods, information and peoples, and of strong interconnections of problems and drawbacks - it is no longer possible to conceive as a selfish and closed "destiny and blood community". On the contrary, in this arising framework, the form and the idea of a "project community" (Castells 1997) are able not only to counter and resist local shocks but also with new capacities to act in an equitable and proactive way coping with the local splitting processes induced by the globally induced forces.

The critical focus and challenge entailed by this matter is how to translate, at least partially, these kinds of grassroots practices and bottom-up initiatives within the framework of the institutional planning and design tools and how it could reshape, in this commitment, the role of the bioregional planner. That especially, in terms of which are the issues and priorities she/he has to cope with in this challenging commitment that very often needs to critically and swiftly act in contexts affected by unbalanced power relationships. All this will be addressed, at least in part, in the next paragraph.

2.2 *The Socially Constructive and Revealing Role of Planning (And Not an Easy One for the Planners)*

As it is not possible for our society to trigger and enhance subsidiarity using only a top-down devolution movement, likewise bioregional planning will hardly unfold its potential without revisioning current technocratic spatial planning practices and institutional forms. It turns out to be worth, in this sense, the recovery of some underpinning issues inherited from the regional planning tradition. About that it firstly comes to the foreground the recovery and development of the educational value and role of regional planning that, drawing also on the RPAA and southern regionalism of E.W. Odum, represents a key factor in promoting place awareness jointly with community commitment. A dimension mainly ignored by current forms of planning.

That direction means employing a requirement of going beyond the best intended informational, communicative, and hearing practices in planning and design tools, to focus ourselves on the requisite cornerstone of firstly developing and empowering open and shared knowledge about territory, place, and city. The aim here would be to enable citizens and inhabitants to develop a critical eye and proactive role toward establishing policies and planning goals as genuine participants in the process.

Furthermore, intertwined with this “Looking Forward” approach, of better engaging citizens, goes together an aim of “reactivating” contextual skillsets and knowledge bases, not yet having been totally forgotten or made inoperative by the current and overwhelming technocratic approach that dominates planning. According to this proposed evolution, the planning role is not so much geared to “explain” applying technical procedures presumed as being at the heart or “very” nature of territorial features and processes; rather it turns out to be also a “revealing” role, that is, one aimed to unravel embodied regional and territory potentialities entrenched in the long run, but not yet expressed, as – quoting again Benton MacKaye – “what that belongs to the ages” (B. MacKaye 1928, cit.) and which are very often cognitive endowments of contextual and ordinary knowledge.

In this framework, the “enabling” value of the planning process relates, first of all, to the structuration of shared and inclusive deliberative process aimed to elicit such a cognitive domain in the context of spatial planning tool formation. Nevertheless, in accordance with the bioregional paradigm, participative planning techniques and practices cannot be considered as neutral technical procedures, that is, it has to take into account current “power asymmetries” and imbalances, either in terms of resource use and distribution or in relation to the socio-spatial arrangements corresponding to those imbalances.

That goes to particularly address the different “voice” possibilities (Hirshmann 1970) that the various social actors are able to exert within the planning field and, especially, the empowerment of the various “weak interest” (e.g., ecosystems, future generations, urban agriculture, etc.) in coping with more structured conditioning of social group and lobbying interests.

Conceived in these terms, a bioregional approach entails a strong promotion and practice of empowering action, and sometimes of advocacy, on behalf of the planner himself/herself. In accordance with engaging that planner role and responsibility, it is not necessarily contoured as a “third” and neutral one in reference to the issues at stake. The participative and deliberative process construction itself also encompasses social demand and a problematic framework requiring reframing as well as addressing arising conflict management issues.

In this sense, what resonates as best fitting – and a little bit comforting – may be Rob Thayer’s words according to which the regional planner role if it “… do not provide professional planner with a road to riches … (it) … can provide considerably more in the way of a moral and ethical job satisfaction for their participants” (Thayer 2003, p. 170).

3 Integrating Spatial Planning and Local Development: Promoting Self-Reliance and Fairness

Indeed, and finally, bioregional planning, considering its interwoven social, ecological, and fairness goals, has also to deal with development and sustaining of the *living in place* issues. Aiming to express and pursue new ways to generate "expansion" and "co-production" to sustain life (Jacobs 2001, cit). Drawing on Berg and Dasmann (Berg and Dasmann 1977), the latter means "… following the necessities and pleasure of life as they are uniquely presented by a particular site, and evolving ways to ensure long-term occupancy of that site." Whereas, substantially, *reinhabitation* is the process by which some humans, either individuals or groups, learn again how to be *living in place*, settling there according to the limits and potentialities of that particular place. This also starting from conditions of disruption due to past or inherited production, exploitive practices, or "lost landscapes" (Power 1996).

In this framework, too, continuity between an RPAA regionalist movement and bioregionalism appears evident. According to MacKaye (1928, cit), indeed, regional planning has to be conceived – starting from human needs and human desires and bequeathed limits of nature. As an activity "revealing" of the potentialities of a region – often not evident to sectoral gaze - and of its various opportunities "to control a single actuality" (MacKaye 1928, cit. p. 153). Planning, then, is not a matter to grasp upon with unique and technically correct answers, in a linear/mechanical process, adhering to a previously defined set of sectorally established issues, but instead to envision some possible co-evolutive pathways and scenarios either at different scales (Sale 1991, cit.) or according with different time thresholds. So it is also – in accordance with bioregionalist claims – a highly "strategic" activity pursuing "… the visualizing within a region of coordinated action for the purpose of general human living" (MacKaye 1928, cit. p. 153).

It is in accordance with these overall coordinates that – we believe – bioregional development and economy discourse can be unfolded and specified. Natural limits become potentialities, in a revealing process hinged upon the study of the long-lasting and regional heritage, inherited in the long term, and of the co-evolutionary process from which such heritage originated. In this kind of discourse also "endogenous recovery" (Gotlieb 1996) or "regenerative" regions and, especially, city regions are worth to be considered and reframed in an innovative way. That is, as heuristic model that denotate opportunities to retrieve the condition of *living-in-place* through development of place-based and proximity economies. Especially by reducing exogenous dependency - in terms of energy, matter and good flows – and also by empowering circular flows as well as deeper self-reliance, although not self-sufficient and closed/autarchic-economies.

Here it rests another challenge for bioregional approach in planning domain. That is, pursuing local bioregional development means not only analyzing and appraising natural and ecosystem limits, depletion and functions. It also seeks for pointing out the opportunities for recovering economies based on the strong and retrieved general interaction between nature and culture, long-lasting spatial patterns, and natural structures. This turns out in "revealing," through this relation, the best regional/local development strategy and scenarios, according to a measure of human well-being, justice, and *living world* stewardship. It entails for the bioregional planner to cope with the endeavor of denoting, representing, and mentoring this integration, either by introducing innovative issues and methods in the field of planning or by supporting and triggering bottom-up participatory practices. It is a new way forward to look to our territorial heritage, as a "genetic pool," representing – in analogy with Roegen's flow-fund model – both the active, ruling reproductive conditions and the matter concerned with the development process itself. Therefore, this idea of local bioregional development calls for new ways to explore and conceive our regional resources, as a model of planning and design aimed to purpose new key issues and recognize grassroots practices for bioregional recovery and co-evolution as well as introducing and proposing new integrative methods of survey and design fitting with this goal. It is not an easy agenda or endeavor for practitioners and "reflexive" bioregional "researchers in action" to accomplish. Some possible "steps forward" and other issues, stemming from facing that challenge, will be explored in Volume II of this book.

References

Becattini, G. (2015). *La coscienza dei luoghi. Il territorio come soggetto corale*. Roma: Donzelli.

Berg, P., & Dasmann, R. (1977). Reinhabiting California. *The Ecologist, 7*(10), 399–401.

Brenner, N., & Schmid, C. (2015). Toward a new epistemology of the urban? *City, 19*(2–3), 151–182.

Castells, M. (1997). *The power of identity. The information age: Economy, society, and clture* (Vol. II). Molden, MA: Blackwell.

Clément, G. (2012). *Jardins, paysage et génie naturel*. Paris: Collége de France.

EDORA-ESPON, (2010). European development opportunities for rural areas. *Draft Final Report, Part A & B,* (Version 1), Luxembourg, https://www.espon.eu/sites/default/files/attachments/EDORA_Draft_Final_Report_Version_2.4_April_2010.pdf. Accessed January 15, 2019.

Gotlieb, Y. (1996). *Development, environment and global dysfunctions. Toward sustainable recovery*. Delray Beach, FL: St.Lucie Press.

Hirshmann, A. (1970). *Exit, voice, and loyalty : Responses to decline in firms, organizations, and states*. Cambridge, MA: Harvard University Press.

Jacobs, J. (2001). *The nature of economies*. New York: Vintage Books.

Jonas, A. E. G. (2012). City-regionalism: Question of distribution and politics. *Progress in Human Geography, 36*(6), 822–829.

Mc Kinnon, D. (2017). Regional inequality, regional policy and progressive regionalism. *Sounding* (online Journal). https://www.lwbooks.co.uk/soundings/65/regional-policy-progressive-regionalism. Accessed January 12, 2020.

Latour, B. (2017). *Où atterrir? Comme s'orienter en politique*. Paris: La Découverte.

MacKaye, B. (1928). *The new exploration. A Philosophy of regional planning*. Urbana_Champaign, IL: University of Illinois Press.

Magnaghi, A. (2010). *Il Progetto Locale. Torino*. eBollati Boringhieri. (II_{th} edition reviewed). (English translation of first edition, (2005) *The Urban villages: A charter for democracy and local self-sustainable*. London: Zed Books).

M'Goonigle, R. M. (1999). Ecological economics and political ecology: Towards a necessary synthesis. *Ecological Economics, 28*, 11–26.

Morgan, K. (2004). Sustainable Regions: governance, innovation and scale. *European Planning Studies, 12*(6), 871–89.

Norgaard, R. B. (1994). *Development betrayed. The end of progress and a coevolutionary revisioning of the future*. London/New York: Routledge.

Ostrom, E. (2013). Regions and regional dynamics. *Governing the Commons. The evolution of institutions fro collective actions*. Cambridge (UK): Cambridge University Press.

Paasi, A. (2002). Place and region: Regional worlds and words. *Progress in Human Geography, 28*(6), 802–811.

Paasi, A. (2009). Regions and regional dynamics. In C. Rumford (Ed.), *Handbook of European studies* (pp. 464–484). London: Sage.

Power, T. M. (1996). *Lost landscape and failed economies. The search for Places*. Washington, DC: Island Press.

Rodrìguez-Pose, A. (2008). The rise of the 'City region' concept and its development policy implications. *European Planning Studies, 16*(8), 1025–1046.

Sale, K. (1991). *Dwellers in the land. The bioregional vision*. Santa Cruz, CL: New Society Publisher.

Thayer, R. L. (2003). *Life place: Bioregional thought and practice*. Berkley: University of California Press.

Wheeler, S. (2002). The new regionalism: Key characteristics of an emerging movement. *Journal of the American Planning Association, 68*(3), 267–278.

Short Glossary

Maria Rita Gisotti

1 Territory/Territorio

The concept of territory, as conceived by the Italian territorialist school, is intended as "the result of long-lasting co-evolutionary processes between human settlement and the natural environment and between culture and nature" (Magnaghi 1998, p. 3; Magnaghi 1990, p. 26). Its origins lie in the cross-fertilisation between spatial planning and other disciplines: three contributions are considered particularly important for the development of this concept. The first of these is the structural interpretation of places and regions adopted by Italian historical geographers such as Lucio Gambi and Emilio Sereni (who in turn had been inspired by Marc Bloch and Fernand Braudel of the French Annales school). "When we talk about territory" – Gambi states – "we don't evoke an abstract space, but a space defined and determined by specific features or, rather, by a system of relationships that unifies these features" (Gambi 1986, p. 103). The "fairly mature awareness" (ivi) that inhabitants possess of the uniqueness of the region in which they dwell, presides over the construction of that territory. Sereni develops a similar concept, interpreting anthropogenic action as based on "awareness" and a "systematic" vision (Sereni 2001, I ed.1961). The historical-geographic approach is further developed by Claude Raffestin (Raffestin 1984), Angelo Turco's (Turco 1988) reflections on the territorialisation process (which they divide into three main phases) and Massimo Quaini and Claudio Greppi's thoughts on landscapes.

The second important contribution comes from Saverio Muratori and the Italian school of planning typology.[1] Their study of enduring rules for constructing the

[1] Saverio Muratori, Italian architect and historian, 1910–1973. Founder of the outstanding school of urban morphology and architectural typology studies (see Cataldi 2002).

M. R. Gisotti (✉)
Architecture Department-Dida, Florence University, Florence, Italy
e-mail: mariarita.gisotti@unifi.it

D. Fanfani, A. Matarán Ruiz (eds.), *Bioregional Planning and Design: Volume I*,
https://doi.org/10.1007/978-3-030-45870-6_12

built environment at different scales resulted in the definition of a territorial type (an element – together with building type, urban fabric and urban organism – that structures anthropogenic space): this element is defined as a "… concept of territory, appropriate to a given historical period and place that the inhabitants of that place instinctively understand and follow; it is a spontaneous awareness of the area in which they live that encompasses how they experience that territory, how they decide where to settle and where to set up their productive activity" (Caniggia, Maffei 1979, p. 238).

"Awareness" of the relationships that connect territorial structures characterises this conceptualisation of territory; more recently, Giuseppe Dematteis (Dematteis 1995) affirmed that this awareness provided an "implicit" set of guidelines for territory design. The third contribution to enrich the concept of territory comes from critical reflections which Françoise Choay (1973) has described as "humanistic"; these reflections are greatly influenced by the writings and work of Lewis Mumford and of his beloved mentor Patrick Geddes.

Geddes' heritage in territorialist thought is articulated on different levels: one relates to the uniqueness of a place that "…has a true personality; and with this shows some unique elements a personality too much asleep it may be, but which it is the task of the planner, as master artist, to awaken" (Geddes 1915, p. 397); another relates to the city conceived as a "living being, in constant relation to its environment; and with the advantages of this, its limitations too" (ibidem, p. 264); and a third level refers to the "political", collective and community dimensions involved in creating/developing a sense of place. "Eutopia, then, lies in the city around us; and it must be planned and realised, here or nowhere, by us as its citizens each a citizen of both the actual and the ideal city seen increasingly as one" (ibidem p. vii). To sum up, the territorialist approach conceives territory as a co-evolutionary, collective, structural construct, as the expression of an updated relationship between the physical, built and social environment.

2 Territorial Heritage/Patrimonio Territoriale

The concept of territorial heritage stems from a structural interpretation of territory[2]: the definition, provided in the Tuscany Region Spatial Planning Act, L. 65/2014 Rules for territory planning,[3] states that "Territorial heritage includes all long-lasting structures that are the result of co-evolution between the natural environment and human settlements, the value of which is acknowledged for present and future generations". According to this Tuscan law, and the Territorial Regional Plan (PIT)[4] associated with it, these structures refer to four fundamental components

[2] See glosssary entry Territory.

[3] *Norme per il Governo del Territorio.*

[4] *Piano d'Indirizzo Territoriale Regionale* (PIT).

of the territory: hydro-geomorphology, ecosystems, settlements and agroforestry. Allowing for minor lexical variations, most heritage-oriented territorial plans drawn up recently in Italy follow the same approach.

In the "layers" deposited by territorialisation/co-evolution processes, it is possible to identify relationships that interact with parts of these structures which, by virtue of their own "meta-historic rationality" (Baldeschi 2000), appear to be permanent or persistent with respect to transformative historical processes.

These are principles which reflect the morphogenetic role of the territory whose visible interface is represented by the relationships that connect, for instance, soil structure and settlement systems, with the latter usually established in safe areas with stable geo-morphological characteristics. Within this interpretive framework, it is important to note that not all parts of the territory endowed with historic attributes can be considered territorial heritage: areas closely tied to specific social and economic activities that are now extinct or in decline are destined to be preserved only as testimonials.

The heritage approach is then intrinsically dynamic and project oriented; it is somewhat similar to Mumford's "usable past" or to Saverio Muratori's concept of "active history". As the Italian landscape planner and scholar Roberto Gambino has underlined, heritage should not be conceived as an "…inert reservoir of unrelated, heterogeneous 'things' from which to extract whatever is needed from time to time [but rather as] a more-or-less coherent and interconnected system of tangible and intangible historical, cultural and natural heritage, of belonging and relationship networks that connect places and social formations […]. It is here that a survey can discover the 'roots of the future' […] with which to develop territorial plans and projects" (Gambino 2011, p. 140).

The remarkable analytical, interpretive and structural descriptive phase that usually characterises the surveys which underpin the territorialist approach to elaborating strategic scenarios and plans does not aim "to transform the territory into a museum or to copy forms from the past, but rather seeks to obtain guidelines dictated by environmental wisdom for the transformation project" (Magnaghi 2000, p. 64).

A crucial issue is raised at this point, which if not addressed makes it impossible to effectively protect and reproduce territorial heritage: it is essential that all participants in transformative territorial processes (professionals, public administrators, politicians, inhabitants, NGOs) play an active role in recognising the implications of rationality and sustainability (environmental, economic, social) embodied in heritage and in promoting its modernisation as a reservoir of design principles.

3 Structural Invariant/Invariante Strutturale

From an epistemological point of view, the term "invariant" has been borrowed from a wide range of disciplines, ranging from natural sciences to mathematics and linguistics (Saragosa 2011, Maggio 2014). It was first adopted in spatial planning – along with the term "structure" – in the Tuscany Region Law on Spatial Planning n. 5/1995, although a similar term, "territorial invariants", was used in the 1987 Landscape Plan for the Emilia Romagna Region (Bottino 1987, p. 51). The term "structural invariant" was introduced in an innovative disciplinary context where the objective was to provide an alternative to predominantly quantitative/functionalist planning criteria.[5] A structural approach to the territory was developed as a theoretical and operative paradigm capable of addressing sustainable development issues. In addition to the "territorialist school" contribution (Poli 2010), Bernardo Secchi's innovative work on the concept of "territorial structure" should also be mentioned. This concept was applied to Siena's Municipal Plan,[6] drawn up in the early 1990s, and is described in the journal *Urbanistica* (Di Biagi, Gabellini 1990). The Tuscany Planning Law 5/1995 includes the concept of "structural invariants" in its normative apparatus but does not provide a definition. Significant methodological developments for defining this concept came in the following years from working procedures in Tuscany: in 1998 the Territorial Coordination Plan of the Province of Florence identified the basic structural invariant as "the deep structure of the territory, that is, the persistent and resistant underlying structure of settlement and landscape". Territorial Coordination Plans with similar analytical and applicative paradigms were drawn up for three other Tuscan provinces (Arezzo, Prato and Siena) in the same period. The Tuscany Regional Law on Territorial Planning (L. 1/2005) provides a codified normative formulation (albeit a rather confusing one) of structural invariants. Despite the somewhat flawed definition – its formulation employs a repetitive (though not strictly tautological) mechanism to define the invariants and the related concept of the Territory Statute – this law introduces an important development because it highlights the relational value of structural invariants and their role in providing performance parameters for functions associated with sustainable territorial systems (e.g. settlements and landscape patterns, hydrogeomorphological structure, ecological networks, etc.) which enable the sustainable reproduction of the territory. This development represents a fundamental reappraisal of the concept of "structural invariant" in a dynamic and design sense, subtracting it, at least in theory, from erroneous interpretations that focus only on the term "invariant", considering the objects that fall within this category to be "frozen" and in need of static conservative action only (e.g. listed heritage). The Spatial Planning Regional Law 65/2014 that identifies structural invariants as "the specific features, the generative principles and the rules that assure the reproduction of qualifying and identitary components of the territorial heritage" concludes the development of the concept of "structural variant" in Tuscany.

This concept has been applied in some other Italian regional contexts, especially in regional territorial/landscape plans (Gisotti 2016; Marson 2016) as in the Tuscan

[5] There were a number of innovative regional initiatives in this period that were designed to provide an alternative to the outdated 1949 National Planning Act.

[6] Urban Development Plan.

Territorial Regional Plan (PIT), in Calabria (QTRP)[7], Friuli Venezia Giulia (PPR)[8] and Apulia (PPTR) plans.[9] The Apulia plan, in particular, introduces a rigorous distinction – essential for ensuring an effective application and articulation of regulatory and protection levels – between the structures that make up the territorial palimpsest and the "invariant rules" that underpin the reproduction of territorial heritage (Barbanente 2015).

4 Territorial Statute/Statuto del Territorio

The concept of Territory Statute is inseparable from that of Structural Invariant. It first appeared in the Tuscany Regional Planning Law 5/1995 with the title of Place Statute.[10] The definition was ambiguous, but it contributed – along with some other regional Italian disciplinary and normative advancements, such as the "founding description" in the Liguria Regional Planning Law 36/1997 – to a radical rethinking of the approach to and contents of regional and local plans. These plans ceased to be "containers" for future infrastructure and development and became documents focussed on establishing a shared awareness and acknowledgement of resources and values to be mobilised and enhanced for sustainable development goals. A year after Law 5/95 was approved, Mario Cusmano (Cusmano 1996, p. 12) enriched the initial definition of the Statute of Places, by introducing a meaningful interpretation of the concept of Territory Statute which he defined as a "charter of rights and duties toward a collective good which, in turn, is a product and heritage of the action of a collectivity and of single actors".

Similarly, Alberto Magnaghi calls the Statute a "constitutional act for local development": "a project for a socially shared future" (Magnaghi 2000, p. 125). Considering the wide range of reflections that this notion entails, it is worth underlining at least two of them: the first one regards citizen participation in planning process issues and the second one the use of innovative forms and techniques for plan representation. With regard to citizen participation, the process of recognising the invariant rules required for planning the transformation of the territory needs to be dialogical and inclusive; negotiation is also essential so that conflict, whilst unavoidable, can enrich the construction processes of the plan planning processes and the strategic scenarios arising therefrom (Fanfani 2007). Planning experience has demonstrated that it is impossible for the process of acknowledging territorial transformation rules to be negotiated using consensus building and mediating the issues posed by different social actors. In this process, conflicts have to be assumed as an unavoidable dimension, stemming from either a power imbalance within

[7] QTRP-Quadro Territoriale Regionale Paesaggistico (Regional Territorial Landscape Framework).

[8] PPR-Piano Paesaggistico Regionale.(Regional Landscape Plan).

[9] PPTR-Piano Paesaggistico Territoriale Regionale (Regional Territorial Landscape Plan).

[10] Statuto dei Luoghi.

society or from the relevance of the issues at stake (Fanfani 2007). In this regard, reflections on the statutory planning model and its implementation have resulted in a vast and diversified set of research/implementation practices – University education, where the echoes of Geddesian influence are clear and strong, has played a role in this – which aim to create a new role for local society in territorial planning and design processes (Paba et al. 2009).

The other major research front opened by the aforementioned disciplinary normative specifications and innovations was the codification of the so-called identity and statutory representation. In 2010 Roberto Gambino stated: "A new idea of the territory – which embodies a new idea of the relationship with places – requires new representations" (Gambino 2010, p. 73). The transition from territory conceived as a blank sheet, to territory seen as a dense stratified subject, rich in assets, to be translated into invariant rules shared in the "constitutional" paper as represented by the Statute, has also used the enormous potential offered by the Geographical Information System (GIS) and its related tools to produce atlases, heritage maps and scenario visions that are more readily understood than traditional cartography and are able to stimulate the social production processes within the territory (Lucchesi 2005).

References

Baldeschi, P. (2000). *Il Chianti fiorentino. Un progetto per la tutela del paesaggio*. Roma-Bari: Laterza.

Barbanente, A. (2015). Il Piano paesaggistico della Regione Puglia. *Sentieri Urbani, 17*, 46–53.

Bottino, F. (1987). Dal vincolo al Piano. *Urbanistica, 87*, 48–53.

Caniggia, G., & Maffei, G. L. (1979). *Composizione architettonica e tipologia edilizia. 1 Lettura dell'edilizia di base*. Venezia: Marsilio.

Cataldi, G. (2002). Saverio Muratori and the Italian School of Planning Typology. *Urban Morphology, 1*(6), 3–14.

Choay, F. (1973). *La città. Utopie e realtà*. Torino: Einaudi (first ed. 1965).

Cusmano, M. G. (1996). Il territorio del piano. *Paesaggio urbano, 3*, 10–12.

Dematteis, G. (1995). *Progetto implicito. Il contributo della geografia umana alle scienze del territorio*. Milano: Franco Angeli.

Di Biagi, P., Gabellini, P. (Ed.) (1990). Il nuovo piano regolatore di Siena. In *Urbanistica* 99, 31–88.

Fanfani, D. (2007). Gli scenari strategici nel dibattito internazionale e nell'approccio statutario ed identitario del governo del territorio: un modello interpretativo. In A. Magnaghi (Ed.), *Scenari strategici. Visioni identitarie per il progetto di territorio* (pp. 33–46). Firenze: Alinea.

Gambi, L. (1986). La costruzione dei piani paesistici. *Urbanistica, 85*, 102–105.

Gambino, R. (2010). Interpretazione strutturale e progetto di territorio. In D. Poli (Ed.), *Contesti. Città, territori, progetti. 2, Il progetto territorialista*. Firenze: All'insegna del Giglio. (Special Issue).

Gambino, R. (2011). Patrimonio e senso del paesaggio (riconoscere il patrimonio territoriale). In G. Paolinelli (Ed.), *Habitare. Il paesaggio nei piani territoriali*. Milano: Franco Angeli.

Geddes, P. (1915). *Cities in evolution. An introduction to the town planning movement and to the study of civics*. London: Williams & Norgate.

Gisotti, M. R. (2016). Dal vincolo al progetto. Il quadro della pianificazione paesaggistica in Italia e una proposta per un modello operativo. In A. Magnaghi (Ed.), *La pianificazione paesaggistica in Italia. Stato dell'arte e innovazioni* (pp. 1–35). Firenze: Firenze University Press.

Lucchesi, F. (2005). *Il territorio, il codice, la rappresentazione. Il disegno dello statuto dei luoghi*. Firenze: Firenze University Press.

Maggio, M. (2014). *Invarianti strutturali nel governo del territorio*. Firenze: Firenze University Press.

Magnaghi, A. (Ed.). (1990). *Il territorio dell'abitare. Lo sviluppo locale come alternativa strategica*. Milano: Franco Angeli.

Magnaghi, A. (Ed.). (1998). *Il territorio degli abitanti. Società locali e autosostenibilità*. Milano: Dunod.

Magnaghi, A. (2000). *Il progetto locale*. Torino: Bollati Boringhieri (first english translation Magnaghi, A. (2005). *The urban village: A charter for democracy and local self-sustainable development*. London: Zed Books).

Marson, A. (Ed.). (2016). *La struttura del paesaggio. Una sperimentazione multidisciplinare per il Piano della Toscana*. Bari: Laterza.

Paba, G., Pecoriello, A. L., Perrone, C., & Rispoli, F. (2009). *Partecipazione in Toscana. Interpretazioni e racconti*. Firenze: Firenze University Press.

Poli, D. (Ed.) (2010). Il progetto territorialista, *Contesti. Città, territori, progetti*, 2, Firenze. (Special Issue).

Raffestin, C. (1984). Territorializzazione, deterritorializzazione, riterritorializzazione e informazione. In A. Turco (Ed.), *Regione e Regionalizzazione* (pp. 69–82). Milano: Franco Angeli.

Saragosa, C. (2011). *Città tra passato e futuro. Un percorso critico sulla via di Biopoli*. Roma: Donzelli Editore.

Sereni, E. (2001). *Storia del paesaggio agrario italiano*. Roma-Bari: Laterza (first ed. 1961).

Turco, A. (1988). *Verso una teoria geografica della complessità*. Milano: Unicopli.

The manufacturer's authorised representative in the EU is Springer
Nature Customer Service Centre GmbH, Europaplatz 3, 69115 Heidelberg,
Germany. If you have any concerns regarding our products, please
contact ProductSafety@springernature.com

Printed and bound by CPI Group (UK) Ltd, Croydon, CR0 4YY
28/09/2026
02224089-0004